AF757200

RENAL TUMOR

Edited by **Jindong Chen**

Renal Tumor
http://dx.doi.org/10.5772/56083
Edited by Jindong Chen

Contributors
Tetsuo Fujita, Masatsugu Iwamura, Kazumasa Matsumoto, Kazunari Yoshida, Mirjana Rajer, Carolin Eva Hach, Stefan Siemer, Stephan Buse, Akihiro Tojo, Luis Miguel Anton Aparicio, Luis Leon, Martin Lazaro, Javier Afonso, Sergio Vazquez Estevez, Urbano Anido, Ovidio Fernandez, Manuel Ramos, María Carmen Areses Manrique, Henryk Zielinski, Tomasz Syrylo, Stanislaw Szmigielski, Archil Chkhotua, Ryoiti Kiyama, Vasiliki Michalaki, Sina Vatandoust, Thean Hsiang Tan, Michail Charakidis

Published by InTech
Janeza Trdine 9, 51000 Rijeka, Croatia

Copyright © 2013 InTech
All chapters are distributed under the Creative Commons Attribution 3.0 license, which allows users to download, copy and build upon published articles even for commercial purposes, as long as the author and publisher are properly credited, which ensures maximum dissemination and a wider impact of our publications. After this work has been published by InTech, authors have the right to republish it, in whole or part, in any publication of which they are the author, and to make other personal use of the work. Any republication, referencing or personal use of the work must explicitly identify the original source.

Notice
Statements and opinions expressed in the chapters are these of the individual contributors and not necessarily those of the editors or publisher. No responsibility is accepted for the accuracy of information contained in the published chapters. The publisher assumes no responsibility for any damage or injury to persons or property arising out of the use of any materials, instructions, methods or ideas contained in the book.

Publishing Process Manager Viktorija Zgela
Typesetting InTech DTP Team
Cover InTech Design Team

Additional hard copies can be obtained from orders@intechopen.com

Renal Tumor, Edited by Jindong Chen
p. cm.
ISBN 978-953-51-0981-5

We are IntechOpen, the world's leading publisher of Open Access books

Built by scientists, for scientists

4,200+
Open access books available

116,000+
International authors and editors

125M+
Downloads

151
Countries delivered to

Our authors are among the
Top 1%
most cited scientists

12.2%
Contributors from top 500 universities

CLARIVATE ANALYTICS BOOK CITATION INDEX INDEXED

WEB OF SCIENCE™

Selection of our books indexed in the Book Citation Index
in Web of Science™ Core Collection (BKCI)

Interested in publishing with us?
Contact book.department@intechopen.com

Numbers displayed above are based on latest data collected.
For more information visit www.intechopen.com

For EU product safety concerns:
IN TECH d.o.o., Prolaz Marije Krucifikse Kozulić 3, 51000 Rijeka, Croatia,
info@intechopen.com or visit our website at intechopen.com.

Meet the editor

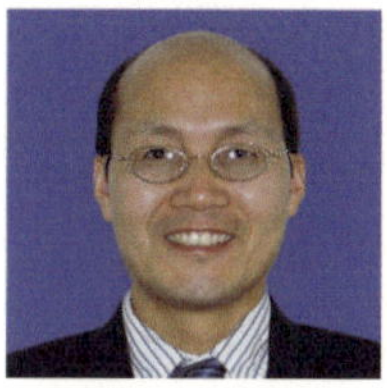

Jindong Chen, Ph.D., Research Associate Professor, Laboratory Co-director, AACR active member, Kidney Cancer Laboratory, Department of Urology, University of Rochester Medical Center, New York, USA. Upon graduation from Laboratory of Cancer Genetics, Department of Molecular Medicine, Karolinska Institute, Sweden, he has been working on kidney cancer since 2000. Upon graduation, he has served as Postdoctoral Fellow, Research Scientist at Van Andel Research Institute, USA; Senior Scientist at National Cancer Centre Singapore. He identified two kidney cancer-related genes, NORE1 and LSAMP by positional cloning strategy, and was awarded in 94th AACR annual meeting. In addition, he was also involved in cloning of another kidney cancer-related gene HRPT2. Afterward, he has successfully developed a few FLCN (BHD) and HRPT2 conditional knockout mouse models and was again awarded in the 100th AACR annual Meeting for generating the first renal tumor-developing FLCN knockout mouse model.

Contents

Preface

Renal cell carcinoma (RCC) is the most common type (>80%) of kidney cancer that arises from the cells of the renal tubules. Although RCC is relatively rare and only represents approximately 3% of all adult cancer, an alarming increase in incidence has been observed in the past five decades. Worldwide, approximately 150,000 new cases are diagnosed with RCC each year, and around 95,000 affected people die from the disease annually. While patients with early, localized RCC have a good prognosis, those with advanced disease (metastatic RCC) do not respond to most traditional therapeutic approaches, and survival for such patients is often less than 1 year. Unfortunately, most patients are diagnosed with advanced RCC, which causes anti-RCC treatment more challenging. Even so, with the advent and improvement of edge-cutting biomedical techniques, a significant amount of new information concerning the epidemiology, molecular genetics, immunologic characteristics, and therapy for patients with these tumors has appeared. Through the integration of molecular-based technologies, systematic tissue procurement and medical informatics, research data can rapidly be translated into useful diagnostic and treatment strategies. In fact, the increasing understanding of the pathogenesis of RCC has led to the development of novel targeted agents. New anti-RCC drugs have now been approved and commercially available, some potential drugs are also under clinical trial.

Here, to provide urologist and kidney cancer researchers with updated knowledge of RCC biology, current treatment practices, and novel treatment strategies, experts from all over the world, combining their our experience, explored and reviewed the latest developments in molecular genetics, surgery, and novel therapeutic strategies for renal tumors and organized into this book Renal Tumor. This book contains 11 chapters in three parts, covering the roles of partial nephrectomy, radical nephrectomy, and laparoscopy, as well as the latest developments in molecular genetics and immune dysfunction, signal transduction, and anti-RCC drugs associated with the diseases. Also discussed are imaging and screening for RCC, its diagnosis, paraneoplastic syndromes, and prognostic factors in metastatic disease.

It is hoped that Renal Tumor will offer all physicians treating kidney cancer as well as researchers current practical knowledge about the nature, diagnosis, prognosis, management and treatment of this difficult disease.

Finally, thanks to all the authors who have contributed their valuable time to write all the chapters. Without their efforts and dedication, the formation of this book would never be possible.

Jindong Chen, Ph.D.
Research Associate Professor, Co-director,
Kidney Cancer Research Laboratory, Department of Urology
University of Rochester Medical Center, Rochester, NY, USA

Section 1

Molecular Biology of Renal Tumor

Chapter 1

Genetics of Renal Tumors

Ryoiti Kiyama, Yun Zhu and Tei-ichiro Aoyagi

Additional information is available at the end of the chapter

http://dx.doi.org/10.5772/54588

1. Introduction

Kidney and urinary tract cancers accounted for a total of 16936 cases and 6764 deaths in 2007 in Japan (Matsuda et al., 2012), which is roughly 2% of all cancers. Renal cell carcinoma (RCC) is the most common type of kidney cancer, and is classified into three major subtypes, clear cell RCC, papillary RCC and chromophobe RCC, representing 80, 10, and 5% of all RCCs, and the majority of renal tumors are sporadic although 2-4% are hereditary (Hagenkord et al., 2011).

A number of genes have been studied in association with renal tumors, including those involved in tumorigenesis, and the progression and outcome of the cancer, by means of mutational searches, gene expression profiling, proteomics/metabolomics and pathological/clinical studies. The genes can be classified into several categories, such as familial, sporadic, epigenetic and quantitative, depending on the timing of their expression, and the factors affecting their effects, such as microRNA (miRNA) and metabolites have emerged. Since tumorigenesis is believed to be initiated with genetic/epigenetic modulations of at least several genes, but not a single gene alone, the balance among these cancer-related genes is considered to be more important than the contribution of a dramatic change caused by a single gene. Thus, an extensive and competitive search for oncogenes and tumor suppressor genes based on the search for their mutations was immediately accompanied by the search for interacting proteins/factors at the mutation sites. This indicates that lineages of gene functions, or signaling pathways, are important to understanding tumorigenesis, as well as the progression and outcome of the cancer. Although such pathways are not fully understood, it is important to summarize the latest knowledge of genes and their functions in terms of the coordinated functions of genes to achieve a basic understanding of cancer and to use the information obtained for diagnostics/therapeutics.

Here, we summarize and discuss the genes associated with renal tumors (Section 2) and then show one of them, *Kank1*, from gene-function networks or signaling pathways (Section 3). We

INTECH
open science | open minds

© 2013 Kiyama et al.; licensee InTech. This is a paper distributed under the terms of the Creative Commons Attribution License (http://creativecommons.org/licenses/by/3.0), which permits unrestricted use, distribution, and reproduction in any medium, provided the original work is properly cited.

also discuss a methodology for collecting information on multiple gene functions with a simple pathological system (Section 4).

2. Genes associated with renal tumors

While kidney cancer ranked 9th in 2002 in the European Union and the United States (Baldewijns et al., 2008), its mortality rate was not high in Japan (12th in 2002 and 2007: Matsuda et al., 2012). Although this difference could be attributable to risk factors such as smoking, hypertension and long-term dialysis, there might be a contribution of genes associated with the cancer. In spite that RCC shows a poor survival rate (less than 19%) for patients with metastasis, molecular pathological tests, such as those dividing good and poor prognosis groups, have not been established (Stewart et al., 2011). A lack of such effective tests may be one of the reasons why the mortality rate in Japan has been gradually increasing from 1.8% (2002) to 2.0% (2007).

A large majority of RCC cases are sporadic and only 2-4% are hereditary. There are cases where gene expression profiling cannot distinguish between them (Beroukhim et al., 2009), suggesting common genetic factors between them. Several genes are known to be associated with RCC, such as *VHL*, *TSC1* and *TSC2*, which play different roles in the mechanism of cancer and so have different advantages in diagnostics/therapeutics. The information about genes can be categorized by the levels of genomics, transcriptomics, proteomics and others including metabolomics, and used to understand the mechanism of cancer, to support diagnostic or therapeutic processes. In this section, we focus on the roles and merits of these genes.

2.1. Genes associated with tumorigenesis

Since a majority of sporadic cancers originate from a recessive mutation that causes a loss of function of a particular type of gene, loss of heterozygosity (LOH) is an important step in the disabling of a functional gene (or a wild-type allele) to give a mutated and cancer phenotype. Such genes are termed tumor suppressor genes, and so far, more than 100 have been reported (Fearon, 2002; Polinsky, 2007). Among them, twenty well-characterized genes showed both familial and sporadic phenotypes (Sherr, 2004). Since a cancer phenotype can be revealed by morphological changes, growth stimulation, gaining immortality and/or others, there are quite a few functions associated with tumor suppressor genes. Thus, it is easier to examine tumorigenesis in association with genomic status, mutations and/or epigenetic modifications, by analyzing the loci specific to RCC.

2.1.1. VHL gene

The gene best known to be associated with RCC is the von Hippel-Lindau (*VHL*) gene, whose inactivation accounts for nearly 100% of hereditary cases and sporadic clear cell RCC cases (Baldewijns et al., 2008). This gene was found by positional cloning from the locus associated with the VHL disease, a familial syndrome accompanying cancer in the eye, brain, spinal cord,

http://dx.doi.org/10.5772/54588

kidney, pancreas and adrenal glands. The *VHL* gene encodes the 30-kDa protein VHL, 213 amino acid residues long, and is implicated in the regulation of hypoxia-inducible factors (HIFs) (Maher et al., 2011). The VHL protein forms a complex with elongin B, elongin C and cullin-2, and the complex has ubiquitin ligase E3 activity and is involved in the ubiquitination and degradation of HIFα, the α subunits of transcription factors HIF-1 and HIF-2, which form a dimer with HIFβ and regulate the transcription of hypoxia-inducible genes such as those for VEGF (vascular endothelial growth factor), PDGF (platelet derived growth factor) and TGFα (transforming growth factor α) (Kondo and Kaelin, 2001; Kaelin, 2009; Fig. 1). However, the cancer found in VHL disease is sporadic and the lifetime risk of RCC in VHL disease patients is about 70% (Maher et al., 2011). So, it is reasonable to assume that additional genes are involved in RCC and the mutations in *VHL* are not the definitive cause of RCC, which is one of the reasons to explore new genes and genetic loci (see below). Meanwhile, the status of the *VHL* gene is important for the treatment of VHL disease and kidney cancer patients. HIF-responsive gene products, such as VEGF and PDGF, activate the angiogenesis of tumors and therefore are good therapeutic targets. Inhibitors of VEGF and PDGF, sunitinib and sorafenib, have been approved by the US Food and Drug Administration (Kaelin, 2009).

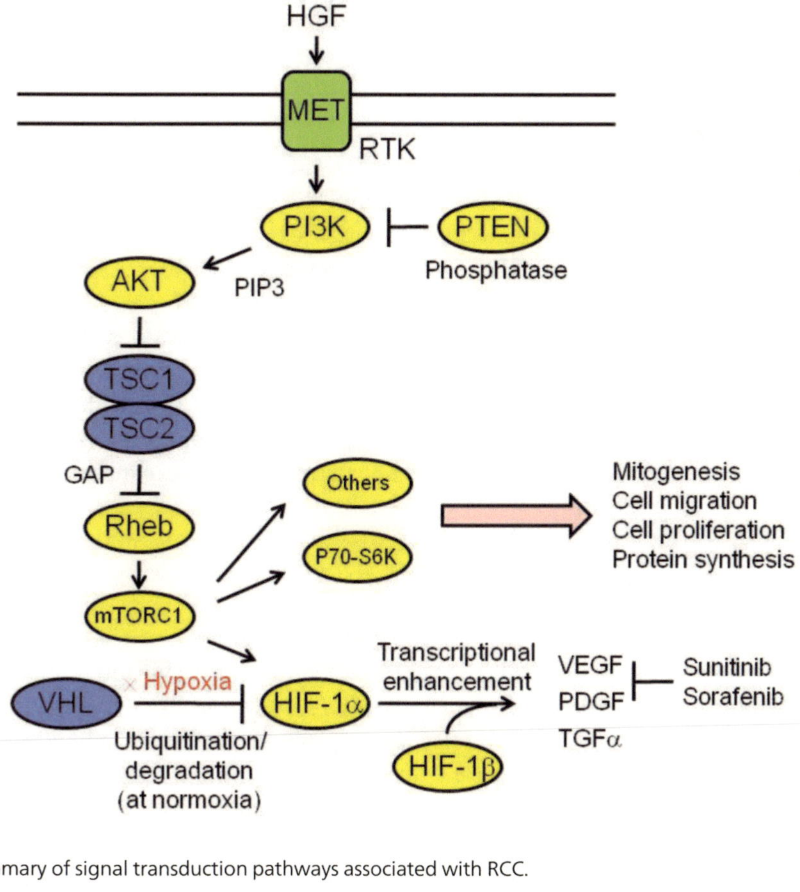

Figure 1. Summary of signal transduction pathways associated with RCC.

2.1.2. MET gene

The *MET* protooncogene was found in hereditary papillary RCC without mutations in the *VHL* gene (Schmidt et al., 1997). *MET* encodes a membrane receptor (MET) for hepatocyte growth factor (HGF). MET has tyrosine kinase activity, and HGF activates this kinase activity and initiates signaling for mitogenesis and migration (Fig. 1). While aberrantly active MET triggers tumor growth, angiogenesis and metastasis, such cases are relatively rare (~5%) among sporadic papillary RCC, suggesting other genes to play a major role in the tumorigenesis (Baldewijns et al., 2008).

2.1.3. TSC1/TSC2 genes

Two tumor suppressor genes, *TSC1* and *TSC2*, were found in a study of tuberous sclerosis complex (TSC), which is known to develop into various types of RCCs, including clear cell RCC, papillary RCC and chromophobe RCC (Borkowska et al., 2011). The TSC1 and TSC2 proteins form a heterodimer and inhibit the mammalian target of rapamycin (mTOR; a key signaling mediator for cell growth), by inactivating a small GTPase Rheb (an activator of mTOR) as a GTPase-activating protein (GAP) (Linehan et al., 2010; (Fig. 1). However, mutations are not frequently found in sporadic RCC (Parry et al., 2001) and therefore its role is not completely clear yet.

2.1.4. PBRM1 gene

Several genes, *UTX* (or *KDM6A*), *JARID1C* (or *KDM5C*) and *SETD2*, were found in close association with clear cell RCC by a recent technology of the next-generation sequencing (Dalgliesh et al., 2010). As these genes are related with the methylation status of lysine residues of hitone H3, further mutation studies were conducted to identify a SWI/SNF chromatin remodeling complex gene, *PBRM1*, to be frequently (over 40%) mutated in clear cell RCC (Varela et al., 2011). *PBRM1* is mapped to chromosome 3p21 and encodes the BAF180 protein, a chromatin targeting subunit of a SWI/SNF chromatin remodeling complex, which regulates replication, DNA repair and cell proliferation/differentiation. Knock-down of this gene enhanced colony formation and migration of cancer cells, suggesting this gene to be a tumor suppressor gene. Further studies are needed to reveal a mechanism of cancer involving *PBRM1* and to find its clinical application.

2.1.5. Genes related to hereditary renal cancer syndromes

Approximately 2-4% of RCC cases are hereditary and some genes have been identified as the genes responsible for hereditary renal cancer (HRC) syndromes (Verine et al., 2010). Apart from the genes already mentioned above (*VHL, MET, TSC1* and *TSC2*), several more genes have been described in association with HRC syndromes, including *FH* and *FLCN* genes. *FH* is the gene responsible for a HRC syndrome, hereditary leiomyomatosis and renal cell cancer (HLRCC), in which affected individuals often develop cutaneous and uterine leiomyoma and an aggressive form of papillary RCC (Linehan et al., 2004). The *FH* gene encodes an enzyme (FH) catalyzing the conversion of fumarate to malate in the tricarboxylic acid (Krebs) cycle.

From the analysis of their mutations, this gene is considered as a tumor suppressor gene (Sudarshan et al., 2007). Although the mechanism that leads *FH* alterations to cancer is not clearly understood, there is a link between fumarate dysregulation and impaired HIF hydroxylation (Isaacs et al., 2005).

FLCN, on the other hand, is the gene responsible for Birt-Hogg-Dubé (BHD) syndrome, which is a rare autosomal dominant disease including kidney tumors, predominantly chromophobe RCC. Mutations in this gene were found in approximately 80% of BHD kindreds and loss of expression of this gene were frequently found in kidney tumors from BHD patients, suggesting this gene to be a tumor suppressor gene (Baldewijns et al., 2008).

2.1.6. Other genes

Several genes were recently implicated in association with RCC, including *BAP1*, *SETD2* and *NF2*, by means of advanced technologies such as the next-generation sequencing, a microarray-based analysis and a mouse transgene analysis. *BAP1* plays a role of a tumor suppressor and encodes a nuclear deubiquitinase, which is inactivated in 15% of clear cell RCC cases (Peña-Llopis et al., 2012). Mutations in *BAP1* anticorrelates with those in another tumor suppressor gene, *PBRM1*, and these mutations comprise a subtype of clear cell RCC (70% of all clear cell RCC cases). The BAP1 protein may work with host cell factor-1 (HCF-1), a scaffold protein, to regulate transcription factors and suppress cell proliferation.

SETD2 was found by the analysis of accumulated transcripts containing premature termination codons and encodes a histone methyltransferase, which is responsible for trimethylation of the lysine residue at position 36 of histone H3 and may play a role in suppressing tumor development (Duns et al., 2012).

NF2 was identified as a tumor suppressor gene by the analysis of knock-out mice (Morris and McClatchey, 2009). The mice developed kidney tumors in 6-10 months with characteristics of hyperactive epidermal growth factor receptor (EGFR) signaling. Merlin, the *NF2* gene product, was implicated in suppressing tumorigenesis by inhibiting hyperactivated EGFR signaling.

2.2. Genes implicated in diagnostic markers and therapeutic targets

The recurrence of RCC is 20 to 40%, depending on the stage and grade of tumor (Chin et al., 2006). So, it is important to understand the genes (and their products) associated with progression/metastasis to predict the outcome of cancer. The classification of RCC subtypes is apparently not possible by a single marker, but could be done using combinations of markers such as vimentin, epithelial cell adhesion molecule (EpCAM), glutathione S-transferase α (GSTα), carbonic anhydrase II (CA II), cytokeratin 7 (CK7) and cluster of differentiation 10 (CD10) (Stewart et al., 2011).

Important prognostic markers for RCC represent specific cellular signaling pathways, such as the VHL and mTOR pathways. The VHL pathway gives several well-studied markers, such as VHL, HIFs, VEGF and carbonic anhydrase 9 (CAIX), although their applicability is sometimes questionable (Stewart et al., 2011). HIF-responsive gene products are potential markers representing angiogenesis (VEGF, PDGF, SDF, CXCR4, TGFβ and CTGF), glucose uptake and metabolism (HK2 and PDK4), pH control (CAIX and CAXII), invasion/metastasis (MMP1, SDF, CXCR4 and c-Met), and proliferation and survival (TGFα) (Smaldone and Maranchie, 2009).

Another pathway for potential makers is the mTOR pathway (Fig. 1). The main cascade of this pathway is PI3K/AKT/mTOR, which mediates signals by activating phosphoinositide 3-kinase (PI3K) through kinases such as receptor tyrosine kinases to generate phosphatidylinositol (3,4,5)-trisphosphate (PIP3), which further activates AKT via phosphorylation and phospho-AKT activates mTOR complex 1 (mTORC1) through inhibition of the TSC1/TSC2 complex (Allory et al., 2011). Then, mTORC1 phosphorylates proteins such as P70-S6 kinase and activates protein synthesis and cell proliferation. Importantly, HIF-1α expression is dependent on mTORC1 signaling (Toschi et al., 2008). Potential markers in this pathway include P70-S6 kinase, PTEN (a phosphatase that decreases PIP3) and phospho-AKT.

2.3. Mutation sites and LOH loci

A comprehensive analysis of RCC genomes has been done through genomic (Hatano et al., 2001; Cifola et al., 2008), transcriptomic (Takahashi et al., 2001; Takahashi et al., 2003; Cifola et al., 2008) and proteomic/metabolic (Perroud et al., 2006; Raimondo et al., 2012) approaches. We used a genome-subtraction technique, or the in-gel competitive reassociation method (Kiyama et al., 1995; Rodley et al., 2003), for cloning the sites of LOH that occurred in a RCC genome by subtracting normal DNA from cancer DNA of the same patient (Hatano et al., 2001). The minimum size of LOH (caused by hemizygous deletions) detected by this method was roughly 50 kb. This resolution was made possible by *Mse*I, which recognizes TTAA, a sequence appearing frequently in human genomic DNA, and completely digests genomic DNA to sizes mostly below 1 kb. Such a high resolution has not been used even in recent genome-wide association studies (see Jacobs et al., 2012, for example). A total of 187 clones were mapped on the chromosomes and a total of 44 candidate regions, where at least two clones were mapped within 5 Mb, were selected and analyzed for mapping the sites of LOH in 61 cancer cases (Table 1). Among them, we found interesting LOH sites at 5q32-q34, 6q21-q22, 8p12 and 9p24, whose frequencies are relatively high among RCC and whose lengths are less than ~10 Mb (Hatano et al., 2001; Sarkar et al., 2002; Fig. 2). A tumor suppressor gene, *Kank1*, was found at 9p24 after extensive analysis of the LOH site by examining the loss of function upon its mutation; the loss of expression of the gene at mRNA and protein levels in RCC, and the loss of suppression of tumor growth in renal tumor cells (Sarkar et al., 2002).

2.4. Chromosomal abberations in RCC

Chromosomal abberations are often observed in RCC (Ross et al., 2012). Deletions of chromosome 3p, where the *VHL* gene resides, are found in most sporadic and familial clear cell RCCs. Distinctive abnormalities were reported for papillary RCC, where, in contrast to clear cell RCC, most of the tumors are characterized by trisomy of chromosomes 7 and 17 along with loss of Y, while the 3p arm is intact. In Xp11.2 RCC, the gene fusion was observed between the *TFE3* gene on the X chromosome and either of *ASPL* (17q25), *PRCC* (1q21), *PSF* (1q34), *NonO* (Xq12) and *CLTC* (17q23) (Kuroda et al., 2012). All of the gene fusions result in overexpression of the TFE3 protein, a transcription factor. Among them, the translocation of t(X;17)(p11.2q25), which fuses the *ASPL* and *TFE3* genes, is most frequently observed. Meanwhile, there are some unclassified cases, such as those where trisomy 7/17 in areas typical of papillary RCC and both trisomy 7/17 and 3p loss in areas with clear cell RCC were observed (Ross et al., 2012).

2.5. Exploration of new genetic markers

Even though a number of genetic markers have been reported, they are not currently used for the diagnosis of RCC. As discussed in Section 1, this is because understanding a single gene or a few genes is not enough for a diagnosis of sufficient reliability. For diagnosing more complex and more specific states of diseases or disease phenotypes, groups of markers that are able to more accurately distinguish the phenotypes are needed. Such markers should be derived from the direct process of the disease and therefore would represent the signal transduction that occurs within the cell. There are several new technologies which might open the door to a more comprehensive understanding of RCC especially at the level of cellular signaling: array-based genome-wide association studies, microRNA (miRNA) studies and next-generation sequencing-based expression profiling.

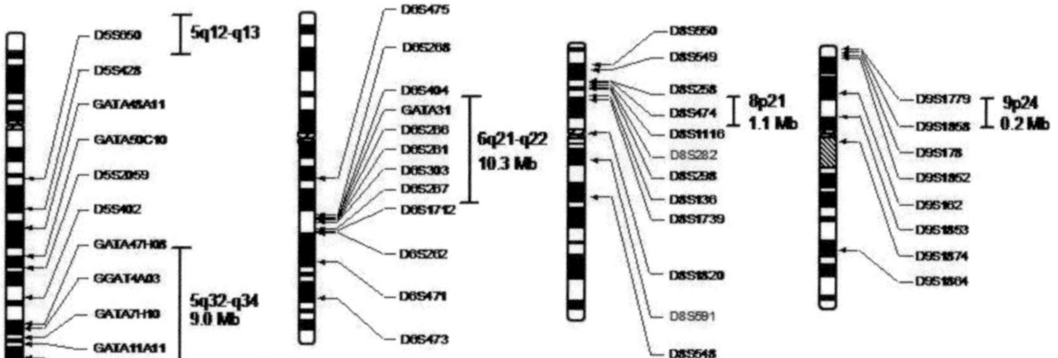

Figure 2. Significant LOH regions in RCC. LOH regions of less than ~10 Mb were identified as the minimum overlapping regions of LOH by subtraction cloning of mutated regions followed by the quantitative allelic analysis of over 60 RCC cases using microsatellite markers (see Hatano et al., 2001; Sarkar et al., 2002).

Location	LOH	(%)
3p22-p23	15/16	(93.8)
3p21.2-p21.3	21/23	(91.3)
3q13.3-q21	13/31	(41.9)
5q12-q13.1	10/31	(32.3)
5q13.1-q14	7/28	(25.0)
5q23.3	10/27	(37.0)
5q31.3-q32	7/28	(25.0)
5q32-q34	14/30	(46.7)
6q22.3	9/34	(26.5)
7p12-p14	5/32	(15.6)
7q11.23	7/33	(21.2)
7q22.1-q31.2	5/38	(13.2)
8p12	5/29	(17.2)
8q13	6/34	(17.6)
9p21-p22	5/20	(25.0)
9p12-q11	6/33	(18.2)
9q31	8/41	(19.5)
11q13.3-q14.1	5/28	(17.9)
11q22.3	2/17	(11.8)
14q11.2-q12	9/26	(34.6)
14q13-q21	10/34	(29.4)
14q24.1-q31	12/36	(33.3)
14q32.1-q32.3	7/22	(31.8)
15q23	5/28	(17.9)
18p11.1-q11.2	8/35	(22.9)
18q22	7/39	(17.9)
Xq26-q28	3/4	(75.0)

Table 1. Summary of LOH at significant locations among 44 sites. For details, see Hatano et al. (2001) and Sarkar et al. (2002). Only the loci in which more than 10 % of RCC patients had LOH are shown. The LOH analysis is applicable to only female patients for the cluster at Xq26-q28. There were a total of 44 clusters containing more than two of 187 clones analyzed within 5 Mb. The locations of the clusters other than those shown above are as follows: 1p31.1, 1p13.3-p22.3, 1p13.3-q12, 1q12-p21.1, 2p21-p22, 2p12-q11.2, 4p14, 4p13.3-p21.1, 4q22, 4q32, 10p14-p15.1, 10p12.1-p12.2, 12q13.3-q15, 13q13-q14.1, 13q14.2-q14.3, 16q12.1-q12.2, and 20p11.2-p12.

Recent advances in high-resolution genomic arrays have enabled us to analyze 1,000 or more disease cases efficiently, and thus to give statistically significant loci associated with the diseases. Such an approach was applied to the study of RCC. A genome-wide association study

http://dx.doi.org/10.5772/54588

based on more than 5,000 RCC cases revealed two loci, 2p21 and 11q13.3, to be associated with RCC susceptibility (Purdue et al., 2011). Although the authors claimed these sites to be previously unidentified, both of the loci were actually identified in 2001 (Hatano et al., 2001; Table 1). While the association is statistically significant, the frequencies among RCC cases are not very high (less than 20%), and therefore, it is doubtful that these sites alone can be used for diagnosis. The candidate genes in these loci which contribute to the association are *EPAS1* encoding hypoxia-inducible factor-2α (HIF2α) and *SCARB1* encoding a scavenger receptor. While HIF2α was known to be associated with RCC though it has not yet been used clinically, SCARB1 is new and its association with RCC may indicate a new signaling pathway. The array-based genome-wide association technique was also applied to the study of copy-number variations (Krill-Burger et al., 2012).

The study of miRNA is rapidly providing as new information about disease phenotypes. MiRNA, a group of short non-coding RNA with lengths of 19-22 nucleotides, differs from mRNA in that it has a role in gene function, and, while information about mutations is important for mRNA, quantity is mostly emphasized for miRNA. So, while there are cases where mRNA bearing a mutation without a change in its quantity contributes to a disease phenotype, there would be few such cases for miRNA. Naturally, the linkage of a disease to a genomic location reveals in most cases a mutation in a gene. This may indicate that miRNA contributes to quantitative change as a group as a result of changes in transcriptional efficiency caused by alterations to the transcriptional machinery or genomic location/status, or by epigenetic modifications. In contrast to mRNA, however, the quantity of miRNA can be controlled rapidly and specifically, and thus, miRNA could be more advantageous for the rapid control of the amount of specific proteins, which is important in signal transduction. Such cases were reported for TGFβ, WNT, Notch and EGF signaling in association with homeostasis, cancer, metastasis, fibrosis and stem cell biology (Inui et al., 2010), and VHL-signaling and VEGF-signaling in association with RCC (Fendler et al., 2011). Several miRNAs were reported to be induced or repressed by VHL-induced hypoxia in RCC and regulate the PI3K/AKT/mTOR pathway and Wnt signaling/β-catenin pathway to control cell proliferation, tumorigenesis and other cellular functions (Redova et al., 2011).

Next-generation sequencing technology was applied to genome-wide expression profiling of miRNA related to clear cell RCC (Osanto et al., 2012). By analyzing 22 RCCs, 100 miRNA differentially expressed between clear cell RCC and matched normal tissues were found. While the biological relevance of these novel miRNAs is unknown, they may be potential diagnostic markers or targets for therapeutics.

3. Kank family genes and renal tumors

3.1. Structure of *Kank*-family genes

The human *Kank1* gene was found as a candidate tumor suppressor gene for renal tumors at 9p24, and encodes a protein containing ankyrin-repeats at the C-terminus and coiled-coil motifs near the N-terminus (Sakar et al., 2002). Based on domain and phylogenetic analyses,

Kank2, *Kank3* and *Kank4* were found to form a family with *Kank1* (Zhu et al., 2008). Five repeats of the ankyrin-repeat motif comprise the basic structure of all Kank proteins (Fig. 3A). In addition, each Kank protein contains different combinations of four types of coiled-coil motifs. They also have a conserved region close to the N-terminus, named the KN-motif (Zhu et al., 2008; Fig. 3A), which contains a leucine-rich region and an arginine-rich region.

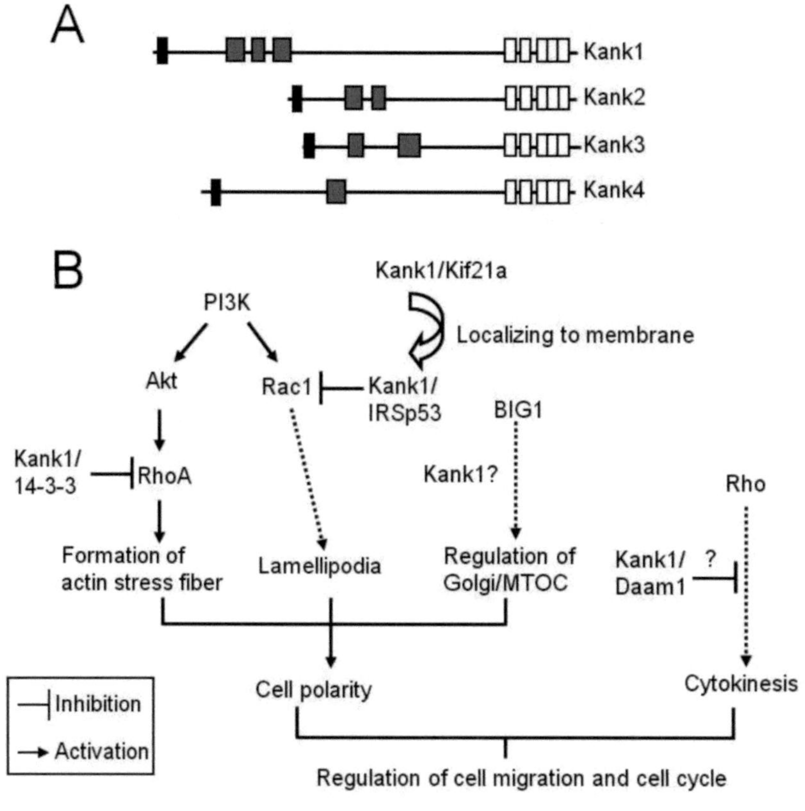

Figure 3. (A) Schematic structure of human Kank family proteins. Black boxes indicate the Kank N-terminal (KN) motif. Gray boxes indicate coiled-coil motifs. White boxes indicate the ankyrin-repeat (ANK) motifs. (B) A hypothetical model of Kank1 functions. Kank1 is transported to areas of membrane ruffling, such as lamellipodia, through association with Kif21a. Kank1 regulates RhoA and Rac1 activities through interaction with 14-3-3 in PI3K/Akt signaling and IRSp53 in Rac1 signaling, respectively. These interactions negatively regulate the formation of actin stress fibers and lamellipodia, and finally decrease cell migration. Kank1 and BIG1 may exist in a multimolecular complex that affects Golgi/MTOC orientation and regulates cell polarity during directed migration. Kank1 may inhibit Rho activation by binding to Rho-regulating proteins, like Daam1, which may result in negative regulation of cytokinesis.

Yeast-two hybrid or mass-spectrometrical studies have shown that Kank1 can directly bind to several proteins, such as 14-3-3 proteins, insulin receptor substrate (IRS) p53, Kif21a and Disheveled-associated activator of morphogenesis 1 (Daam1). Kank1 binds to IRSp53 and Daam1 at its coiled-coil domain (Kakinuma et al., 2011). In addition, there is a 14-3-3-binding motif, serine at position 167, located between the first and second coiled-coil motifs. Kif21a is a unique protein found to interact with the ankyrin-repeat domain of Kank1 (Kakinuma et al., 2008 & 2009; Roy et al., 2009; Suzuki et al., unpublished data). Although the function of the KN-motif is not clear, it contains several potential motifs for a nuclear localization signal (NLS) and nuclear export signal (NES). These signals may contribute to nucleo-cytoplasmic shuttling of Kank1, and further affect the subcellular distribution of β-catenin (Wang et al., 2006; Previdi et al., 2010).

3.2. Functions of *Kank*-family genes

Some studies have demonstrated that *Kank*-family genes are related to various cell functions. VAB-19, an ortholog of the Kank1 protein in *C. elegans*, was reported to occur with components of an epidermal attachment structure. It plays an antagonistic role in the regulation of actin cytoskeleton and halts basement membrane opening associated with cell invasion and tissue remodeling (Ding et al., 2003; Ihara et al., 2011). The deletion of *Kank1* is associated with parent-of-origin-dependent inheritance of familial cerebral palsy (Lerer et al., 2005). There have also been reports that *Kank1* was fused with the gene for platelet-derived growth factor receptor β (PDGFRβ) and that the fusion protein was a vital regulator of hematopoietic cell proliferation (Medves et al., 2010 & 2011). Meanwhile, *Kank1* expression was down-regulated in patients with polycythemia vera, suggesting this gene to be related to myeloproliferative disorders (Kralovics et al., 2005). Some studies have described about the functions of other *Kank*-family members. Kank2, found as a novel podocyte-associated protein, may contribute to the regulation of actin dynamics in podocyte foot processes in the renal filter physiology and diseases (Xu et al., 2011). In addition, NBP, an ortholog of Kank3 in zebrafish, interacts with Numb, an adaptor protein implicated in various basic cellular processes, through the PTB domain, which is well conserved among vertebrate *Kank* genes. In embryogenesis, NBP accumulates at the cell periphery during gastrulation and, later in the development, is concentrated at the basal poles of differentiated cells. These findings suggest a role for NBP in regulating cell adhesion and tissue integrity (Boggetti et al., 2012).

Kank1 may contribute to several regulatory activities, such as regulation of the actin cytoskeleton, cell migration and the cell cycle through interactions with the proteins described above (Sakar et al., 2002; Kakinuma et al., 2008 & 2009; Roy et al., 2009; Suzuki et al., unpublished data; summarized in Fig. 3B). Kank1 regulates the Rac1-dependent formation of lamellipodia and the activity of RhoA, resulting in the inhibition of cell migration. This function is mediated through two binding partners of Kank1, 14-3-3 and IRSp53. Kank1 binds to the Akt-phosphrylation motif of 14-3-3θ, 14-3-3γ, 14-3-3η and 14-3-3ε. Interaction between these two proteins is enhanced by growth factors such as insulin and epidermal growth factor (EGF) (Kakinuma et al., 2008). This interaction regulates the activation of RhoA through the PI3K/Akt signaling pathway. When a 14-3-3 binding motif is phosphorylated by Akt, 14-3-3 is separated from an activation complex for RhoA, and binds to Kank1 resulting in the inhibition of RhoA activities, and thereby decreases the formation of actin stress fibers and inhibition of cell migration (Kakinuma et al., 2008). The coiled-coil domain of IRSp53, which is the site for the interaction with active Rac1, binds to Kank1. Endogenous Kank1 and IRSp53 are co-localized at the site of membrane protrusions such as lamellipodia, which are needed for cell migration. Overexpression of Kank1 inhibits the formation of lamellipodia induced by active Rac1 in NIH3T3 cells, and knockdown of Kank1 enhances the formation. Therefore, Kank1 negatively regulates membrane protrusions at the leading edge of cells, by inhibiting the association between active Rac1 and IRSp53 (Roy et al., 2009). Taken together, Kank1 regulates cell migration through inhibition of IRSp53 in Rac1 signaling and inactivation of RhoA activity through PI3K/Akt signaling (Fig. 3B). As the Kank1 locus shows loss of heterozygosity in RCC and the expression of the Kank1 gene is suppressed in RCC, Kank1 may contribute to the malignant transformation of cells such as metastasis.

Kank1 regulates cell migration by inhibiting Rac1 signaling and RhoA activity as described above. To fulfill this function, Kank1 needs to be located at the leading edge of cells and affect the neighboring membrane. Because Kank1 has no membrane-targeting motif or membrane protein to associate with, some proteins may help transport Kank1 to the site of membrane ruffling. Kank1 interacts with the third and fourth coiled-coil domains of KIF21a, a member of the Kif4-class superfamily of kinesin motors that acts as a plus-end kinesin motor (Marszalek et al., 1999; Kakinuma et al., 2009), at its ankyrin-repeat domain. Overexpression of Kif21a or one of the Kif21a mutants (R954W) enhances the translocation of Kank1 to the membrane. In contrast, knockdown of Kif21a decreases the amount of Kank1 at the membrane (Yamada et al., 2005; Kakinuma et al., 2009). Although the mechanisms involved need further study, translocation of Kank1 mediated by Kif21a may affect cell migration (Fig. 3B). Kank1 is also functionally associated with a protein, brefeldin A-inhibited guanine nucleotide-exchange 1 (BIG1), a binding partner of Kif21a. Although there is no direct interaction between these two proteins, they may exist in a multimolecular complex that maintains the orientation of the Golgi/microtubule-organizing center (MTOC) and regulates cell polarity during directed migration. Furthermore, a protein complex containing BIG1, Kif21a and Kank1 may contribute to directed transport along microtubules (Li et al., 2011).

Overexpression of Kank1 suppresses the cell cycle and cell growth (Sakar et al., 2002). We observed that the overexpression of Kank1 blocked cytokinesis and generated binucleated cells. We also found co-localization of endogenous Kank1 with Rho, a key molecule required in cytokinesis for regulating the constriction of the contractile ring, at the contractile ring during cytokinesis of NIH3T3 cells (Kamijo et al., 2006; Li et al., 2010; Kakinuma et al., 2011; Suzuki et al., unpublished data). The coiled-coil domain of Kank1 binds to another protein, Daam1 (Suzuki et al., unpublished data). Daam1 belongs to a novel protein family containing formin homology domains and has been implicated in the regulation of cell polarity associated with the Wnt/Frizzled/Rho signaling pathway (Jantsch-Plunger V et al., 2000; Kosako H et al., 2000). Although the mechanism is still not clear, Kank1 may block cytokinesis by regulating Rho activity through the interaction with Daam1 (Fig. 3B). Therefore, it may reveal a new mechanism of regulation of cytokinesis and tumor suppression.

3.3. *Kank*-family genes and renal tumors

The *Kank1* gene was found at 9p24 by a comprehensive analysis of human chromosomes for loss of heterozygosity (LOH) in RCC (Sakar et al., 2002). Kank1 family proteins localize at the area of cytoplasma in renal tubular cells and glandular cells of some digestive and endocrine organs (Roy et al., 2005). Kank family genes show different expression patterns at the mRNA and protein levels in normal and tumor kidney tissues and some kidney tumor cell lines (Zhu et al., 2008; Wang et al., 2005). Loss of expression of *Kank1* in RCC was confirmed by Western blotting, RT-PCR and immunohistochemical analyses (Sakar et al., 2002, Roy et al., 2005). In addition, immunostaining in RCC showed decreased expression of Kank1 in high grade tumors (Zhu et al., 2011). Therefore, the *Kank* family genes may be related to renal carcinoma, and function as tumor suppressors.

A growth inhibitory effect of Kank1 has been reported. Overexpression of *Kank1* in HEK293 cells resulted in cell cycle arrest at G_0/G_1. On the other hand, growth suppression of tumor cells was caused by *Kank1* gene expression using nude mice abdominally injected with HEK293 cells stably expressing *Kank1* (Sakar et al., 2002). These findings demonstrated that Kank1 can regulate the growth of cells and can also regulate the abnormal growth of cancer cells. Kank1 may exert its growth inhibitory effect by regulating Rho activity mediated via its association with Daam1, resulting in abnormal nuclear division, and thus blocking the cytokinesis of cancer cells (Suzuki et al., unpublished data). According to recent studies, Kank1 can negatively regulate the formation of actin stress fibers and cell migration (Kakinuma et al., 2008; Roy et al., 2009). When cells need to control migration, Kank1 could be transferred to the leading edge of the moving cells' membranes, mediated by Kif21a, and co-localized with IRSp53. Kank1 may bind to IRSp53 competing with active Rac1, and thus inhibits integrin-induced cell spreading and the formation of lamellipodia. Simultaneously, Kank1 may inactivate RhoA, which is controlled by binding with 14-3-3, inhibit the formation of actin stress fibers and ultimately inhibit cell migration. Loss of expression of Kank-family proteins may enhance cell migration in renal cell carcinoma. Since enhancement of cell migration is related to metastasis, Kank-family proteins might be related to the malignancy of renal cell carcinoma.

According to studies to date, the Kank1 protein may act as a tumor suppressor through inhibition of cell migration and cell cycle. These functions are facilitated by several proteins interacting with Kank1, including 14-3-3, IRSp53, Kif21a and Daam1. Further studies of the interactions of these proteins will help us to understand clearly the role of Kank family proteins in tumorigenesis.

3.4. Clinical study of *Kank1* gene in renal cancer patients

3.4.1. Genetic and clinical characteristics of renal tumors

Kidney cancer accounts for about 4% of adult cancers, with an estimated 64,770 new cases annually in the US (Siegel et al., 2012). Of kidney cancers, 92% are pathologically diagnosed as RCC. This "RCC" has interesting and unique characteristics when investigated from a clinical view point. Although 95% of patients with T1-T2 RCC survived 5 to 10 years, among those with metastatic disease the 5 year survival rate was 26% (DeCastro and McKiernan, 2008). Renal cancer is resistant to conventional chemotherapeutic agents and also to radiation therapy. Many cancer-related genes have been found in renal cancer, including a multi-drug resistance gene (Walsh et al., 2009), anti-apoptotic genes (Bilim et al., 2009), and radiation resistant components (Kransny et al., 2010). The most characteristic genomic structure in renal cancer is the *VHL*-related hypoxia-inducible factor gene and its cascades shown in hereditary RCC and sporadic RCC cases (Linehan et al., 2011). The down-regulation in expression of *Kank1*, our main theme, was also found from the study of renal cancer and normal renal tubular cells (Sarkar et al., 2002), as we mentioned in other sections. The current WHO classification of RCC in 2004 (Deng and Melamed, 2012) follows the earlier Heidelberg and Rochester classifications, recognizing the heterogeneity of RCC, and describes distinct types of RCC with unique morphologic and genetic characteristics. The most popular histological type, clear cell RCC, accounts for 80 % of all RCC cases. Compared with clear cell RCC, papillary RCC (10%) and chromophobe RCC (5%) are more benign. Collecting duct (bellini) (1%) type or other rare sarcomatous types of RCCs are more aggressive (Deng and Melamed, 2012). However, once metastasis occurs, papillary and choromophobe RCCs are more resistant to immunological and new molecular targeting agents than clear cell RCC (Chowdhury et al., 2011). These clinical features characterize the complexity of the clinical categorization of RCC.

Kank1 was found by a genome subtraction method among the genes at 9p24 susceptible to RCC (Sarkar et al., 2002). A devoted study revealed that *Kank1* belongs to a four-member family, has splice variants, and plays a role in cell migration, intracellular transport and cell division, suggesting that *Kank1* has a kind of tumor suppressor function (Kakinuma et al., 2009). In this section, the expression of the Kank1 protein in renal cancer specimens resected from RCC patients is indicated using immunohistochemical methods, and the relationship between the expression and tumor pathology, patient status, and clinical outcomes is examined.

3.4.2. Expression of Kank1 protein in renal cancer and autologous normal kidney

1. Expression of *Kank1* in RCC

We tried to find a RCC-related gene at 9p24, which lead to the discovery of *Kank1*. Of nine ESTs analyzed in the 9p24 region, only three (WI-17492, WI-12779 and WI-19184) were expressed in the kidney. The *Kank1* gene was associated with WI-12779. This *Kank1*-associated EST lost its expression in six out of eight cancer cases. Kank1 expression was examined in 5 matched normal kidney and cancer pairs by Western blotting using an anti-Kank1 antibody, which was obtained as mentioned below. Reduced or loss of Kank1 expression in cancer was observed in all 5 cases.

2. Immunohistochemical study of *Kank1* expression in RCC and the relationship between its expression and clinical-pathological outcomes

One hundred and five formalin-fixed paraffin-embedded slides including normal renal tubular cells and RCC were subjected to immunohistological staining for Kank1 with a monoclonal antibody. An anti-Kank1 (total Kank1) antibody was generated by a previously reported method (Roy et al., 2005). In brief, amino acids 406 to 580 of the Kank1 protein were fused in-frame with the glutathione S-transferase gene in the vector pGEX. After induction of the fusion protein in *E. coli*, it was purified and used to immunize mice. A mouse hybridoma cell producing an anti-Kank1 antibody was selected and amplified for further use.

The histological subtypes of RCC analyzed here were as follows; 92 clear cell RCCs, 11 papillary RCCs, 5 chromophobe RCCs and 7 other histological types. We compared all histological subtypes with clear cell RCC. The evaluation of positivity of staining was done by two independent examiners, who decided that the sample was positive when more than 30 % of cells were stained with the antibody, weakly positive (±) when 5 to 30 % cells were stained, and negative when less than 5 % cells were stained. The 2004 WHO histological classification (Eble et al., 2004), 2002 TNM classification (Edge et al., 2010) and Fuhrman nuclear grade (Fuhrman et al., 1982) were used in this study. Kaplan-Meyer cause-specific survival was determined and statistical difference in positivity was evaluated by the Kluskal-Wallis test using Stat View™ software following the instructions.

Representative examples of positive and negative staining for the Kank1 protein in clear cell RCC and positive staining in normal renal tubular cells are indicated in Fig. 4. Normal renal tubules usually expressed Kank1. Of 92 clear cell RCCs, Kank1 was positive in 47 cases (52%). Kank1 was weakly positive (less than 30% of cells) in 14 cases (15%). Kank1 was negative in 29 cases (33%). The results grouped by clinical outcome (clear cell RCC) and histology are summarized in Table 2. There was no relation or special tendency between the staining results and clinical results on Kank1 expression. Kank1 was expressed in 87.5% of other histological RCC subtypes.

		Kank1		
		(+)	(±)	(-)
Clear cell	Alive without cancer	29	11	18
	Alive with cancer	7	1	4
	Dead	11	2	7
Others	16 alive, 7 dead	21	2	1

Table 2. Immunohistological staining of Kank1 antibody classified by clinical outcome (clear cell RCC) and histological subtypes. Sums of the numbers of patients do not match all the evaluated numbers due to inavailabilty of follow-up to judge the clinical outcome.

There were no differences in the survival curves for clear cell RCC among the groups (Fig. 5). However, when the positivity rate was evaluated among the groups divided by the Furman nuclear grade, a highly malignant grade of clear cell RCC showed high Kank1 positivity ($p < 0.05$), while the others did not (Table 3). In clear cell RCC, 42% of grade 1 tumors were Kank1 negative, while 80% of grade 3 tumors were Kank1 positive. In other histological types, there was no apparent difference among nuclear grades (most of them showed Kank1). When sub-divided by pathological T stages, higher T stages of clear cell RCC showed a tendency to express Kank1 ($p = 0.07$) (Table 4). Other factors such as patient's age, gender and the size of the tumor (largest diameter) had no relation to the expression of Kank1 in clear cell and other RCCs (data not shown).

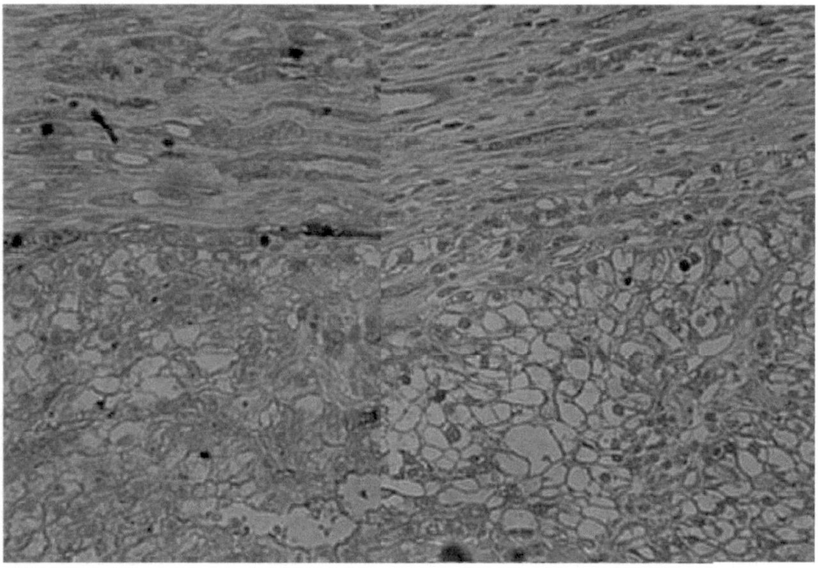

Figure 4. Immunohistochemical analysis of Kank1 protein in clear cell RCC. There was a case of positive staining of Kank1 protein in both normal renal tubular cells (upper left) and clear cell RCC (lower left), while another case indicates negative staining of Kank1 in clear cell RCC (lower right) while it was positive in the normal renal cells (upper right) (reduced from 40x images).

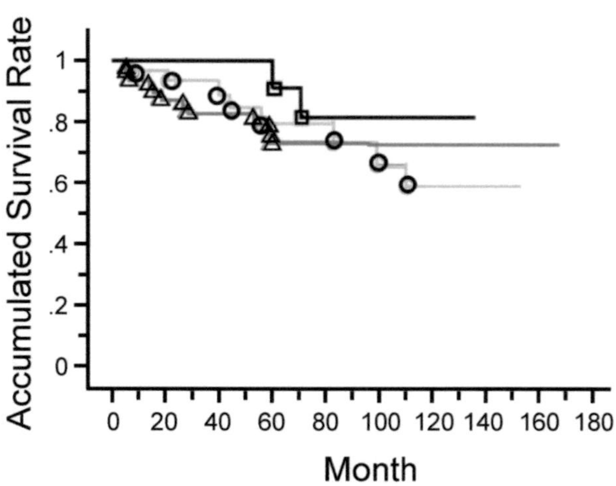

Figure 5. Kaplan-meyer's overall survival curve of RCC patients classified by Kank1 positivity (○ psitive; △ weakly positive; □ negative). None of these survival curves showed statistical differences.

		Kank1		
		(+)	(±)	(-)
Clear cell RCC	grade 1	9	6	11
	grade 2	31	6	19
	grade 3	8	2	0
Others	grade 1	5	0	0
	grade 2	12	1	1
	grade 3	5	1	0

Table 3. Results of Kank1 staining classified by histological grade.

		Kank1		
		(+)	(±)	(-)
Clear cell RCC	pT1	27	10	17
	pT2	5	2	8
	pT3	14	2	4
	pT4	2	0	0
Others	pT1	11	1	1
	pT2	5	0	0
	pT3	5	0	0
	pT4	1	1	0

Table 4. Results of Kank1 staining classified by pathological stage.

3.4.3. Meaning of Kank1 expression and clinical outcome

Many RCC cells showed inactivation of the *Kank1* gene as shown here. This inactivation presumably occurs at the early stage of carcinogenesis in normal renal tubular cells. Because hemizygous methylation of *Kank1* was observed in many cancer cells (Sarkar et al., 2002), inactivation of *Kank1* could be caused in both alleles by an epigenetic modification such as methylation, rather than by mutations.

Concerning the genetic abnormality of RCC, mutations in the *VHL* gene are most prevalent especially in clear cell RCC (Arai and Kanai, 2011). While *VHL* mutations can be found quite often in sporadic clear cell RCC, they are not significant in other RCC histological subtypes or benign oncocytoma. *VHL* mutations affect the activation of hypoxia-inducible factors, and investigation of this pathway will contribute to a new molecular targeting therapy for RCC (Suwaki et al., 2011). The difference in *VHL* mutations among the RCC histological subtypes suggests a difference in carcinogenesis for each histological subtype, though the origin of the cancer is always a renal tubular cell.

Given that the alteration of *Kank1* expression occurred at the early stage of carcinogenesis, our findings that *Kank1* expression differed among the histological subtypes of RCC might reflect a difference in cancer development (Kim et al., 2005). In clear cell RCC, the loss of *Kank1* expression occurred at a high rate in the lower grade tumors, and the expression was reoccurred as the malignant grade increased. Although the reason for this is not clear, it is presumed that epigenetic modifications such as methylation might have been removed when the malignant grade increased, and consequently, the expression reoccurred (Kisseljova and Kisseljov, 2005). There was no difference in *Kank1* expression between the samples obtained from the groups of patients who survived or not (Table 2). This may reflect the fact that histological grade does not necessarily contribute to clinical outcome, but clinical stage (i.e. the presence of metastasis) is more crucial to obtaining a good prognosis (RCC patients diagnosed at the early stage have more than a 90% five year survival rate) (Lane and Kattan, 2008). The discordance of T stage (tumor size) and the malignant grade on *Kank1* expression could also be supposed for the same reason. A similar result was found for the expression of *CDKN2A* encoding a growth suppressor protein, which is located at 9p21 and close to *Kank1* (9p24) (unpublished data). Although the loss of *Kank1* expression resulted in increased proliferation and poor differentiation in *in vitro* study (Sarkar et al., 2002), our results about the *in vivo* expression of *Kank1* in clinical cases proved that reduced expression does not necessarily reflect a high grade malignancy or poor clinical outcome. These contradictory experimental and clinical results are very interesting, because they suggest that malignant transformation of a normal renal tubular cell has many genetic alterations and clinical outcome is contributed to by many factors in RCC.

4. Prospect of using Kank family genes in genetic diagnosis and gene therapy for renal tumors

4.1. Future diagnostics for RCC

The lack of clinical impact of the current diagnostic markers for RCC apparently requires progress in methodology, biology and pathology (Stewart et al., 2011). The progress in methodology needs the quality of the methods to satisfy the specificity, stability and biological relevance of the markers for diagnosis. For this, sufficient numbers, tens to thousands, of markers would be needed and such markers could be obtained only through cellular signaling analyses. There are quite a number of potential protein and genetic markers for diagnosis and therapeutic targets of RCC based on the information of signal transduction (see Section 2), and more information would be added in the future. While sampling is easier for DNA and RNA-based assays, protein assays such as immunohistochemistry and more advanced mass-spectrometry techniques have problems of contamination and degradation/modification at sampling and processing. In immunohistochemisty, protein cross-linking at the preparation steps disturbs antibody binding. Sampling of homogenously expressed proteins is crucial for the stability of assays, but would not be possible for most sampling cases as the tissue itself is not homogenous. However, diagnosis even for such cases could be possible with markers sufficiently distinguishing heterogenously expressed proteins in different parts of the diseased tissue. In all cases, a statistical significance analysis should be included as a standard evaluation step for quality control of multi-marker systems such as DNA microarrays (Shi et al., 2010).

Biologically relevant markers will be made available in the future based on the analysis of signal transduction, because, as shown in Fig. 1 (Section 2), there are a number of markers available even within a single signaling pathway and there are sufficient numbers of different pathways affected by the disease, which will contribute to the stability of assays. As discussed, the VHL and mTOR pathways have drawn much attentions to prognosis/diagnosis and therapeutic targets for RCC, but there are more pathways such as the Myc and FLCN pathways and pathways related to VEGF, PDGF and TGFα, and some are specific to subtypes of RCC (Linehan et al., 2010; Allory et al., 2011).

Meanwhile, pathologically relevant markers will also be made available in the future, although the situation is different from other technologies due to the technical limit in the number of markers to examine simultaneously.

4.2. A new fluorescence-based immunohistochemical technique

One obstacle to improving immunohistochemistry is the availability of markers. Immunostaining is a relatively simple technique and thus can be used in unequipped laboratories and hospitals, because the preparation, storage and handling of samples are relatively simple. However, ordinary immunostaining is based on single-dye (or single-marker) colorimetric techniques such as the alkaline phosphatase-based method. This is because of a lack of multi-dye (or multi-marker) colorimetric techniques due to expensive devices and, especially, inavailability of stable fluorescent dyes. Fluorescent dyes have been used in many technologies although this has not happened yet in immunohistochemistry because of the lack of their sufficient stability. Stable fluorescent dyes are thus needed for progress in immunohistochemistry.

We reported applications of a new fluorescent dye, Fluolid, for DNA microarray assays and immunohistochemistry (Zhu et al., 2011). Fluolid dyes, including Fluolid-Orange, show stability against heat and excess light compared with other dyes (Fig. 6) and thus can be stored for more than a year without losing fluorescence (data not shown). So, multi-color immunohistochemistry with stable fluorescent dyes will change the pathological diagnostics in several ways: long-term storage of stained sections, simultaneous multi-marker detection and handling of fluorescently stained sections. Heat and light stable fluorescent dyes will enable us to store fluorescently stained sections at room temperature for a long time, which will be important for follow-up studies by microdissection of specific regions.

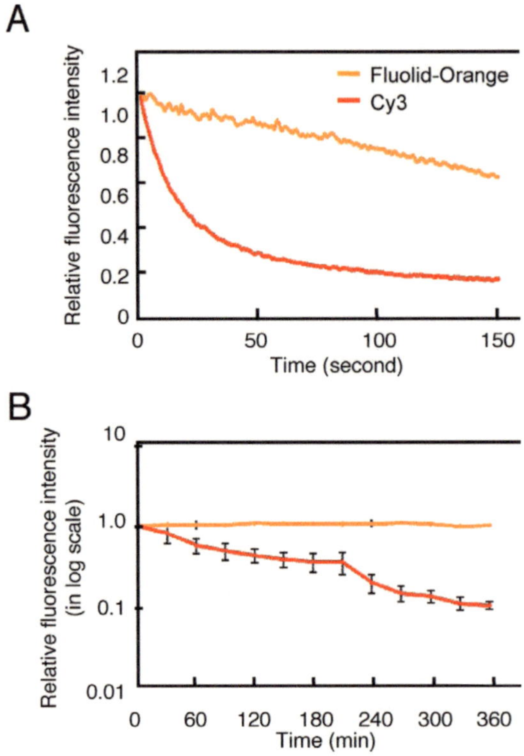

Figure 6. Stability of fluorescently labeled IgG. (A) Photostability of Fluolid-Orange- or Cy3-labeled IgG under irradiation for up to 150 sec with a laser beam at 488 nm. (B) Heat stability. Fluolid-Orange- or Cy3-labeled IgG was left in an environment of 100ºC and fluorescence was measured every 30 min. For details, see Zhu et al. (2011).

4.3. Future therapeutics

As discussed in Section 4.1, future diagnosis will be based on sufficient numbers of protein markers possibly obtained from signal transduction pathways, which will give a statistically significant decision even for cases where no decisive markers, such as disease-causing mutations or constitutive active proteins, are available. In the case of future therapeutics, multiple targets will also be considered to be an effective strategy. Signal transduction-based targeted therapeutics have already been developed for some diseases and drugs such as imatinib or Gleevec/Glivec, a small molecule inhibitor against activated tyrosine kinase activity by the Bcr-Abl fusion gene used for the treatment of chronic myelogenous leukemia, are available (Radford, 2002). Other monoclonal antibody-based drugs such as trastuzumab or Herceptin, which blocks a growth factor receptor HER2/neu (c-erbB-2) to treat breast cancer, and panitumumab or Vectibix, which blocks HER1 to treat colorectal cancer, have been developed based on signal-transduction. Although these drugs are effective, continuous use will sometimes generate drug-resistant cancer (Schenone et al., 2011). So, treatment with multiple targeting drugs will be important in future therapeutics and the same is true for the matched diagnostics about multiple targets.

Acknowledgements

This research has been supported by a Special Coordination Fund for Promoting Science and Technology (Encouraging Development of Strategic Research Centers), a Knowledge Cluster Initiative program and a Grant-in-aid for Basic Areas from the Ministry of Education, Culture, Sports, Science and Technology, Japan.

Author details

Ryoiti Kiyama[1*], Yun Zhu[1] and Tei-ichiro Aoyagi[2]

*Address all correspondence to: kiyama.r@aist.go.jp

1 Biomedical Research Institute, National Institute of Advanced Industrial Science and Technology, Ibaraki, Japan

2 Ibaraki Medical Center, Tokyo Medical University, Ibaraki, Japan

References

[1] Allory, Y., Culine, S., and de la Taille, A. (2011). Kidney cancer pathology in the new context of targeted therapy. Pathobiology 78 (2), 90-98.

[2] Arai, E., and Kanai, Y. (2011). Genetic and epigenetic alterations during renal carcinogenesis. Int. J. Clin. Exp. Pathol. 4, 58-73.

[3] Baldewijns, M.M., van Vlodrop, I.J., Schouten, L.J., Soetekouw, P.M., de Bruïne, A.P., and van Engeland, M. (2008). Genetics and epigenetics of renal cell cancer. Biochim. Biophys. Acta 1785 (2), 133-155.

[4] Beroukhim, R., Brunet, J.P., Di Napoli, A., Mertz, K.D., Seeley, A., Pires, M.M., Linhart, D., Worrell, R.A., Moch, H., Rubin, M.A., Sellers, W.R., Meyerson, M., Linehan, W.M., Kaelin, W.G. Jr., and Signoretti, S. (2009). Patterns of gene expression and copy-number alterations in von-hippel lindau disease-associated and sporadic clear cell carcinoma of the kidney. Cancer Res. 69 (11), 4674-4681.

[5] Bilim, V., Ougolkov, A., Yuuki, K., Naito, S., Kawazoe, H., Muto, A., Oya, M., Billadeau, D., Motoyama, T., and Tomita,Y. (2009). Glycogen synthase kinase-3: a new therapeutic target in renal cell carcinoma. Br. J. Cancer 101, 2005-2014.

[6] Boggetti, B., Jasik, J., Takamiya, M., Strähle, U., Reugels, A.M., and Campos-Ortega, J.A. (2012). NBP, a zebrafish homolog of human Kank3, is a novel Numb interactor essential for epidermal integrity and neurulation. Dev. Biol. 365 (1), 164-174.

[7] Borkowska, J., Schwartz, R.A., Kotulska, K., and Jozwiak, S. (2011). Tuberous sclerosis complex: tumors and tumorigenesis. Int. J. Dermatol. 50 (1), 13-20.

[8] Chin, A.I., Lam, J.S., Figlin, R.A., and Belldegrun, A.S. (2006). Surveillance strategies for renal cell carcinoma patients following nephrectomy. Rev. Urol. 8 (1), 1-7.

[9] Chowdhury, S., Matrana, M.R., Tsang, C., Atkinson, B., Choueiri, T.K., and Tannir, N.M. (2011). Systemic therapy for metastatic non-clear cell renal cell carcinoma: recent progress and future directions. Hematol. Oncol. Clin. North Am. 25, 853-869.

[10] Cifola, I., Spinelli, R., Beltrame, L., Peano, C., Fasoli, E., Ferrero, S., Bosari, S., Signorini, S., Rocco, F., Perego, R., Proserpio, V., Raimondo, F., Mocarelli, P., and Battaglia, C. (2008). Genome-wide screening of copy number alterations and LOH events in renal cell carcinomas and integration with gene expression profile. Mol. Cancer 14, 7:6.

[11] Dalgliesh, G.L., Furge, K., Greenman, C., Chen, L., et al. (2010). Systematic sequencing of renal carcinoma reveals inactivation of histone modifying genes. Nature 463 (7279), 360-363.

[12] DeCastro, G.J., and McKiernan, J.M. (2008). Epidemiology, clinical staging, and presentation of renal cell carcinoma. Urol. Clin. North Am. 35, 581-592.

[13] Deng, F.M., and Melamed, J. (2012). Histological variants of renal cell carcinoma: Does tumor type influence outcome? Urol. Clin. North Am. 39, 119-132.

[14] Ding, M., Goncharov, A., Jin, Y., and Chisholm, A.D. (2003). C. elegans ankyrin repeat protein VAB-19 is a component of epidermal attachment structures and is essential for epidermal morphogenesis. Development 130 (23), 5791-5801.

[15] Duns, G., van den Berg, E., van Duivenbode, I., Osinga, J., Hollema, H., Hofstra, R.M., and Kok, K. (2010). Histone methyltransferase gene SETD2 is a novel tumor suppressor gene in clear cell renal cell carcinoma. Cancer Res. 70 (11), 4287-4291.

[16] Eble, J.N., Sauter, G., Epstein, J.I., and Sesterhenn, I.A. (2004). Classification of Tumours. In "Pathology and genetics of tumors of the urinary system and male genital organs", IARC Press.

[17] Edge, S.B., Byrd, D.R., Compton, C.C., Fritz, A.G., Greene, F.L., and Trotti, A. (2010). "AJCC cancer staging manual", 7th edition,Springer (NY).

[18] Fearon, E.R. (2002) Tumor suppressor genes. In "The Genetic Basis of Human Cancer", (eds, Vogelstein, B., and Kinzler, K.W.), McGraw-Hill, 197-206.

[19] Fendler, A., Stephan, C., Yousef, G.M., and Jung, K. (2011). MicroRNAs as regulators of signal transduction in urological tumors. Clin. Chem. 57 (7), 954-968.

[20] Fuhrman, S.A., Lasky, L.C., and Limas, C. (1982). Prognostic significance of morphologic parameters in renal cell carcinoma. Am. J. Surg. Pathol. 6, 655-663.

[21] Hagenkord, J.M., Gatalica, Z., Jonasch, E., and Monzon, F.A. (2011). Clinical genomics of renal epithelial tumors. Cancer Genet. 204 (6), 285-297.

[22] Hatano, N., Nishikawa, N.S., McElgunn, C., Sarkar, S., Ozawa, K., Shibanaka, Y., Nakajima, M., Gohiji, K., and Kiyama, R. (2001). A comprehensive analysis of loss of heterozygosity caused by hemizygous deletions in renal cell carcinoma using a subtraction library. Mol. Carcinog. 31 (3), 161-170.

[23] Ihara, S., Hagedorn, E.J., Morrissey, M.A., Chi, Q., Motegi, F., Kramer, J.M., and Sherwood, D.R. (2011). Basement membrane sliding and targeted adhesion remodels tissue boundaries during uterine-vulval attachment in Caenorhabditis elegans. Nat. Cell Biol. 13 (6), 641-651.

[24] Inui, M., Martello, G., and Piccolo, S. (2010). MicroRNA control of signal transduction. Nat. Rev. Mol. Cell Biol. 11(4), 252-263.

[25] Isaacs, J.S., Jung, Y.J., Mole, D.R., Lee, S., Torres-Cabala, C., Chung, Y.L., Merino, M., Trepel, J., Zbar, B., Toro, J., Ratcliffe, P.J., Linehan, W.M., and Neckers, L. (2005). HIF overexpression correlates with biallelic loss of fumarate hydratase in renal cancer: novel role of fumarate in regulation of HIF stability. Cancer Cell 8 (2), 143-153.

[26] Jacobs, K.B., Yeager, M., Zhou, W., Wacholder, S., et al. (2012). Detectable clonal mosaicism and its relationship to aging and cancer. Nat. Genet. 44(6), 651-658.

[27] Jantsch-Plunger, V., Gönczy, P., Romano, A., Schnabel, H., Hamill, D., Schnabel, R., Hyman, A.A., and Glotzer, M. (2000). CYK-4: A Rho family gtpase activating protein (GAP) required for central spindle formation and cytokinesis. J. Cell Biol. 149 (7), 1391-1404.

[28] Kaelin, W.G. Jr. (2009). Treatment of kidney cancer: insights provided by the VHL tumor-suppressor protein. Cancer 115 (10 Suppl.), 2262-2272.

[29] Kakinuma, N., and Kiyama, R. (2009). A major mutation of KIF21A associated with congenital fibrosis of the extraocular muscles type 1 (CFEOM1) enhances translocation of Kank1 to the membrane. Biochem. Biophys. Res. Commun. 386 (4), 639-644.

[30] Kakinuma, N., Roy, B.C., Zhu, Y., Wang, Y., and Kiyama, R. (2008). Kank regulates RhoA-dependent formation of actin stress fibers and cell migration via 14-3-3 in PI3K-Akt signaling. J. Cell Biol. 181(3), 537-549.

[31] Kakinuma, N., Zhu, Y., Ogaeri, T., Suzuki, J.I., and Kiyama, R. (2011). Functions of Kank1 and carcinogenesis. In "Tumor Suppressors", Chapter 9, Nova Science Publishers, 161-173.

[32] Kakinuma, N., Zhu, Y., Wang, Y., Roy, B.C., and Kiyama, R. (2009). Kank proteins: structure, functions and diseases. Cell Mol. Life Sci. 66 (16), 2651-2659.

[33] Kamijo, K., Ohara, N., Abe, M., Uchimura, T., Hosoya, H., Lee, J.S., and Miki, T. (2006). Dissecting the role of Rho-mediated signaling in contractile ring formation. Mol. Biol. Cell 17 (1), 43-55.

[34] Kim, H.C., Roh, S.A., Ga, I.H., Kim, J.S., Yu, C.S., and Kim, J.C. (2005). CpG island methylation as an early event during adenoma progression in carcinogenesis of sporadic colorectal cancer. J. Gastroenterol. Hepatol. 20, 1920-1926.

[35] Kisseljova, N.P., and Kisseljov, F.L. (2005). DNA demethylation and carcinogenesis. Biochemistry (Moscow) 70, 743-752.

[36] Kiyama, R., Inoue, S., Ohki, R., Kikuya, E., Yokota, H., and Oishi, M. (1995). A differential cloning procedure for rearranged or altered genomic DNA based on in-gel competitive reassociation. Adv. Biophys. 31, 151-161.

[37] Kondo, K., and Kaelin, W.G. Jr. (2001). The von Hippel-Lindau tumor suppressor gene. Exp. Cell Res. 264 (1), 117-125.

[38] Kosako, H., Yoshida, T., Matsumura, F., Ishizaki, T., Narumiya, S., and Inagaki, M. (2000). Rho-kinase/ROCK is involved in cytokinesis through the phosphorylation of myosin light chain and not ezrin/radixin/moesin proteins at the cleavage furrow. Oncogene 19 (52), 6059-6064.

[39] Kralovics, R., Teo, S.S., Buser, A.S., Brutsche, M., Tiedt, R., Tichelli, A., Passamonti, F., Pietra, D., Cazzola, M., and Skoda, R.C. (2005). Altered gene expression in myeloproliferative disorders correlates with activation of signaling by the V617F mutation of Jak2. Blood 106 (10), 3374-3376.

[40] Krasny, L., Shimony, N., Tzukert, K., Gorodetsky, R., Lecht, S., Nettelbeck, D.M., and Haviv, Y.S. (2010). An in-vivo tumor microenvironment model using adhesion to type collagen reveals Akt-dependent radiation resistance in renal cancer cells. Nephrol. Dial. Transplant. 25, 373-380.

[41] Krill-Burger, J.M., Lyons, M.A., Kelly, L.A., Sciulli, C.M., Petrosko, P., Chandran, U.R., Kubal, M.D., Bastacky. S.I., Parwani, A.V., Dhir, R., and LaFramboise, W.A. (2012). Renal cell neoplasms contain shared tumor type-specific copy number variations. Am. J. Pathol. 180 (6), 2427-2439.

[42] Kuroda, N., Mikami, S., Pan, C.C., Cohen, R.J., Hes, O., Michal, M., Nagashima, Y., Tanaka, Y., Inoue, K., Shuin, T., and Lee, G.H. (2012). Review of renal carcinoma associated with Xp11.2 translocations/TFE3 gene fusions with focus on pathobiological aspect. Histol. Histopathol. 27 (2), 133-140.

[43] Lane, B.R., and Kattan, M.W. (2008). Prognostic models and algorithms in renal cell carcinoma. Urol. Cin. North Am. 35, 613-625.

[44] Lerer, I., Sagi, M., Meiner, V., Cohen, T., Zlotogora, J., and Abeliovich, D. (2005). Deletion of the ANKRD15 gene at 9p24.3 causes parent-of-origin-dependent inheritance of familial cerebral palsy. Hum. Mol. Genet. 14 (24), 3911-3920.

[45] Li, C.C., Kuo, J.C., Waterman, C.M., Kiyama, R., Moss, J., and Vaughan, M. (2011). Effects of brefeldin A-inhibited guanine nucleotide-exchange (BIG) 1 and KANK1 proteins on cell polarity and directed migration during wound healing. Proc. Natl. Acad. Sci. USA 108 (48), 19228-19233.

[46] Li, J., Wang, J., Jiao, H., Liao, J., and Xu, X. (2010). Cytokinesis and cancer: Polo loves ROCK'n' Rho(A). J. Genet. Genomics 37 (3), 159-172.

[47] Linehan, W.M., Srinivasan, R., and Schmidt, L.S. (2010). The genetic basis of kidney cancer: a metabolic disease. Nat. Rev. Urol. 7 (5), 277-285.

[48] Linehan, W.M., Vasselli, J., Srinivasan, R., Walther, M.M., Merino, M., Choyke, P., Vocke, C., Schmidt, L., Isaacs, J.S., Glenn, G., Toro, J., Zbar, B., Bottaro, D., and Neckers, L. (2004). Genetic basis of cancer of the kidney: disease-specific approaches to therapy. Clin. Cancer Res. 10 (18 Pt 2), 6282S-6289S.

[49] Linehan, W.M., Srinivasan, R., and Schmidt, L.S. (2011). Genetic basis of kidney cancer. In "Comprehensive textbook of genitourinary oncology", 4th edition, (eds, Scardino, P.T., Linehan, W.M., Zelefsky, M.J., and Vogelzang, N.J.), Lippincott Williams and Wilkins, 677-685.

[50] Maher, E.R., Neumann, H.P., and Richard, S. (2011). von Hippel-Lindau disease: a clinical and scientific review. Eur. J. Hum. Genet. 19 (6), 617-623.

[51] Marszalek, JR., Weiner, JA., Farlow, SJ., Chun, J., and Goldstein, L.S. (1999). Novel dendritic kinesin sorting identified by different process targeting of two related kinesins: KIF21A and KIF21B. J. Cell Biol. 145 (3), 469-479.

[52] Matsuda, T., Marugame, T., Kamo, K.I., Katanoda, K., Ajiki, W., Sobue, T., and the Japan Cancer Surveillance Research Group. (2012). Cancer Incidence and Incidence Rates in Japan in 2006: Based on Data from 15 Population-based Cancer Registries in the Monitoring of Cancer Incidence in Japan (MCIJ) Project. Jpn. J. Clinical Oncol. 42, 139-147.

[53] Medves, S., Duhoux, F.P., Ferrant, A., Toffalini, F., Ameye, G., Libouton, J.M., Poirel, H.A., and Demoulin, J.B. (2010). KANK1, a candidate tumor suppressor gene, is fused to PDGFRB in an imatinib-responsive myeloid neoplasm with severe thrombocythemia. Leukemia 24 (5), 1052-1055.

[54] Medves, S., Noël, L.A., Montano-Almendras, C.P., Albu, R.I., Schoemans, H., Constantinescu, S.N., and Demoulin, J.B. (2011). Multiple oligomerization domains of KANK1-PDGFRβ are required for JAK2-independent hematopoietic cell proliferation and signaling via STAT5 and ERK. Haematologica 96 (10), 1406-1414.

[55] Morris, Z.S., and McClatchey, A.I. (2009). Aberrant epithelial morphology and persistent epidermal growth factor receptor signaling in a mouse model of renal carcinoma. Proc. Natl. Acad. Sci. USA 106 (24), 9767-9772.

[56] Osanto, S., Qin, Y., Buermans, H.P., Berkers, J., Lerut, E., Goeman, J.J., and van Poppel, H. (2012). Genome-wide microRNA expression analysis of clear cell renal cell carcinoma by next generation deep sequencing. PLoS One 7 (6), e38298.

[57] Parry, L., Maynard, J.H., Patel, A., Clifford, S.C., Morrissey, C., Maher, E.R., Cheadle, J.P., and Sampson, J.R. (2001). Analysis of the TSC1 and TSC2 genes in sporadic renal cell carcinomas. Br. J. Cancer 85 (8), 1226-1230.

[58] Peña-Llopis, S., Vega-Rubín-de-Celis, S., Liao, A., Leng, N., et al. (2012). BAP1 loss defines a new class of renal cell carcinoma. Nat. Genet. 44 (7), 751-759.

[59] Perroud, B., Lee, J., Valkova, N., Dhirapong, A., Lin, P.Y., Fiehn, O., Kültz, D., and Weiss, R.H. (2006). Pathway analysis of kidney cancer using proteomics and metabolic profiling. Mol. Cancer 5:64.

[60] Polinsky, K.R. (Ed.) (2007). "Tumor Suppressor Genes", Nova Science Publishers.

[61] Previdi, S., Maroni, P., Matteucci, E., Broggini, M., Bendinelli, P., and Desiderio, M.A. (2010). Interaction between human-breast cancer metastasis and bone microenvironment through activated hepatocyte growth factor/Met and beta-catenin/Wnt pathways. Eur. J. Cancer 46 (9), 1679-1691.

[62] Purdue, M.P., Johansson, M., Zelenika, D., Toro, J.R., et al. (2011). Genome-wide association study of renal cell carcinoma identifies two susceptibility loci on 2p21 and 11q13.3. Nat. Genet. 43 (1), 60-65.

[63] Radford, I.R. (2002). Imatinib. Novartis. Curr. Opin. Investig. Drugs 3 (3), 492-499.

[64] Raimondo, F., Salemi, C., Chinello, C., Fumagalli, D., Morosi, L., Rocco, F., Ferrero, S., Perego, R., Bianchi, C., Sarto, C., Pitto, M., Brambilla, P., and Magni, F. (2012). Proteomic analysis in clear cell renal cell carcinoma: identification of differentially expressed protein by 2-D DIGE. Mol. Biosyst. 8 (4), 1040-1051.

[65] Redova, M., Svoboda, M., and Slaby, O. (2011). MicroRNAs and their target gene networks in renal cell carcinoma. Biochem. Biophys. Res. Commun. 405 (2), 153-156.

[66] Rodley, P., Hatano, N., Nishikawa, N.S., Roy, B.C., Sarkar, S., and Kiyama, R. (2003). A differential genomic cloning method for cancer study: an outline and applications. Recent. Res. Dev. Mol. Biol. 1, 13-27.

[67] Ross, H., Martignoni, G., and Argani, P. (2012). Renal cell carcinoma with clear cell and papillary features. Arch. Pathol. Lab. Med. 136 (4), 391-399.

[68] Roy, B.C., Aoyagi, T., Sarkar, S., Nomura, K., Kanda, H., Iwaya, K., Tachibana, M., and Kiyama, R. (2005). Pathological characterization of Kank in renal cell carcinoma. Exp. Mol. Pathol. 78 (1), 41-48.

[69] Roy, B.C., Kakinuma, N., and Kiyama, R. (2009). Kank attenuates actin remodeling by preventing interaction between IRSp53 and Rac1. J. Cell Biol. 184 (2), 253-267.

[70] Sarkar, S., Roy, B.C., Hatano, N., Aoyagi, T., Gohji, K., and Kiyama, R. (2002). A novel ankyrin repeat-containing gene (Kank) located at 9p24 is a growth suppressor of renal cell carcinoma. J. Biol. Chem. 277 (39), 36585-36591.

[71] Schenone, S., Bruno, O., Radi, M., and Botta, M. (2011). New insights into small-molecule inhibitors of Bcr-Abl. Med. Res. Rev. 31 (1), 1-41.

[72] Schmidt, L., Duh, F.M., Chen, F., Kishida, T., et al. (1997). Germline and somatic mutations in the tyrosine kinase domain of the MET proto-oncogene in papillary renal carcinomas. Nat. Genet. 16 (1), 68-73.

[73] Sherr, C.J. (2004). Principles of tumor suppression. Cell 116 (2), 235-246.

[74] Shi, L., Campbell, G., Jones, W.D., Campagne, F., et al. (2010). MAQC Consortium. The MicroArray Quality Control (MAQC)-II study of common practices for the development and validation of microarray-based predictive models. Nat. Biotechnol. 28 (8), 827-838.

[75] Siegel, R., Naishadham, D., and Jemal, A. (2012). Cancer statistics, 2012. C.A. Cancer J. Clin. 62, 10-29.

[76] Smaldone, M.C., and Maranchie, J.K. (2009). Clinical implications of hypoxia inducible factor in renal cell carcinoma. Urol. Oncol. 27 (3), 238-245.

[77] Stewart, G.D., O'Mahony, F.C., Powles, T., Riddick, A.C., Harrison, D.J., and Faratian, D. (2011). What can molecular pathology contribute to the management of renal cell carcinoma? Nat. Rev. Urol. 8 (5), 255-265.

[78] Sudarshan, S., Pinto, P.A., Neckers, L., and Linehan, W.M. (2007). Mechanisms of disease: hereditary leiomyomatosis and renal cell cancer--a distinct form of hereditary kidney cancer. Nat. Clin. Pract. Urol. 4 (2), 104-110.

[79] Suwaki, N., Vanhecke, E., Atkins, K.M., Graf, M., et al. (2011). A HIF-regurated VHL-PTP1B-Src signaling axis identifies a therapeutic target in renal cell carcinoma. Sci. Transl. Med. 3 (85), 85ra47.

[80] Takahashi, M., Rhodes, D.R., Furge, K.A., Kanayama, H., Kagawa, S., Haab, B.B., and Teh, B.T. (2001). Gene expression profiling of clear cell renal cell carcinoma: gene identification and prognostic classification. Proc. Natl. Acad. Sci. USA 98 (17), 9754-9759.

[81] Takahashi, M., Yang, X.J., Sugimura, J., Backdahl, J., Tretiakova, M., Qian, C.N., Gray, S.G., Knapp, R., Anema, J., Kahnoski, R., Nicol, D., Vogelzang, N.J., Furge, K.A., Kanayama, H., Kagawa, S., and The, B.T. (2003) Molecular subclassification of kidney tumors and the discovery of new diagnostic markers. Oncogene 22 (43), 6810-6818.

[82] Toschi, A., Lee, E., Gadir, N., Ohh, M., and Foster, D.A. (2008). Differential dependence of hypoxia-inducible factors 1 alpha and 2 alpha on mTORC1 and mTORC2. J. Biol. Chem. 283 (50), 34495-34499.

[83] Varela, I., Tarpey, P., Raine, K., Huang, D., et al. (2011). Exome sequencing identifies frequent mutation of the SWI/SNF complex gene PBRM1 in renal carcinoma. Nature 469 (7331), 539-542.

[84] Verine, J., Pluvinage, A., Bousquet, G., Lehmann-Che, J., de Bazelaire, C., Soufir, N., and Mongiat-artus, P. (2010). Hereditary renal cancer syndromes: an update of a systematic review. Eur. Urol. 58 (5), 701-710.

[85] Walsh, N., Larkin, A., Kennedy, S., Connolly, L., Ballot, J., Ooi, W., Gullo, G., Crown, J., Clynes, M., and O'Driscoll, L. (2009). Expression of multidrug resistance markers ABCB1 (MDR-1/P-gp) and ABCC1 (MRP-1) in renal cell cacinoma. BMC Urology 9:6.

[86] Wang, Y., Kakinuma, N., Zhu, Y., and Kiyama, R. (2006). Nucleo-cytoplasmic shuttling of human Kank protein accompanies intracellular translocation of beta-catenin. J. Cell Sci. 119, 4002-4010.

[87] Wang, Y., Onishi, Y., Kakinuma, N., Roy, B.C., Aoyagi, T., and Kiyama, R. (2005). Alternative splicing of the human Kank gene produces two types of Kank protein. Biochem. Biophys. Res. Commun. 330 (4), 1247-1253.

[88] Xu, X., Patrakka, J., Sistani, L., Uhlen, M., Jalanko, H., Betsholtz, C., and Tryggvason, K. (2011). Expression of novel podocyte-associated proteins sult1b1 and ankrd25. Nephron. Exp. Nephrol. 117 (2), e39-46.

[89] Yamada, K., Hunter, D.G., Andrews, C., and Engle, E.C. (2005). A novel KIF21A mutation in a patient with congenital fibrosis of the extraocular muscles and Marcus Gunn jaw-winking phenomenon. Arch. Ophthalmol. 123 (9), 1254-1259.

[90] Zhu, Y., Kakinuma, N., Wang, Y., and Kiyama, R. (2008). Kank proteins: a new family of ankyrin-repeat domain-containing proteins. Biochim. Biophys. Acta 1780 (2), 128-133.

[91] Zhu, Y., Ogaeri, T., Suzuki, J.I., Dong, S.J., Aoyagi, T.I., Mizuki, K., Takasugi, M., Isobe, S.I., and Kiyama, R. (2011). Application of Fluolid-Orange-labeled probes for DNA microarray and immunological assays. Biotechnol. Lett. 33, 1759-1766.

Chapter 2

Signaling Pathways and Biomarkers in Renal Tumors

Tetsuo Fujita, Masatsugu Iwamura,
Kazumasa Matsumoto and Kazunari Yoshida

Additional information is available at the end of the chapter

http://dx.doi.org/10.5772/53787

1. Introduction

Sunitinib malate (Sutent, Pfizer inc., New York, NY) is an orally administered, multitargeted inhibitor of tyrosine kinases, including vascular endothelial growth factor (VEGF) receptor, platelet-derived growth factor (PDGF) receptor, stem cell factor receptor (KIT), fms-like tyrosine kinase (FLT) -3, CSF-1R, and RET. Since the introduction of sunitinib for patients with advanced renal tumor [1], significant objective responses of sunitnib have been revealed [2-6]. In a randomized, multicenter, phase III trial enrolled 750 patients with previously-untreated metastatic renal tumor to receive either sunitinib or interferon (IFN) -α, sunitinib was superior to IFN-α in the objective response rate (47% *vs* 12%), progression-free survival time (11.0 *vs* 5.0 months), and overall survival time (26.4 *vs* 21.8 months) [3, 4]. Also in a Japanese, multicenter, phase II trial enrolled 51 patients with first-line and pretreated metastatic clear-cell renal tumor to recieve sinitinib, significant responses of sunitinib have been reported that objective response rate was 52.9%, the median progression-free survival time was 12.2 and 10.6 months, and the median overall survival time was 33.1 and 32.5 months in first-line and pretreated patients, respectively [5, 6]. Sunitinib is approved worldwide for first-line treatment of advanced clear-cell renal tumor. However, approximately half of patients with advanced renal tumor do not see clinical benefits from sunitinib treatment. A prognostic marker is needed for selecting patients who will benefit most from sunitinib.

It has been advocated that the necessity of determining molecular and clinical biomarkers that may predict efficacy of sunitinib. The identification of biomarkers to predict response is urgently needed. This chapter provides a brief overview of the signaling pathways of renal tumors and introduces biomarkers to predict response to sunitinib of clinical variables.

INTECH
open science | open minds

© 2013 Fujita et al.; licensee InTech. This is a paper distributed under the terms of the Creative Commons Attribution License (http://creativecommons.org/licenses/by/3.0), which permits unrestricted use, distribution, and reproduction in any medium, provided the original work is properly cited.

2. Signaling pathways in renal tumors

Renal tumors originates from the tubular structures of the kidney and is calssified into four major histological cell types. Clear-cell renal tumor is the most common type, accounting for approximately 75% of all renal tumors. Other types are followed by papillary renal tumor (approximately 15%), chromophobe renal tumor (approximately 5%), and renal oncocytoma (approximately 5%) [7].

The most important molecular disorder in renal tumors involves the von Hippel-Lindau (VHL) tumor suppressor gene, which is responsible for clear-cell renal tumors. The protein production of the *VHL* gene, which is located on chromosome 3p25, prevents angiogenesis and suppresses tumors [7]. Inactivating the phosphorylated VHL protein activates hypoxia-inducible factor (HIF) and the induction of VEGF in clear-cell renal tumors. Mesenchymal-epithelial transition factor (MET) and fumarate hydratase (FH) are responsible for papillary renal tumors. While chromophobe renal tumors, Birt-Hogg-Dube (BHD) tumor suppresor gene is mutated [8]. The inherited renal tumor genes *VHL, MET, FH, folliculin, succinate dehydrogenase,* tuberous sclerosis complex (TSC) 1, and *TSC2* are all involved in metabolic pathways related to oxygen, iron, energy, and nutrient sensing [9].

Alterations in proto-oncogenes and tumor suppressor genes leads to dysregulated signal transduction that underlies the abnormal growth and proliferation of cancer cells. Signaling proteins that are centrally located in important cancer-associated signaling networks can serve as therapeutic targets [10].

2.1. Angiogenetic signaling pathways

Renal tumors are frequnently characterized by hypoxic conditions. Hypoxia and compensatory hyperactivation of angiogenesis are thought to be particularly important in renal tumors, given the highly vascularized nature and the specific association of mutation in *VHL*, a critical regulator of the hypoxic response. Hypoxic signaling is mediated by HIF. Increased expression of HIF target genes is implicated in promoting cancer, inducing both changes within the tumor and changes in the growth of adjacent endothelial cells to promote blood vessel growth. The expression level of VEGF in renal tumors is known to strongly correlate with microvessel density [10].

2.2. PI3K/AKT/mTOR pathway

Mammalian target of rapamycin (mTOR) and protein kinase B (AKT) are key oncogenic process including cell proliferation, survival, and angiogenesis. PI3K promotes the generation of phosphatidylinositol-3, 4, 5-triphosphate. Signaling from VEGF and PDGF through AKT activates mTOR. Components of this PI3K/AKT/mTOR pathway are constitutively activated in renal tumors compared to normal renal tissues [11].

http://dx.doi.org/10.5772/53787

2.3. HGF/MET pathway

Changes in expression and activity of hepatocyte growth factor (HGF) and its receptor c-MET have been associated with renal tumors. HGF binding to MET leads to phosphorylation of two tyrosine residues at the C-terminus of MET, which leads to the recruitment of adapter proteins and activation of PI3K/AKT pathway to promote renal tumor growth and metastasis [12].

3. Biomarkers of response to sunitinib in renal tumors

3.1. Prognostic model

In the cytokine era, Motzer et al. [13] reported Memorial Sloan-Kettering Cancer Center (MSKCC) risk classification, which is based on data from 463 patients with advanced renal tumor who were treated with IFN-α cytokine therapy as first-line systemic therapy. The MSKCC risk classification extracted five variable risk factors for short survival: low Karnofsky performance status (PS) (< 80%), high lactate dehydrogenase (> 1.5 times the upper limit of normal), low serum hemoglobin, high corrected serum calcium (> 10 mg/dL), and time from initial renal tumor diagnosis to IFN-α therapy of less than one year. Each patient was assigned to one of three risk groups: those with zero risk factors (favorable risk), those with one or two risk factors (intermediate risk), and those with three or more risk factors (poor risk). The median time to death was 30, 14, and 5 months in the favorable, intermediate, and poor-risk groups, respectively [13]. These five risk criteria are now most frequently used prognostic model for patients with advanced renal tumor.

In the era of targeted therapy, Heng et al. [14] reported a new prognostic model that added platelet and neutrophil counts to the MSKCC model from a large multicenter study of 645 patients with metastatic renal tumor who were treated with targeted therapy. This study included three groups of patients: 396 patients treated with sunitinib, 200 patients treated with sorafenib, and 49 patients treated with bevacizumab. Four of the five adverse prognostic factors according to the MSKCC risk classification–low hemoglobin, high corrected serum calcium, low Karnofsky PS, and time from the initial renal tumor diagnosis to the start of treatment of less than one year–emerged as independent predictors of poor survival. Additionally, platelets greater than the upper limit of normal range, and neutrophils greater than the upper limit of normal range, emerged as independent adverse prognostic factors. MSKCC model with the addition of platelet and neutrophil counts can be incorporated into patient care of targeted therapies [14].

3.2. C-reactive protein

C-reactive protein (CRP), a non-specific inflammatory acute-phase protein, is a representative marker of systemic inflammatory response. CRP levels correlate with the production of proinflammatory cytokines, such as interleukin (IL) -6 [15], and with tumor progression [16, 17]. It has been recognized as an important prognostic marker in the cytokine era. Atzpodien et al. [16] reported data from 425 patients who received cytokine-based home therapy. On multivariate analysis, elevated CRP (≥ 1.1 mg/dL) was a poor prognostic factor, and Kaplan-Meier analysis demonstrated that patients with elevated CRP had significantly worse overall survival [16]. Casamassima et al. [17] reported that normal CRP (≤ 0.8 mg/dL) was the most independent prognostic factor for 110 patients treated with IL-2-based immunotherapy. Ramsey et al. [18] investigated the Glasgow Prognostic Score, which is based on a combination of hypoalbuminemia and elevated CRP (> 1.0 mg/dL). They found that CRP was independently associated with cancer-specific survival in 119 patients receiving immunotherapy [18]. Saito et al. [19] described that CRP kinetics have an impact on survival in patients with metastatic renal tumor treated with immunotherapy and/or metastasectomy. A decrease of CRP level during treatment predicts better prognosis in patients with metastatic renal tumor, and prolonged normalized CRP period is associated with prolonged survival [19].

Variable	Univariate		Multivariate	
	Odds Ratio (95% Confidence Interval)	*P*-value	Odds Ratio (95% Confidence Interval)	*P*-value
Pretreatment				
Age	0.988 (0.920–1.061)	0.7410		
Gender	0.573 (0.139–2.355)	0.4384		
ECOG PS0	4.200 (0.884–19.947)	0.0598		
MSKCC non-poor	0.150 (0.026–0.864)	0.0206	0.632 (0.058–6.850)	0.7042
First-line	0.879 (0.238–3.249)	0.8468		
Normal CRP	17.600 (1.961–157.970)	0.0011	13.525 (1.111–164.602)	0.0163
Adverse events				
Hypertension	3.667 (0.954–14.094)	0.0523		
HFS	6.500 (1.537–27.490)	0.0069	2.272 (0.324–15.930)	0.4104
Stomatitis	3.200 (0.826–12.404)	0.0844		
Diarrhea	1.375 (0.368–5.136)	0.6347		
Altered taste	8.250 (1.498–45.436)	0.0064	4.422 (0.533–36.655)	0.1517
Fatigue	5.133 (1.131–23.303)	0.0238	1.572 (0.192–12.841)	0.6740
Leukopenia	8.333 (0.867–80.130)	0.0337	5.436 (0.190–155.246)	0.2717
Anemia	1.771 (0.392–8.003)	0.4559		
Thrombocytopenia	758.701 (0.000)	0.0670		
Increased creatinine	2.182 (0.566–8.415)	0.2505		
TSH abnormalities	2.812 (0.734–10.774)	0.1255		

Table 1. Univariate and multivariate logistic regression analyses for selected variables

In the targeted therapy era, Fujita et al. [20] recently reported that CRP is an independent prognostic indicator for patients with advanced renal tumor treated with sunitinib. A total of

41 consecutive patients between December 2008 and August 2011 were enrolled in this study. All patients had histologically proven clear-cell renal tumor. Non-tumor variables which were selected from pretreatment characteristics and treatment-related adverse events were analyzed on univariate and multivariate logistic regression analysis. Pretreatment characteristics were age, gender, Eastern Cooperative Oncology Group (ECOG) PS 0, MSKCC non-poor (favorable and intermediate) risk, first-line treatment, and normal CRP. Treatment-related adverse events were hypertension, hand-foot skin reaction (HFS), stomatitis, diarrhea, altered taste, fatigue, leukopenia, anemia, thrombocytopenia, increased creatinine, and thyroid-stimulating hormone (TSH) abnormalities. On univariate analyses among pretreatment characteristics, MSKCC non-poor risk classification and normal CRP level were significantly correlated with response to treatment ($P = 0.0206$ and 0.0011, respectively). Among adverse events, HFS, altered taste, fatigue, and leukopenia were significantly corralated with response to treatment ($P = 0.0069$, 0.0064, 0.0238, and 0.0337, respectively). Variable values in the multivariate analysis included MSKCC non-poor risk classification, normal CRP, HFS, altered taste, fatigue, and leukopenia. After adjusting for differences in these variables, normal CRP was independently associated with response to treatment ($P = 0.0163$).

Patients were grouped into two cohorts: those with normal CRP levels (≤ 0.30 mg/dL) and those with elevated CRP levels (> 0.30 mg/dL), according to the normal values provided by the manufacturer. The cohort with normal CRP comprised 10 males and 3 females (total 13 patients; 31.7%) with a median age of 63 years (range 46–77 years). The elevated CRP cohort comprised 20 males and 8 females (total 28 patients; 68.3%) with a median age of 64 years (range 36–80 years). MSKCC risk classification was favorable for 15.4% of the normal CRP cohort and intermediate for 86.4%. In contrast, in the elevated CRP cohort, MSKCC risk classification was favorable for 21.4%, intermediate for 46.4%, and poor for 32.2%. The difference in risk classification between the two groups was statistically significant ($P = 0.0377$). There were no statistically significant differences in any other pretreatment variables and tumor characteristics. The rate of partial response plus stable disease to treatment was 84.6% for the normal CRP cohort and 35.7% for the elevated CRP cohort. The higher response rate observed in the normal CRP cohort was statistically significant ($P = 0.0022$).

	Normal CRP (≤ 0.30 mg/dL)	**Elevated CRP (> 0.30 mg/dL)**	***P*-value**
	13 (31.7%)	28 (68.3%)	
Gender (*n* (%))			0.7118
Male	10 (76.9)	20 (71.4)	
Female	3 (23.1)	8 (28.6)	
Age (years)			0.5953
Median	63	64	
Range	46–77	36–80	
Mean ± standard deviation	64.8 ± 9.0	63.2 ± 9.1	

	Normal CRP (≤ 0.30 mg/dL)	**Elevated CRP (> 0.30 mg/dL)**	***P*-value**
ECOG PS (*n* (%))			0.0595
0	12 (92.3)	18 (64.3)	
≥ 1	1 (7.7)	10 (35.7)	
MSKCC risk classification (*n* (%))			0.0377
Favorable	2 (15.4)	6 (21.4)	
Intermediate	11 (84.6)	13 (46.4)	
Poor	0 (0)	9 (32.2)	
Prior nephrectomy (*n* (%))			0.2767
Yes	12 (92.3)	22 (78.6)	
No	1 (7.7)	6 (21.4)	
T stage (*n* (%))			0.8187
T1 or T2	6 (46.2)	14 (50.0)	
≥ T3	7 (53.8)	14 (50.0)	
Grade (*n* (%))			0.6628
1 or 2	9 (69.2)	17 (60.7)	
3	3 (23.1)	8 (28.6)	
Prior immunotherapy (*n*)			0.2482
IFN-α	9	14	
IL-2 and IFN-α	3	6	
Prior targeted therapy (*n*)			0.8651
Sorafenib	5	10	
Metastatic sites (*n*)			
Lung	12	21	
Bone	2	12	
Lymph nodes	3	7	
Brain	1	3	
Pancreas	–	4	
Adrenal	–	4	
Skin	–	3	
Kidney	–	2	
Local	–	2	
Liver	–	2	

http://dx.doi.org/10.5772/53787

	Normal CRP (≤ 0.30 mg/dL)	Elevated CRP (> 0.30 mg/dL)	*P*-value
Prostate	1	–	
No. metastatic sites (*n* (%))			0.1929
1	6 (46.1)	8 (28.6)	
≥ 2	6 (46.1)	20 (71.4)	
Treatment (*n* (%))			0.2122
First-line	3 (23.1)	13 (46.4)	
Second-line	6 (46.1)	6 (21.4)	
Third-line	4 (30.8)	9 (32.2)	
Responses (*n* (%))			0.0022
Partial response plus stable disease	11 (84.6)	10 (35.7)	

Table 2. Patient characteristics grouped by CRP level

The median progression-free survival time for the elevated CRP cohort was 6.0 months. In contrast, the median progression-free survival time for the normal CRP cohort was significantly longer, at 19.0 months (log-rank $P = 0.0361$).

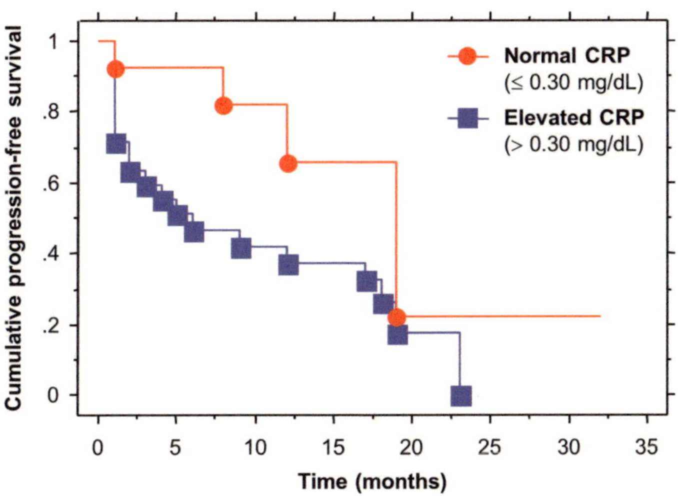

Figure 1. Kaplan-Meier progression-free survival for patients grouped by CRP level

CRP is a significant independent prognostic indicator for patients with advanced renal tumor treated with sunitinib. Pretreatment CRP level could be a useful biomarker for response to sunitinib treatment [20].

3.3. Selected adverse events

Sunitinib has been related a variety of adverse events, key notable clinical adverse events included diarrhea (61%), fatigue (54%), hypertension (30%), stomatitis (30%), HFS (29%), and asthenia (20%) [4]. Laboratory abnormalities also found that included leukopenia (78%), anemia (79%), increased creatinine (70%), and thrombocytopenia (68%) [4]. If adverse events depends on the degree of systemic exposure to sunitinib, on which clinical efficacy also depends, adverse events might be potential predictors of sunitinib efficacy [21]. Several authors have described the correlation between sunitinib responses and selected treatment-related adverse events.

3.3.1. Hypertension

Hypertension is commonly associated with targeted therapy. It develops when VEGF stimulates production of nitric oxide and prostacyclins in vascular endothelial cells [22, 23], vasodilatory mechanisms become inhibited, and peripheral vascular resistance increases, leading to increased blood pressure.

Rini et al. [24] demonstrated that sunitinib-associated hypertension is associated with improved clinical outcomes without clinically significant increases in hypertension-associated adverse events. This analysis included large pooled data from four clinical trilas of 4915 patients with metastatic renal tumor who were treated with sunitinib. Sunitinib-induced hypertension had significantly better outcomes than those without treatment-induced hypertension in the objective response rate (54.8% *vs* 8.7%), the median progression-free survival time (12.5 *vs* 2.5 months), and the median overall survival time (30.9 *vs* 7.2 months, $P<$ 0.001 for all) [24].

Bono et al. [25] reported that sunitinib-induced hypertension was associated with frequent tumor response ($P = 0.001$), significantly longer disease progression time ($P = 0.0003$), and overall survival time ($P = 0.001$). On multivariate analysis including the variables of pretreatment hemoglobin, pretreatment calcium level, PS, time from diagnosis to onset of metastasis, and treatment-related hypertension, hypertension was an independent predictor of progression-free survival ($P = 0.0030$) [25].

Szmit et al. [26] reported that patients who developed hypertension related to sunitinib treatment experienced significantly longer progression-free survival time and overall survival time compared to those who did not hypertension ($P< 0.00001$). Patients treated with at least 3 antihypertensive agents experienced significantly longer progression-free survival time ($P = 0.00002$) and overall survival time ($P = 0.00001$) compared either with patients who received one or two medications or with patients who received no medications [26].

Rixe et al. [27] reported that appearance or worsening hypertension was found to be the single independent predictor of a better clinical response to sunitinib on multivariate analysis using logistic regression model ($P = 0.009$). Furthermore, grade 3 hypertension was correlated with a better outcome ($P = 0.03$). The appearance of hypertension, particularly grade 3, was associated with higher treatment response to sunitinib in metastatic renal tumors. Early and intensive antihypertensive therapy with the goal of maintaining the sunitinib use may improve response rate in those patients [27].

Overall, hypertension related to sunitinib was a positive predictive factor associated with significantly better objective response rate, longer progression-free survival and overall survival in patients with metastatic renal tumor treated with sunitinib.

3.3.2. Hypothyroidism

Treatment-related hypothyroidism has been reported a useful predictor of progression-free survival for metastatic renal tumors undergoing treatment with sunitinib [28]. In the 52 patients with metastatic renal tumor treated with sunitinib, 13 patients (25.0%) developed hypothyroidism during treatment. Subclinical hypothyroidism was defined as serum TSH above the upper limit of normal, with total triiodothyronine (T3) and thyroxine (T4) within normal limits. Clinical hypothyroidism was defined as low serum T3 and T4 together with elevated TSH. Hypothyroidism was associated with a longer progression-free survival time ($P = 0.032$). Hormone replacement with 1-thyroxine did not have an influence on survival [28].

3.4. Others

Han et al. [29] reported the initial tumor enhancement on contrast-enhanced computed tomography (CT) could be useful as a clinical predictor during targeted therapy in 198 metastatic lesions of 46 patients. On multivariate analyses, tumor enhancement and enhancement pattern were associated with objective responses ($P = 0.003$ and 0.028, respectively). Additionally, tumor enhancement was associated with tumor size reduction ($P = 0.004$). On Cox proportional hazards models, only tumor enhancement was associated significantly with the time to size reduction and progression-free survival time ($P = 0.03$ and 0.015, respectively). Tumor enhancement on contrast-enhanced CT was associated with tumor size reduction, time to response, and time to progression of individual metastases in patients with metastatic renal tumor who received targeted therapy [29].

Kayani et al [30] revealed prognostic significance of ^{18}F-fluorodeoxyglucose-positron emission tomography (FDG-PET)/CT as a biomarker of response to sunitinib. A total of 44 patients with newly diagnosed untreated metastatic renal tumor were enrolled in this study. ^{18}F-FDG-PET/CT scans were conducted before, after 4 weeks, and after 16 weeks of sunitinib given. On multivariate analysis, a high SUV_{max} and an increased number of PET-positive lesions correlated with shorter overall survival. The early metabolic responses are associated with a pharmacodynamic effect of drug and it is not until later identification with acquired resistance occurs [30].

Yuasa et al. [31] reported that initial tumor size is inversely associated with the tumor reduction rate of individual metastatic sites and primary tumors in patients with metastatic renal tumor who underwent targeted therapy. A data from 139 metastatic and 16 primary lesions treated with targeted agents were analyzed. Both univariate and multivariate linear regression analyses revealed that only the initial tumor size was associated with the rate of reduction in individual tumors ($P< 0.001$) [31].

Abel et al. [32] reported that early 10% decrease in tumor diameter of the primary tumor was predictive of improved overall survival in patients with metastatic renal tumor treated with sunitinib. In 75 consecutive treatment-naive patients, median overall survival time for patients without minor primary tumor response, with minor primary tumor response after 60 days, and with early minor primary tumor response was 10.3, 16.5, and 30.2 months, respectively. On multivariate analysis, early minor response was an independent predictor of improved overall survival ($P = 0.031$) [32].

High visceral fat area could be a predictive biomarker from shorter survival in patients given first-line antiangiogenic agents including sunitinib for metastatic renal tumors [33]. In 113 study population, 46 patients received sunitinib as first-line therapy. Visceral fat area was measured retrospectively on the available CT scans performed before sunitinib initiation at the level of the umbilicus with the patient in the supine position. ImageJ software was used to measure pixels with densities in the -190 Hounsfield units to -30 Hounsfield units range to delineate the visceral compartment and to compute the cross-sectional area of each in cm^2. On multivariate analysis, high visceral fat area was independently associated with shorter time to progression and overall survival. Visceral fat area measured before starting first-line targeted therapy is likely to be a simple predictive biomarker in patients with metastatic renal tumor [33].

Finally, hyponatremia seem to represent significant predictive factor for cancer-specific survival in metastatic renal tumors treated with targeted therapy as first-line therapy [34]. A total of 87 patients treated with targeted therapy including sunitinib, severe (≤ 134 mEq/L) and mild (135-137 mEq/L) hyponatremia was shown to be significantly associated with cancer-specific survival time ($P = 0.001$ and 0.013, respectively). In 38 patients treated wth sunitinib, 4 patients (10.5%) developed severe hyponatremia and 8 patients (21.1%) developed mild hyponatremia. Hyponatremia could be easily and readily determined and might be an important prognostic factor [34].

4. Conclusions

Candidate biomarkers to predict response to sunitinib have been shown. Among clinical factors, CRP is a significant independent prognostic indicator for sunitinib. Severe adverse events, hypertension and hypothyroidism also recognized as biomarkers of favorable efficacy. Additionally, tumor enhancement, SUV_{max} on FDG/PET-CT, tumor size, visceral fat area and hyponatremia have been revealed clinical significance of sunitinib responses. Although further investigation will be required, these biomarkers can be utilized to measure therapeutic response and design treatment strategies for advanced renal tumors treated with sunitinib.

http://dx.doi.org/10.5772/53787

Author details

Tetsuo Fujita*, Masatsugu Iwamura, Kazumasa Matsumoto and Kazunari Yoshida

*Address all correspondence to: tfujita@cd5.so-net.ne.jp

Department of Urology, Kitasato University School of Medicine, Japan

References

[1] Motzer, R. J, Michaelson, M. D, Redman, B. G, Hudes, G. R, Wilding, G, Figlin, R. A, Ginsberg, M. S, Kim, S. T, Baum, C. M, DePrimo, S. E, Li, J. Z, Bello, C. L, Theuer, C. P, George, D. J, & Rini, B. I. (2006). Activity of SU11248, a multitargeted inhibitor of vascular endothelial growth factor receptor and platelet-derived growth factor receptor, in patients with metastatic renal cell carcinoma. *Journal of Clinical Oncology*, 24(1), 16-24.

[2] Motzer, R. J, Rini, B. I, Bukowski, R. M, Curti, B. D, George, D. J, Hudes, G. R, Redman, B. G, Margolin, K. A, Merchan, J. R, Wilding, G, Ginsberg, M. S, Bacik, J, Kim, S. T, Baum, C. M, & Michaelson, M. D. (2006). Sunitinib in patients with metastatic renal cell carcinoma. *JAMA*, 295(21), 2516-2524.

[3] Motzer, R. J, Hutson, T. E, Tomczak, P, Michaelson, M. D, Bukowski, R. M, Rixe, O, Oudard, S, Negrier, S, Szczylik, C, Kim, S. T, Chen, I, Bycott, P. W, Baum, C. M, & Figlin, R. A. (2007). Sunitinib versus interferon alfa in metastatic renal-cell carcinoma. *New England Journal of Medicine*, 356(2), 115-124.

[4] Motzer, R. J, Hutson, T. E, Tomczak, P, Michaelson, M. D, Bukowski, R. M, Oudard, S, Negrier, S, Szczylik, C, Pili, R, Bjarnason, G. A, Garcia-del-Muro, X, Sosman, J. A, Solska, E, Wilding, G, Thompson, J. A, Kim, S. T, Chen, I, Huang, X, & Figlin, R. A. (2009). Overall survival and updated results for sunitinib compared with interferon alfa in patients with metastatic renal cell carcinoma. *Journal of Clinical Oncology*, 27(22), 3584-3590.

[5] Uemura, H, Shinohara, N, Yuasa, T, Tomita, Y, Fujimoto, H, Niwakawa, M, Mugiya, S, Miki, T, Nonomura, N, Takahashi, M, Hasegawa, Y, Agata, N, Houk, B, Naito, S, & Akaza, H. (2010). A phase II study of sunitinib in Japanese patients with metastatic renal cell carcinoma: insights into the treatment, efficacy and safety. *Japanese Journal of Clinical Oncology*, 40(3), 194-202.

[6] Tomita, Y, Shinohara, N, Yuasa, T, Fujimoto, H, Niwakawa, M, Mugiya, S, Miki, T, Uemura, H, Nonomura, N, Takahashi, M, Hasegawa, Y, Agata, N, Houk, B, Naito, S, & Akaza, H. (2010). Overall survival and updated results from a phase II study of sunitinib in Japanese patients with metastatic renal cell carcinoma. *Japanese Journal of Clinical Oncology*, 40(12), 1166-1172.

[7] Linehan, W. M, Pinto, P. A, Srinivasan, R, Merino, M, Choyke, P, Choyke, L, Coleman, J, Toro, J, Glenn, G, Vocke, C, Zbar, B, Schmidt, L. S, Bottaro, D, & Neckers, L. (2007). Identification of the genes for kidney cancer: opportunity for disease-specific targeted therapeutics. *Clinical Cancer Research*, 13(2 Pt 2), 671s EOF-679s EOF.

[8] Gad, S, Lefèvre, S. H, Khoo, S. K, Giraud, S, Vieillefond, A, Vasiliu, V, Ferlicot, S, Molinié, V, Denoux, Y, Thiounn, N, Chrétien, Y, Méjean, A, Zerbib, M, Benoît, G, Hervé, J. M, Allègre, G, Bressac-de Paillerets, B, Teh, B. T, & Richard, S. (2007). Mutations in BHD and TP53 genes, but not in HNF1beta gene, in a large series of sporadic chromophobe renal cell carcinoma. *British Journal of Cancer*, 96(2), 336-340.

[9] Linehan, W. M, Srinivasan, R, & Schmidt, L. S. (2010). The genetic basis of kidney cancer: a metabolic disease. *Nature Reviews Urology*, 7(5), 277-285.

[10] Banumathy, G, & Cairns, P. (2010). Signaling pathways in renal cell carcinoma. *Cancer Biology & Therapy*, 10(7), 658-664.

[11] Lin, F, Zhang, P. L, Yang, X. J, Prichard, J. W, Brown, R. E, & Lun, M. (2006). Morphoproteomic and molecular concomitants of an overexpressed and activated mTOR pathway in renal cell carcinoma. *Annals of Clinical & Laboratory Science*, 36(3), 283-293.

[12] Eder, J. P, Vande Woude, G. F, Boerner, S. A, & LoRusso, P. M. (2009). Novel therapeutic inhibitors of the c-Met signaling pathway in cancer. *Clinical Cancer Research*, 15(7), 2207-2214.

[13] Motzer, R. J, Bacik, J, Murphy, B. A, Russo, P, & Mazumdar, M. (2002). Interferon-alfa as a comparative treatment for clinical trials of new therapies against advanced renal cell carcinoma. *Journal of Clinical Oncology*, 20(1), 289-296.

[14] Heng, D. Y, Xie, W, Regan, M. M, Warren, M. A, Golshayan, A. R, Sahi, C, Eigl, B. J, Ruether, J. D, Cheng, T, North, S, Venner, P, Knox, J. J, Chi, K. N, Kollmannsberger, C, McDermott, D. F, Oh, W. K, Atkins, M. B, Bukowski, R. M, Rini, B. I, & Choueiri, T. K. (2009). Prognostic factors for overall survival in patients with metastatic renal cell carcinoma treated with vascular endothelial growth factor-targeted agents: results from a large, multicenter study. *Journal of Clinial Oncology*, 27(34), 5794-5799.

[15] Blay, J. Y, Negrier, S, Combaret, V, Attali, S, Goillot, E, Merrouche, Y, Mercatello, A, Ravault, A, Tourani, J. M, Moskovtchenko, J. F, Philip, T, & Favrot, M. (1992). Serum level of interleukin 6 as a prognosis factor in metastatic renal cell carcinoma. *Cancer Research*, 52(12), 3317-3322.

[16] Atzpodien, J, Royston, P, Wandert, T, & Reitz, M. (2003). Metastatic renal cercinoma comprehensive prognostic system. *British Journal of Cancer*, 88(3), 348-353.

[17] Casamassima, A, Picciariello, M, Quaranta, M, Berardino, R, Ranieri, C, Paradiso, A, Lorusso, V, & Guida, M. (2005). C-reactive Protein: a biomarker of survival in patients with metastatic renal cell carcinoma treated with subcutaneous interleukin-2 based immunotherapy. *Journal of Urology*, 173(1), 52-55.

[18] Ramsey, S, Lamb, G. W, Aitchison, M, Graham, J, & McMillan, D. C. (2007). Evaluation of an inflammation-based prognostic score in patients with metastatic renal cancer. *Cancer*, 109(2), 205-212.

[19] Saito, K, Tatokoro, M, Fujii, Y, Iimura, Y, Koga, F, Kawakami, S, & Kihara, K. (2009). Impact of C-reactive protein kinetics on survival of patients with metastatic renal cell carcinoma. *European Urology*, 55(5), 1145-1154.

[20] Fujita, T, Iwamura, M, Ishii, D, Tabata, K, Matsumoto, K, Yoshida, K, & Baba, S. (2012). C-reactive protein as a prognostic marker for advanced renal cell carcinoma treated with sunitinib. *International Journal of Urology*, 19(10), 908-913.

[21] Yuasa, T, Takahashi, S, Hatake, K, Yonese, J, & Fukui, I. (2011). Biomarkers to predict response to sunitinib therapy and prognosis in metastatic renal cell cancer. *Cancer Science*, 102(11), 1949-1957.

[22] Yang, R, Thomas, G. R, Bunting, S, Ko, A, Ferrara, N, Keyt, B, Ross, J, & Jin, H. (1996). Effects of vascular endothelial growth factor on hemodynamics and cardiac performance. *Journal of Cardiovascular Pharmacology*, 27(6), 838-844.

[23] Wei, W, Jin, H, Chen, Z. W, Zioncheck, T. F, Yim, A. P, & He, G. Q. (2004). Vascular endothelial growth factor-induced nitric oxide- and PGI2- dependent relaxation in human internal mammry arteries: a comparative study with KDR and Flt-1 selective mutants. *Journal of Cardiovascular Pharmacology*, 44(5), 615-621.

[24] Rini, B. I, Cohen, D. P, Lu, D. R, Chen, I, Hariharan, S, Gore, M. E, Figlin, R. A, Baum, M. S, & Motzer, R. J. (2011). Hypertension as a biomarker of efficacy in patients with metastatic renal cell carcinoma treated with sunitinib. *Journal of the National Cancer Institute*, 103(9), 763-773.

[25] Bono, P, Rautiola, J, Utriainen, T, & Joensuu, H. (2011). Hypertension as predictor of sunitinib treatment outcome in metastatic renal cell carcinoma. *Acta Oncologica*, 50(4), 569-573.

[26] Szmit, S, Langiewicz, P, Żołnierek, J, Nurzyński, P, Zaborowska, M, Filipiak, K. J, Opolski, G, & Szczylik, C. (2012). Hypertension as a predictive factor for survival ourcomes in patients with metastatic renal cell carcinoma treated with sunitinib after progression on cytokines. *Kidney Blood Pressure Research*, 35(1), 18-25.

[27] Rixe, O, Billemont, B, & Izzedine, H. (2007). Hypertension as a predictive factor of sunitinib activity. *Annals of Oncology*, 1117 EOF.

[28] Riesenbeck, L. M, Bierer, S, Hoffmeister, I, Köpke, T, Papavassilis, P, Hertle, L, Thielen, B, & Herrmann, E. (2011). Hypothyroidism correlates with a better prognosis in metastatic renal cancer patients treated with sorafenib or sunitinib. *World Journal of Urology*, 29(6), 807-813.

[29] Han, K. S, Jung, D. C, Choi, H. J, Jeong, M. S, Cho, K. S, Joung, J. Y, Seo, H. K, Lee, K. H, & Chung, J. (2010). Pretreatment assessment of tumor enhancement on contrast-

enhanced computed tomography as a potential predictor of treatment outcome in metastatic renal cell carcinoma patients receiving antiangiogenic therapy. *Cancer*, 116(10), 2332-2342.

[30] Kayani, I, Avril, N, Bomanji, J, Chowdhury, S, Rockall, A, Sahdev, A, Nathan, P, Wilson, P, Shamash, J, Sharpe, K, Lim, L, Dickson, J, Ell, P, Reynolds, A, & Powles, T. (2011). Sequential FDG-PET/CT as a biomarker of response to sunitinib in metastatic clear cell renal cancer. *Clinical Cancer Research*, 17(18), 6021-6028.

[31] Yuasa, T, Urakami, S, Yamamoto, S, Yonese, J, Nakano, K, Kodaira, M, Takahashi, S, Hatake, K, Inamura, K, Ishikwa, Y, & Fukui, I. (2011). Tumor size is a potential predictor of response to tyrosine kinase inhibitors in renal cell cancer. *Urology*, 77(4), 831-835.

[32] Abel, E. J, Culp, S. H, Tannir, N. M, Tamboli, P, Matin, S. F, & Wood, C. G. (2011). Early primary tumor size reduction is an independent predictor of improved overall survival in metastatic renal cell carcinoma patients treated with sunitinib. *European Urology*, 60(6), 1273-1279.

[33] Ladoire, S, Bonnetain, F, Gauthier, M, Zanetta, S, Petit, J. M, Guiu, S, Kermarrec, I, Mourey, E, Michel, F, Krause, D, Hillon, P, Cormier, L, Ghiringhelli, F, & Guiu, B. (2011). Visceral fat area as a new independent predictive factor of survival in patients with metastatic renal cell carcinoma treated with antiangiogenic agents. *Oncologist*, 16(1), 71-81.

[34] Kawashima, A, Tsujimura, A, Takayama, H, Arai, Y, Nin, M, Tanigawa, G, Uemura, M, Nakai, Y, Nishimura, K, & Nonomura, N. (2012). Impact of hyponatremia on survival of patients with metastatic renal cell carcinoma treated with molecular targeted therapy. *International Journal of Urology*, doi:10.1111/j.14422042x.

Chapter 3

Imagen Thecniques in Renal-Cell Carcinoma

L. León, M. Ramos, M. Lázaro, S. Vázquez,
M. C. Areses, O. Fernandez, U. Anido, J. Afonso and
L. A. Aparicio

Additional information is available at the end of the chapter

http://dx.doi.org/10.5772/54190

1. Introduction

Over 64000 new renal-cell carcinomas (RCC) are annually detected in the United States, and 13000 people will die from the disease. Most RCC are discovered incidentally on medical imaging and a great percentage of them may be treated by surgery, but one third of patients will present either with locally advanced tumor or with metastases[1]. In addition, another third of patients may develop metastatic disease after initial treatment.

In cancer patients imaging techniques are essential in three aspects. First, at the time of diagnosis and the extension study. Ultrasonography, computed tomography (CT) and magnetic resonance imaging (MRI) are currently available to evaluate renal masses.

Second, since most RCC are now early-stage disease suitable for surgery with curative intent, the patient is candidate to follow-up during years. Early detection of recurrence is vital, because single-organ disease may be trated by metastasectomy. Again, CT and MRI are essential in this setting. Also, these imaging modalities are useful to follow-up people with increased susceptibility for RCC, since we have tools to identify at least a subset of these patients.

And third, imaging techniques are fundamental to evaluate the response to treatment. RECIST criteria, published in 2000 and revised in 2009, has become the most widely accepted guideline for evaluate response [2]. Although RECIST criteria have been proved as a useful tool to asses response in solid tumors, some limitations have been noted. One of these limitations are observed in patients treated with specific targeted therapies [3].

Traditionally, RCC have been remarkably resistant to chemo- and radiotherapy. Over the last decade, there has been an increasing knowledge about pathophysiological processes in RCC

INTECH
open science | open minds

© 2013 León et al.; licensee InTech. This is a paper distributed under the terms of the Creative Commons Attribution License (http://creativecommons.org/licenses/by/3.0), which permits unrestricted use, distribution, and reproduction in any medium, provided the original work is properly cited.

including oncology pathways due to a specific driver mutations: silencing von-Hippel Lindau gene, angiogenesis alterations, evasion of apoptosis or sustained angiogenesis.These features have enabled the emergence of a wide spectrum of novel oncology drugs that are designed to target and interfere with specific aberrant biological pathways. Therefore, morphological criteria may not provide meaningful data in this setting and the incorporation of new imaging techniques (MRI diffusion, perfusion CT, PET scan, etc....) in the diagnosis of extension and assessment of efficacy of this drugs may provide unique physiological data that can be correlated with histopathological changes and may provide functional information.

In this chapter we will review the main techniques of radiological diagnosis and staging, the role of new imaging techniques and we will also discuss the validity of the classical criteria of interpretation of response.

2. Common techniques of characterization of renal lesions

2.1. Ultrasound

Ultrasound (US) is one of the most common techniques used in the initial evaluation of renal lesions. It is a low cost and easy access technique and it also allows avoiding the exposure to ionizing radiation and the use of contrast (Figure 1).

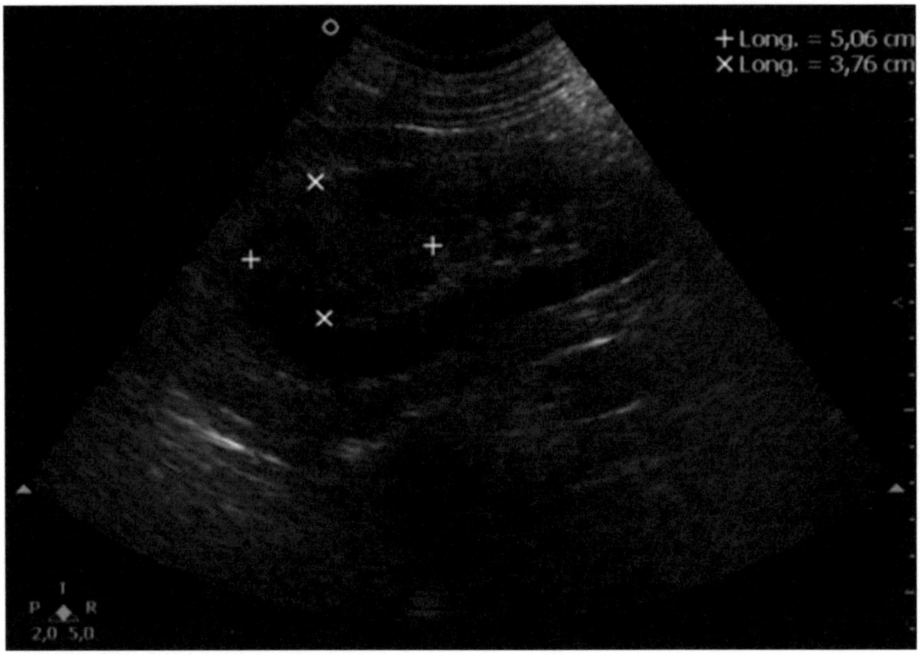

Figure 1. Solid mass in right upper kidney (5 x 3.7 cm).

Although it is an observer-dependent technique, it allows monitoring renal lesions growth and distinguish between cystic and solid lesions. Ultrasonographic features of cystic lesions that allow distinction with malignant lesions or abscesses are:

1. Round morphology, smooth and well-defined walls, separating it from the surrounding parenchyma.

2. There is a strong posterior wall indicating good transmission through the cyst and enhanced transmission beyond the cyst.

3. Absence of internal echoes. The presence of thickened internal septa, calcifications, or mural vascularity indicate malignancy.

One of its limitations is the evaluation and characterization of small lesions. Jamis found that CT detected more renal lesions, especially if they were noncontour deforming. 5% of 2 cm lesions were not detected with CT, an 30% were missed in US. Of lesions under 1 cm, 24% were not detected in TC versus 80% with US [4]. Moreover, given the variability in the echogenicity of malignant kidney, it can be difficult, in the case of isoechoic images, the identification and distinction of these lesions.

In recent years it has become increasingly important the use of contrast-enhanced ultrasound (CEUS). Current CEUS consist of intravenously injected microbubbles that increase the number of reflectors in the vascular space. It has different utilities. It is useful in the differential diagnosis of solid and cystic lesions so as to characterize cystic lesions in benign or malignant [5]. Solid lesions show early arterial enhancement, normally lower than surrounding parenchyma. The delayed enhancement varies and after an arterial phase lesions are isoechoic relative to parenchyma. Often because of intralesional necrosis, there are intralesional areas without contrast enhancement.

It is of particular interest the characterization of complex cystic lesions. Some studies have reported a sensitivity and specificity similar to CT [6] [7]. It can be considered a valid alternative to CT and MRI in monitoring these lesions that need prolonged follow [8]. It may also be useful in detecting small renal masses, improving the accuracy of simple ultrasound, since it allows to observe changes in the thickness of the cortical pyramidal space, not visible in simple US.

2.2. CT scan

Computed tomography (CT) is the modality of choice for the diagnosis and study of extension of renal carcinoma, with a sensitivity greater than 95% (Figure 2) [9]. In addition, the development of multidetector CT has allowed an increase in the rate of detection and diagnosis in early stages [10].

For the evaluation of suspicious lesions, it is advisable to have a specific protocol. This should include a scan without contrast to determine the presence of calcification or fatty tissue within the tumor, and will serve as baseline study to study if these lesions enhance after contrast administration.

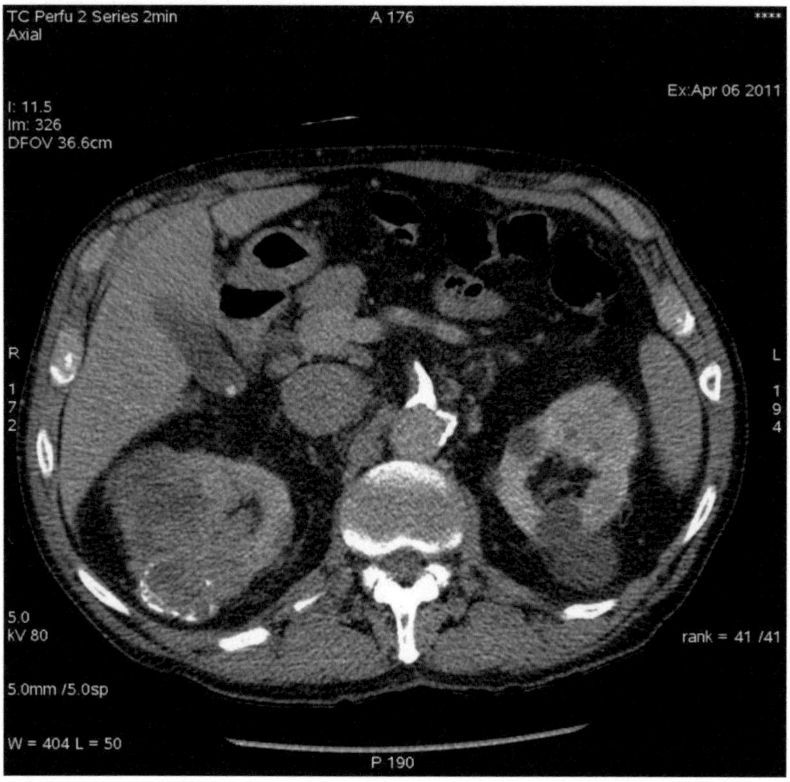

Figure 2. CT scan, right renal cell carcinoma.

The three perfusion renal phases defined in CT diagnosis are: corticomedullary phase, nephrographic phase, and renal elimination phase (or excretory phase) [11].

The images in the corticomedullary phase help to identify the lesion and its vascular supply, being optimal for detecting or excluding tumor invasion of the renal veins [12]. The nephrographic and elimination phase help detecting renal masses, especially those of small size.

The appearance of renal carcinoma in CT varies depending on the size of the tumor vasculature, the extent of necrosis or intratumoral cystic changes. Enhancement of a renal lesion shows that it is hypervascular; this is the most important finding in the evaluation of renal masses, being a useful parameter in differentiating histological subtypes.

Different groups have shown as clear cell carcinoma has a higher contrast enhancement than other histological subtypes, especially papillary carcinomas [13]. Zhang et al show that 90% of the clear cell renal carcinoma are hypervascular and heterogeneous (with solid hypervascular foci and low attenuation foci by necrotic or cystic changes). Seventy five % of papillary carcinomas were hypovascular and 90% had an uniform pattern or peripheral uptake while chromophobe tumors often show a moderate and homogeneous enhancement [10].

Tumors less than 3 cm sometimes have a smooth contour, they are homogeneous and difficult to distinguish from some benign lesions. Renal cystic carcinomas usually have thickened walls and septa, sometimes with calcification. Three-dimensional CT is important in staging renal cell carcinoma, with the objective of identifying patients having a resectable tumor and to define the best therapeutic option. The value of CT is limited to the study of the perirenal fat. Various criteria have been used to describe the appearance of perirenal fat infiltration. Trabeculation of perirenal fat is not a reliable sign of tumor involvement, and is found in approximately 50% of patients with localized tumors T1 and T2. It can be caused by edema, vascular congestion, or prior inflammation [14]. The presence of a nodule uptake in perirenal fat, is considered the most specific finding of perirenal invasion, with high specificity (98%) but low sensitivity (46%) [15].

Helical CT has also been shown to have high accuracy in the diagnosis of renal vein invasion with a negative predictive value of 97% and a positive predictive value of 92% (Figure 3) [16].

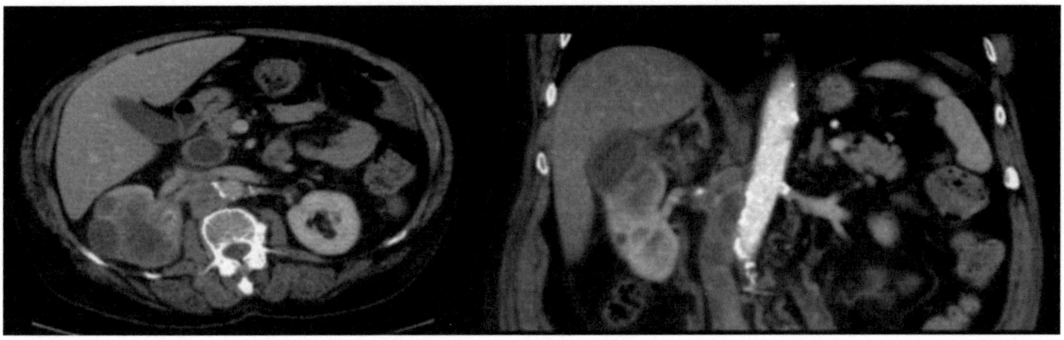

Figure 3. Renal cell carcinoma with thrombosis of the inferior cava vein.

The adrenal evaluation is important because if no abnormalities are detected on CT, adrenalectomy can be avoided. CT has a high negative predictive value in the detection of adrenal involvement by RCC. When the adrenal gland is enlarged, displaced or not displayed an adrenalectomy should be considered [17].

The study of lymph node is based primarily on its size. It is considered that a lymph node could be metastatic when its diameter is greater than 1 cm. However this approach has a limited specificity and sensitivity (between 3 and 43% in different studies) because the size increase may be due to inflammatory changes.

The nodal enhancement pattern helps differentiate between reactive and malignant lymphadenopathy. Metastatic lymph nodes can be enhanced after administration of contrast, especially if the primary tumor is highly vascularized.

Finally, given that CT plays an important role in detecting distant disease, it is necessary to conduct a study of the chest and abdomen in the staging of metastatic disease.

2.3. Magnetic resonance imaging

Magnetic resonance imaging (MRI) is useful when computed tomography cannot be performed, but it has not proved to be superior to CT in the detection or characterization of renal masses. The study should include T1 and T2 sequences and opposed-phase images to detect intratumoral fat. Dynamic study after paramagnetic contrast administration is essential.

Both CT and MRI have high reliability in delineating the extent of intratumoral thrombus, since it could change the surgical approach. However, MRI is more sensitive than CT to differentiate between tumoral and non-tumoral thrombus. The tumoral thrombus is heterogeneous or hyperintense on T2-weighted images, with marked enhancement on the postcontrast images, and, sometimes, it is seen the continuity with the renal tumor. The tumor thrombus is hypointense, not homogeneous and and does not enhance after contrast administration [18].

Also, as discussed below, MRI can help us to distinguish between different histological subtypes of renal cell carcinoma (RCC), and between these ones and benign tumors such as oncocytomas and angiomyolipomas.

Clear cell RCC usually shows a signal intensity similar to that of the renal parenchyma on T1-weighted images and it´s high intensity on T2-weighted images (Figure 4). Central necrosis is common, and it is typically seen as a homogeneus hypointense area in the center of the mass on T1-weighted images, and hyperintense, rarely hypointense, on T2-weighted images [19]. If intratumoral hemorrhage occurs, the appearance of this will depend on the degree of degradation of its components. A hypointense ring, or pseudocapsule, is sometimes seen on both T1 and T2-weighted images, and is due to compression of the adjacent renal parenchyma by the tumor growth. Breakage of this pseudocapsule correlates with advanced stage and higher nuclear grade [20]. This histological subtype tends to be hypervascular, with heterogeneous enhancement during the arterial phase. You can also appreciate renal vein thrombus in more aggressive and advanced tumors. They can also be predominantly cystic, with only a few areas of solid component [21].

The type I papillary RCC is characterized by a homogeneous hyposignal on T2-weighted images, with homogeneous low-level enhancement after contrast administration [22]. Sometimes they show necrosis and hemorrhage. Type II papillary RCC have a more complex appearance, with hemorrhage and necrosis. It is common to see a hemorrhagic cystic mass with enhancing papillary projections at the periphery. In both types is frequent the presence of a fibrous capsule [23].

Chromophobe RCC may show cystic changes within a solid mass. It is not common the presence of necrotic foci, even in large tumors. Its appearance on MR can be identical to those of clear cell RCC [23].

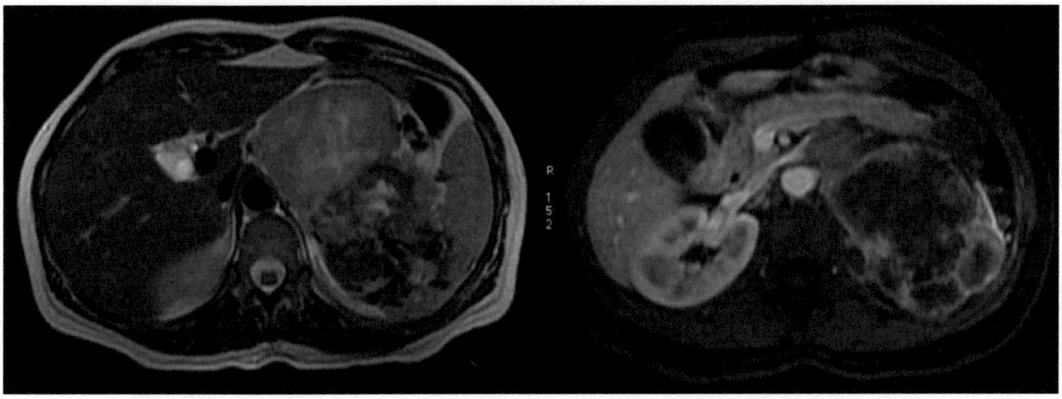

Figure 4. Clear cell RCC. Heterogeneous tumor with focal posterior bleeding. T2 (left side) and T1 sequence (right side) with fast gradient contrast, showing renal vein invasion. Courtesy Dr. Armesto-Pérez.

The MR Imaging appearance of oncocytomas is variable and nonspecific. They are typically spherical and well-defined masses with hyposignal on T1-weighted images and hypersignal on T2-weighted images, in most cases. The central scar, when present, has a stellate appearance with low signal intensity on T1-weighted images and high signal intensity on T2-weighted images, and it may show delayed enhancement after contrast administration. Sometimes are surrounded by a well-defined hypointense capsule [24].

Angiomyolipoma with a predominant fatty component is isointense relative to fat on all MR Imaging sequences and its signal intensity is higher than that of the renal parenchyma on T1-weighted images. Fat-suppression sequences are also useful. Lipid-poor angiomyolipomas are difficult to distinguish from clear cell RCC with current imaging methods, so may occasionally be required histopathological evaluation to establish the correct diagnosis [21].

Diffusion-weighted imaging may be useful in differentiating between RCC and oncocytoma and in the characterization of the different histological subtypes of RCC. Angiomyolipoma, due to the presence of fat, can give false positives, but it is characterized through conventional sequences [25] [26].

The whole-body MRI, at present, is positioning itself as one of the techniques of choice for evaluation of bone marrow in patients with suspected bone metastases with a sensitivity / specificity (> 90%) higher than the radiology conventional CT and bone scans, and similar to PET-CT (Figure 5) [27].

Complement the study with diffusion-weighted imaging, besides allowing a faster interpretation and greater detection of subtle findings could add specificity to the study [28]. This is particularly relevant with the progressive increased use of new anti tumor drugs in which this technique may allow better assessment of tumor response [29].

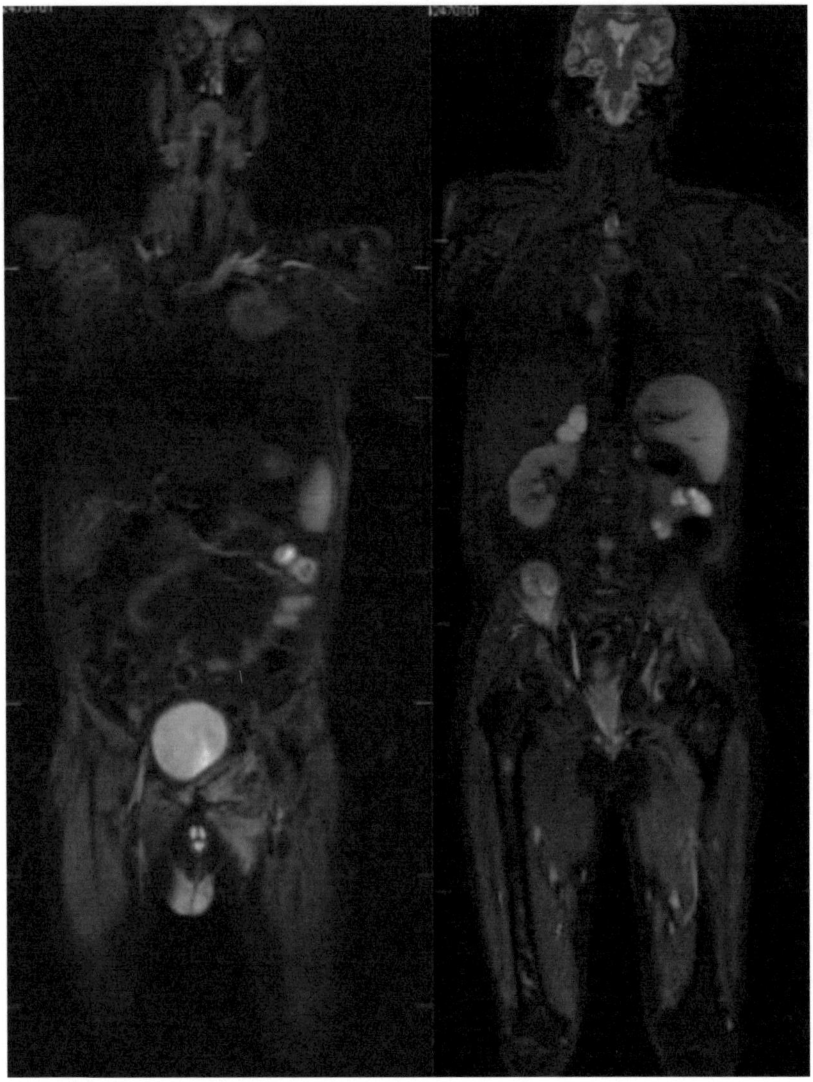

Figure 5. Whole body MRI. Bone, lung and liver metastases. Courtesy Dr. Armesto-Pérez.

2.4. Bone scan

Bone metastases in RCC is reported in 17-37% of patients and its early identification may have prognosis importance because its early intervention leads to significant reduction in patient morbidity. Bone scintigraphy is a very useful tool in diagnosis of bone metastases when those lesions have sufficient osteoblastic reaction (Figure 6). However, bone metastases in RCC usually appear as large expansive lytic lesions, most commonly in the axial skeleton and are poorly visualized in bone scintigraphy [30], showing variable uptake, with a sensitivity between 10-60% in the diagnosis of this metastases in preselected patients with RCC and high probability of skeletal involvement with underestimation of the extension of the extension of the metastatic involvement, being clearly inferior to other techniques such magnetic resonance imaging or PET scan [31]. Because most bone metastases are symptomatic, most of authors recommend the use of bone scintigraphy only in symptomatic patients with or without raised level of alkaline phosphatase [32,33], although others believe that because its poor sensitivity, the routine use of bone scintigraphy in RCC needs to be questioned [34,35].

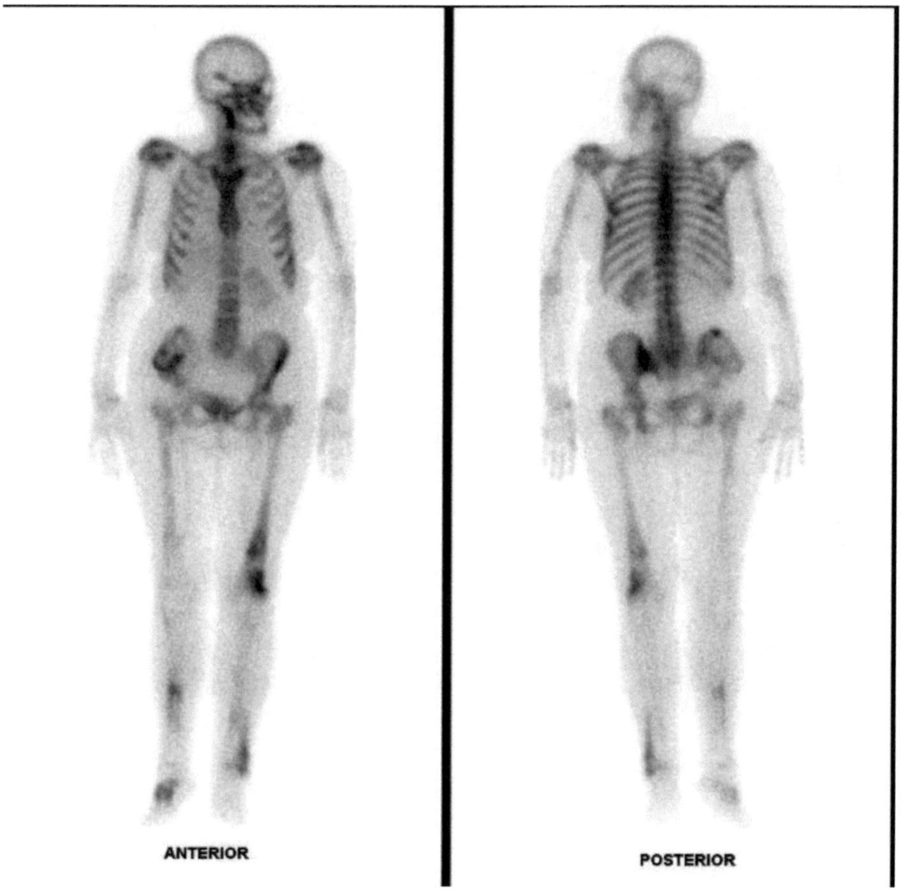

Figure 6. Bone scan of a patient with renal cancer showing metastases in the right tibia, left femur, pelvis and rib cage.

2.5. PET

We can study the PET role of in RCC from three points of view: localized disease, extensive disease and monitoring treatment response.

Localized disease: Most of publications in this patient subset have been made in a retrospective way and many of them studied patients from the PET archive and not from the population of patients with a suspicious kidney mass. More recently we have knows the result of a prospective study that examined 18 patients with renal lesions suspicious for malignancy diagnosed on CT, MRI or ultrasound [36]. In all patients, a FDG-PET/CT was made and diagnosis of malignancy was suspected when intensity on PET was greater than intensity in the renal parenchyma and it was different from the physiological excretion in the collecting system. Patients underwent nephrectomy or surgical resection of the renal mass with the respective histological analysis. PET showed a sensitivity of 46,6% and a specificity of 66,6%. The median diameter and Furhman grade of FDG positive malignant lesions were significantly higher than in FDG-negative malignant lesions (p< 0,05). It is difficult to draw conclusions with a study involving a sample of patients so small, but we can see that about half of the patients could not be diagnosed by PET, so probably we will have to expect better results with this diagnostic technique before introducing it as part of a routine preoperative diagnosis of RCC. A modification of the technique is the immunological PET, using ^{124}I-cG250 (chimeric girentuximab labeled with ^{124}I) because cG250 functions as an epitope of CAIX, a transmembrane enzyme that is almost universally expressed in clear cells RCC cells. With this modality has been observed a 94% sensitivity and 100% specificity, with positive and negative predictive values of 100% and 90% respectively, in a population of 26 patients with renal masses suspicious for malignancy [37].

Extensive disease: Although in the metastatic RCC PET has better sensitivity (63-100%) than in localized disease, some authors believe that FDG-PET currently appears to be too unreliable to recommend is routine use in the staging of RCC, because it is less sensitive than radiological imaging for retroperitoneal lymphadenopathy and bone or lung metastases [38]. However, this technique may have a place detecting recurrence and probably an associated prognostic value (Figure 7). In a recent study, the authors found a sensitivity and specificity of 81% and 71% respectively, for FDG-PET in the diagnosis of recurrence, with correct diagnosis in all cases of intra-abdominal (lymph nodes, local recurrence and adrenal glands) and bone recurrence, with a clear trend for better 5-year survival in PET-negative patients compared with PET-positive patients: 83% versus 46% respectively [39].

Monitoring treatment response: Systemic treatment in metastatic RCC is represented for multikinase inhibitors like sorafenib and sunitinib. This drugs are actives because its capacity of inhibition on the tyrosine kinase receptor VEGF and the platelet-derived growth factor receptor, in the endothelial cells and pericytes. Because expression of Glut (a downstream product of HIF transcriptional activity), it is conceivable that intensity of FDG uptake may be reflective of the magnitude of the entire pathway [40]. In other words, the variable intensity of FDG-PET in RCC may reflect variable strength of the HIF signaling pathway. Kayani et al. studied prospectively 44 treatment naive metastatic RCC. A basal (pretreatment) FDG-PET was made and them repeated it at 4 and 16 weeks of treatment. The most intense lesion of each patient (SUV > 2.5) was used as the index lesion and they defined metabolic response as a decrease of > 20% in SUV and metabolic disease progression as an increase of >20 % or development of new metastatic lesions. In the first comparison (after 4 treatment weeks) they found a metabolic response in 24 (57%) patients but without correlation with the PFS or overall survival. In the second comparison (16 treatment weeks), 12 (28%) patients had metabolic disease progression, which correlated with decreased OS and PFS 8HR: 5.96 [95% CI: 2.43-19-02] and 12,13 [95% CI:3,72-46,51]), respectively [41]. With these results, we can conclude that the FDG-PET probably may be more useful in diagnosing tumor progression than treatment response. Another point that deserves to be examined is whether the cutoff of 20% is appropriate to differentiate responders from those who do not.

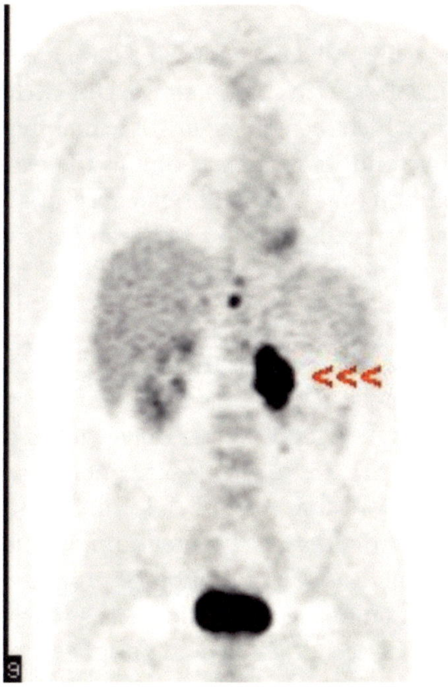

Figure 7. PET scan showing loco-regional recurrence (red arrows), in a patient with a previous left nephrectomy.

3. New techniques in imaging of renal tumors

The introduction of functional imaging techniques have allowed us to study in vivo physiological processes of tissues and tumors. Techniques such as computed tomography (CT) or magnetic resonance (MR) allow us to study tumor perfusion (angiogenesis). Positron emission tomography (PET) scan or spectroscopy RM is useful in the evaluation of tumor metabolism while difusion RM allows the study of the diffusion of water molecules through the diffusion sequences (cellularity) to assess hypoxia phenomena or changes in the lymph nodes function. All these techniques can obtain information on the tumor microenvironment, including levels of oxygenation, tumor cell proliferation or vascularization and open a different dimension in the study of patients: diagnosis, staging, treatment planning, evaluation of response or follow-up [42] [43].

For example, dynamic techniques (MRI or CT) seem most appropriate for assessing antivascular drug response or acting in the VEGF/ PDGFR pathway, such as bevacizumab, whose mechanism of action appears to focus on normalization of tumor vascularization [Jain 2005], while the PET appears to do better in the case of drugs such as cetuximab, acting in the EGFR pathway [44] [45] [46].

3.1. Perfusion-CT

Perfusion CT is based on the temporal change of the attenuation of tissues after intravenous administration of iodinated contrast. This study consists of two phases. The first phase lasts between 40 and 60 seconds in which the enhancement is mainly due to the contrast distribution in the intravascular space and its rapid passage to the extracellular space. This phase requires high temporal resolution (one acquisition per second). In the second phase the contrast enhancement depends on its distribution between intra-and extravascular compartments. In this period the acquisition in more spaced and lasts between 2 and 5 minutes [47] [48] [49,50].

This functional technique can be used to measure a number of parameters including vascular blood flow, blood volume, mean transit time, peak enhancement, time to peak enhancement and capillary permeability. Several studies have validated functional CT data as a biomarker of angiogenesis [47] [51]. There is growing interest on the use of CT perfusion in oncology with multiple applications that may be helpful: differential diagnosis between benign and malignant neoplasms, identifying tumors of unknown origin (with impaired liver perfusion with occult metastatic disease), definition of prognosis (with best response in tumors with more perfusion), monitoring response to treatment and development of new drugs (Figures 8 and 9) [50]. The technique is being applied in multiple tumor types: head and neck, lung, liver, pancreas, colorectal cancer, lymphoma and prostate.

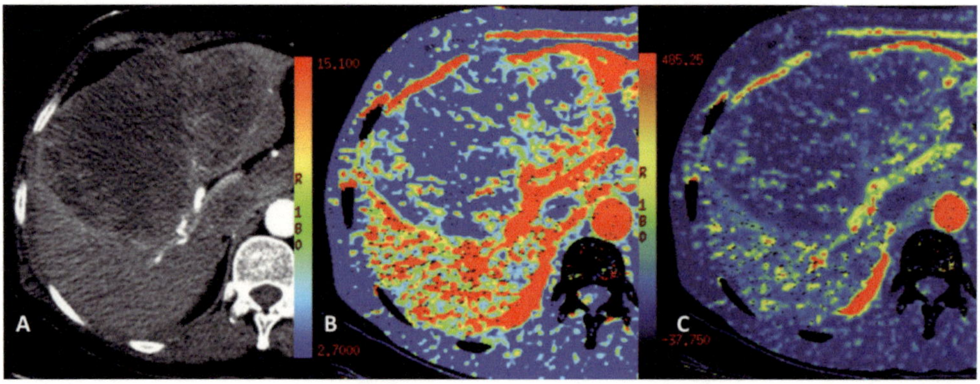

Figure 8. Renal Cancer. Liver metastasis treated with temsirolimus. Axial CT image (A) and blood volume (B) and blood flow (C) parametric maps show low perfusion parameters in metastasis. Courtesy Dr. García Figueiras.

http://dx.doi.org/10.5772/54190

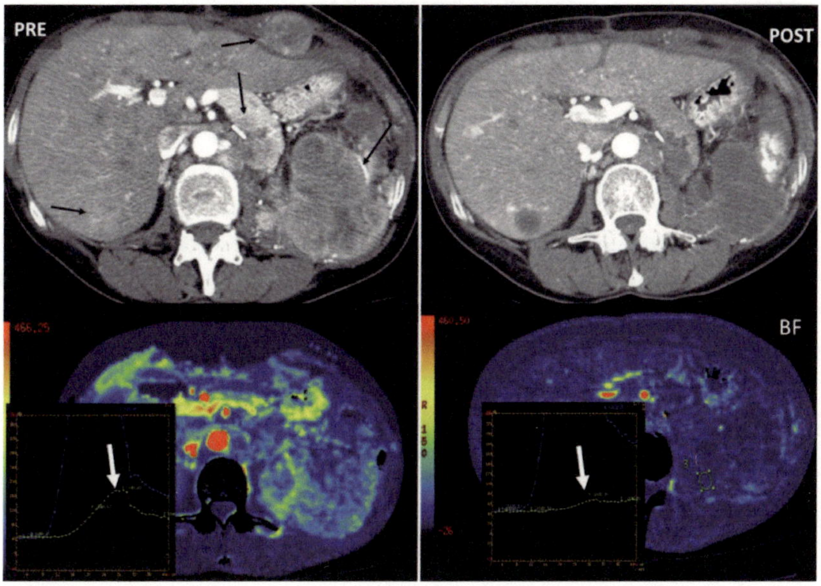

Figure 9. Renal Cancer with diffuse metastatic disease (black arrows) in a 58 year-old female patient. Pre-therapy (left column) and 10 days post-sunitinib (right column). Axial CT images, blood flow (BF) parametric maps, and curves time-density show a partial response with disappearance of some metastatic foci, necrotic changes in many of them, a change in enhancement curve (white arrows) and a BF decrease by 95% in tumor. Courtesy Dr. García Figueiras.

3.2. DCE-MRI

Other functional imaging techniques not specifically focused on the study of angiogenesis, such as diffusion MRI, enabling the study of tumor cellularity and having quantitative parameters such as the apparent diffusion coefficient (ADC). Thus, tumors with high cellularity show low ADC [52] [53]. Moreover, since tumor response is associated with destruction of tumor cells, it is generally associated with increased ADC tumor lesions. The diffusion thus evaluate the apoptotic and necrotic effect but not angiogenesis, main target of new drugs.

Preliminary studies have shown significant changes very early in the flow, blood volume and perfusion with tumor therapy. There is a relationship between changes in Ktrans, Kep and the area under the curve and the response in different tumors, showing a very marked functional changes in the vascular supply to the tumor [54] [55]. Therefore these techniques could be worth to select those patients who will respond to drugs with an early evaluation of the response using functional imaging.

In a subgroup of patients enrolled in the phase II study discontinuation of sorafenib, DCE-MRI was performed before and after initiation of treatment. Radiological response by RECIST criteria was observed in 4/17 patients (ORR 24%), and time to progression was 12.9 months. Ktrans decreased significantly during treatment with sorafenib (60.3% decrease,

95% CI 46.1 to 74.6%). The percentage decrease in Ktrans and change in tumor size was significantly associated with progression-free survival ($p = 0.01$ and 0.05, respectively).

3.3. PET

Finally, molecular techniques such as PET show a limited role in the study of metastatic renal cancer, since this tumor usually has a low activity of glucose metabolism (pathway assessed by 18F-fluorodeoxyglucose, the most widely used radiotracer). Only in cases where the tumor shows an increased metabolism of glucose, PET may be useful in the assessment of the disease and its response to therapy. Other radiotracers that allow the study of important characteristics such as tumor hypoxia, cell proliferation or angiogenesis itself, are still under evaluation and implementation in clinical practice [56]. In an experimentally way it is evaluating the introduction of functional imaging techniques in clinical studies, to develop translational research in oncology imaging applications. In a NCI trial, Dr. Hoffman (University of Utah) is using DCE-MRI and various types of PET (H2150-PET, FDG-PET, FDL-PET) in monitoring response to multi-targeted treatment in renal cancer patients.

4. Response evaluation

4.1. Evaluation of response: Antiangiogenics and mTOR inhibitors

We must consider several issues when assessing the therapeutic response of tumors. The morphological assessment with quantification of changes in size used in the RECIST criteria ("Criteria in Solid Tumors Response") has been our main concern when assessing tumor response [2]. This approach seems true for the use of cytotoxic drugs. However, this assessment is limited, since the macroscopic changes take time to become evident, often are not specific and do not provide information on the physiological and molecular component of tumors [42].

Advances in the field of oncology have led to the development of new drugs in renal cancer as sunitinib, sorafenib, pazopanib, tivoaznib, axitinib, temsirolimus, everolimus and bevacizumab [46]. These drugs (mainly cytostatic) cause little change in lesion size. Therefore, RECIST criteria are not entirely suitable for assessing tumor response, and proper techniques will vary according to the mechanism of action of the drug.

The recent emergence of techniques for the functional study of angiogenesis, such as perfusion CT or dynamic MRI allow obtaining quantitative parameters (blood volume, blood flow mean transit time, ktrans Ve, etc.) and would open a interesting field for assessing tumor response in a more objective [57] [58] [59]. This could open the door to the development of a strategy based on the image for the selection of patients to be treated with antiangiogenic therapies. However, each of these techniques has advantages and disadvantages. Thus, CT perfusion shows the drawback of radiation necessary for conducting the studies, whereas in the case of dynamic MRI the analysis of the results is much more complex.

The functional and molecular imaging techniques could offer clear opportunities in the study of renal tumors, but nevertheless, we must not forget that, for validation as bio-markers, would require completing a qualification and validation process, which would pass through standardization in the collection and analysis of the images and the correlation of the parameters obtained with patient outcomes. Once this is ach-ieved, functional-molecular techniques, especially perfusion CT, could become promis-ing tools in the selection of patients for targeted drug therapy and the assessment of the response [57] [58].

5. Criterios RECIST/MASS/CHOI

Classically, oncology response evaluation is based on comparison of pre and post-treatment tumor volume by studying changes in the diameter of the tumors. RECIST criteria in its original version and its 2009 Update 1.1 are applied routinely in oncology practice [2]. How-ever, it is recognized that the response evaluation focused exclusively on size changes have important limitations, including the importance of excluding changes in tumor metabolism or not considering the appearance of necrosis or fibrosis as a factor which may be related to response to treatment. Furthermore, the introduction of new drugs creates the need for a different evaluation of the tumor and treatment response [46].

The limitations of traditional approaches, as the criteria of the World Health Organiza-tion (WHO) or Response Evaluation Criteria in Solid Tumors (**RECIST**) in the evaluation of targeted therapies have been widely documented [64] [65] [57]. Therapies that act on tumor vascularity may have underestimated clinical benefit by tumor size change since their mechanism of action (more cytostatic that cytotoxic), produces more stabilization than tumoral responses.

Without abandoning the use of size criteria as a key element in the assessment of patients with metastatic renal cancer, some authors have attempted to obtain early information (**EP-TIC**, Early English Post-herapy Imaging Changes) [66] on the prognosis of patients treated with therapy acting at the VEGF pathway. In this regard, it was demonstrated that a 10% decrease in the sum of the largest diameters of the lesions in the first control, provides infor-mation on the subsequent course of patients. Using only tumor size as endpoint criterion would leave aside the use of IV contrast.

Subsequently it was observed a relationship between the degree of tumor enhancement be-fore therapy and the likelihood of response (being higher in those tumors with greater pre-treatment enhancement). Many of these new drugs induce tumor necrosis, causing a dramatic drop in the enhancement of metastatic lesions in the post-therapy evaluation [67]. Based on these observations and on previous experience with gastrointestinal stromal tu-mors treated with imatinib, a set of tumor response criteria based on changes in size and / or density tumor was established: Choi criteria, modified Choi criteria, MASS criteria and SACT criteria (Table 1) [56].

Criterio	Targeted lesions	Complete response	Partial response	Stable disease	Progressive disease
RECIST version 1.1 (2)	Tumor size 10 mm by CT scan	Disappearance of all lesions	Decrease in size 30%	Does not meet criteria for PR or PD	Increase in tumor size 20% (the sum must also demonstrate an absolute increase of at least 5 mm)
	Tumor size 15 mm by chest X-ray	No new lesions	No new lesions		New lesions
	Maximum of 5 target lesions		No PD of non-target lesions		
EPTIC (Early Posttherapy Imaging Changes) (60)	Establishing the prognosis depending on the % size decrease after antiangiogenic therapy Decreased size ≥ 10%= good prognosis.				
Choi Criteria (61) (3)	Tumor size 15 mm	Disappearance of all lesions	A decrease in size 10% or a decrease in tumor attenuation (HU) 15% on CT	Does not meet criteria for CR, PR or PD	Increase in tumor size 10% and does not meet criteria of PR by tumor attenuation
	Maximum of 10 target lesions	No new lesions	No new lesions , no obvious progression of non-measurable disease	No symptomatic deterioration attributed to PD	New lesions
Modified Choi Criteria (62)	Tumor size 15 mm	Disappearance of all lesions	A decrease in size 10% and a decrease in tumor attenuation (HU) 15% on CT	Does not meet criteria for CR, PR or PD	Increase in tumor size 10% and does not meet criteria of PR by tumor attenuation
	Maximum of 10 target lesions	No new lesions	No new lesions , no obvious progression of non-measurable disease	No symptomatic deterioration attributed to PD	New lesions

http://dx.doi.org/10.5772/54190

Criterio	Targeted lesions	Complete response	Partial response	Stable disease	Progressive disease
SCAT Criteria (29)	Tumor size 10 mm		Decrease in tumor size 20%	Does not meet criteria for PR or PD	Increase in tumor size 20%
	Maximum of 10 target lesions		Decrease in tumor size10% and _half of the non-lung target lesions with 20 HU decreased mean attenuation		New metastases, marked central fill-inc of a target lesion or new enhancement in a homogeneously hypoattenuating nonenhancing mass
MASS criteria (63)		Favorable response. No new lesions and any of the following: 1. Decrease in tumor size 20 % 2. One or more predominantly solid enhancing lesions with marked central necrosis or marked decreased attenuation (40 UH)		Does not meet criteria for favorable or unfavorable response	Any of the following: 1. Increase in tumor size of 20 % in the absence of marked central necrosis or marked decreased attenuation 2. New metastases, marked central fill-in, or new enhancement of a previously homogeneously hypoattenuating nonenhancing mass
Functional and molecular image.	No response criteria defined				
CR: complete response. PR: partial response. NC: no changes. PD: progressive disease. RECIST: Response Evaluation Criteria in Solid Tumors. CT: computed tomography. SACT: criteria size and attenuation CT (SACT) criteria. HU: Hounsfield Unit.					

CR: complete response. PR: partial response. NC: no changes. PD: progressive disease. RECIST: Response Evaluation Criteria in Solid Tumors. CT: computed tomography. SACT: criteria size and attenuation CT (SACT) criteria. HU: Hounsfield Unit.

Table 1. CT-based criteria for response evaluation of targeted therapies in renal cell carcinoma.

Each of these criteria has a number of advantages compared to RECIST, but some limitations. So **Choi criteria**, based on the change in size or tumor density on CT (% change in the measured attenuation value at UH), show little advantage over RECIST when establishing the possibility of a long-term response. Furthermore, these show a different utility criteria depending on the type of drug tested, being most useful in the case of sorafenib (which tends to cause more degree of necrosis in lesions) than for sunitinib.

Modified Choi criteria evaluate existing changes in both size and tumor density after treatment. These criteria could differentiate those patients at risk of disease progression, but shows a tendency to classify patients as responders.

SACT criteria (Size and Attenuation CT) differ from the modified Choi criteria that establish an absolute value of change in tumor density (> 20 UH) rather than a % of change. These criteria are more reliable in the case of low attenuation pre-therapy lesions, in which it is easier to obtain a percentage decrease in density.

Finally, the **MASS criteria** (Morphology, Attenuation, Size, and Structure) include morphological and structural elements regardless of the size and density of lesions. These criteria are intended to take into account the extensive necrotic changes frequently associated with tumor response to these drugs [63].

However, both SACT as MASS criteria are complicated and basically useful in differentiating patients with a long progression-free survival (> 250 days) of those showing a rapid progression (<250 days). Overall, we consider that in all these criteria contrast enhancement of lesions plays a major role, so that both imaging protocols (volume of contrast acquisition phase, etc.) or factors such as cardiac function patient can significantly influence the results.

6. Summary

The era of molecular biology have created great expectations on our ability to translate these discoveries into effective treatments for patients. Over the last decade, there has been an increasing knowledge about pathophysiological processes that are common to most tumors including: independence from growth signals, insensitivity to growth-inhibitory signals, evasion of apoptosis, limitless potential for replication, sustained angiogenesis, and tissue invasion and metastasis. These major pathways deregulated in cancer have a key role in tumor development and microenvironment. These features have enabled the emergence of a wide spectrum of novel oncologic drugs that are designed to target and interfere with specific aberrant biological pathways. In general, these agents use different strategies to interfere with specific biological targets, such as blocking growth factors, receptors, or tyrosine kinase (TK) action.

The use of new drugs in the treatment of advanced or metastatic kidney cancer, with different mechanisms of action compared to conventional chemotherapy raises new questions. One of the biggest problems with new drugs are produced in the evaluation of the response, and the incorporation of new imaging techniques (MRI diffusion, perfusion CT, nuclear medicine, etc....) in the diagnosis of extension and assessment of efficacy.

In this chapter we have reviewed the main techniques of radiological diagnosis and staging, the value of new imaging modalities, and discuss the validity of the classical criteria of interpretation of response.

http://dx.doi.org/10.5772/54190

Author details

L. León[1], M. Ramos[2], M. Lázaro[3], S. Vázquez[4], M. C. Areses[5], O. Fernandez[5], U. Anido[1], J. Afonso[6] and L. A. Aparicio[7]

*Address all correspondence to: Aparicio@sergas.es

1 Complexo Hospitalario Universitario de Santiago, Santiago de Compostela, Spain

2 Centro Oncológico de Galica, A Coruña, Spain

3 Complexo Hospitalario Universitario, Vigo, Spain

4 Hospital Universitario Lucus Augusti, Lugo, Spain

5 Complexo Hospitalario Universitario de Ourense, Ourense, Spain

6 Complexo Hospitalario Arquitecto Marcide, Ferrol, Spain

7 Complexo Hospitalario Universitario, A Coruña, Spain

References

[1] Cohen HT, McGovern FJ. Renal-cell carcinoma. N Engl J Med 2005, Dec 8;353(23): 2477-90.

[2] Eisenhauer EA, Therasse P, Bogaerts J, Schwartz LH, Sargent D, Ford R, et al. New response evaluation criteria in solid tumours: Revised RECIST guideline (version 1.1). Eur J Cancer 2009, Jan;45(2):228-47.

[3] Choi H, Charnsangavej C, Faria SC, Macapinlac HA, Burgess MA, Patel SR, et al. Correlation of computed tomography and positron emission tomography in patients with metastatic gastrointestinal stromal tumor treated at a single institution with imatinib mesylate: Proposal of new computed tomography response criteria. J Clin Oncol 2007, May 1;25(13):1753-9.

[4] Jamis-Dow CA, Choyke PL, Jennings SB, Linehan WM, Thakore KN, Walther MM. Small (< or = 3-cm) renal masses: Detection with CT versus US and pathologic correlation. Radiology 1996, Mar;198(3):785-8.

[5] Siracusano S, Bertolotto M, Ciciliato S, Valentino M, Liguori G, Visalli F. The current role of contrast-enhanced ultrasound (CEUS) imaging in the evaluation of renal pathology. World J Urol 2011, Oct;29(5):633-8.

[6] Ascenti G, Mazziotti S, Zimbaro G, Settineri N, Magno C, Melloni D, et al. Complex cystic renal masses: Characterization with contrast-enhanced US. Radiology 2007, Apr;243(1):158-65.

[7] Quaia E, Bertolotto M, Cioffi V, Rossi A, Baratella E, Pizzolato R, Cov MA. Comparison of contrast-enhanced sonography with unenhanced sonography and contrast-enhanced CT in the diagnosis of malignancy in complex cystic renal masses. AJR Am J Roentgenol 2008, Oct;191(4):1239-49.

[8] Park BK, Kim B, Kim SH, Ko K, Lee HM, Choi HY. Assessment of cystic renal masses based on bosniak classification: Comparison of CT and contrast-enhanced US. Eur J Radiol 2007, Feb;61(2):310-4.

[9] Maldazys JD, deKernion JB. Prognostic factors in metastatic renal carcinoma. J Urol 1986, Aug;136(2):376-9.

[10] Zhang J, Lefkowitz RA, Ishill NM, Wang L, Moskowitz CS, Russo P, et al. Solid renal cortical tumors: Differentiation with CT. Radiology 2007, Aug;244(2):494-504.

[11] Kopka L, Fischer U, Zoeller G, Schmidt C, Ringert RH, Grabbe E. Dual-phase helical CT of the kidney: Value of the corticomedullary and nephrographic phase for evaluation of renal lesions and preoperative staging of renal cell carcinoma. AJR Am J Roentgenol 1997, Dec;169(6):1573-8.

[12] Sheth S, Scatarige JC, Horton KM, Corl FM, Fishman EK. Current concepts in the diagnosis and management of renal cell carcinoma: Role of multidetector ct and three-dimensional CT. Radiographics 2001, Oct;21 Spec No:S237-54.

[13] Ruppert-Kohlmayr AJ, Uggowitzer M, Meissnitzer T, Ruppert G. Differentiation of renal clear cell carcinoma and renal papillary carcinoma using quantitative CT enhancement parameters. AJR Am J Roentgenol 2004, Nov;183(5):1387-91.

[14] Zagoria RJ, Bechtold RE, Dyer RB. Staging of renal adenocarcinoma: Role of various imaging procedures. AJR Am J Roentgenol 1995, Feb;164(2):363-70.

[15] Johnson CD, Dunnick NR, Cohan RH, Illescas FF. Renal adenocarcinoma: CT staging of 100 tumors. AJR Am J Roentgenol 1987, Jan;148(1):59-63.

[16] Welch TJ, LeRoy AJ. Helical and electron beam CT scanning in the evaluation of renal vein involvement in patients with renal cell carcinoma. J Comput Assist Tomogr 1997;21(3):467-71.

[17] Gill IS, McClennan BL, Kerbl K, Carbone JM, Wick M, Clayman RV. Adrenal involvement from renal cell carcinoma: Predictive value of computerized tomography. J Urol 1994, Oct;152(4):1082-5.

[18] Trinidad C, Martinez C, Delgado C. Tumores urológicos. Imagen en oncología.. In: Madrid: Ed Médica PAnamericana; 2009. p. 67-78.

[19] Eilenberg SS, Lee JK, Brown J, Mirowitz SA, Tartar VM. Renal masses: Evaluation with gradient-echo gd-dtpa-enhanced dynamic MR imaging. Radiology 1990, Aug; 176(2):333-8.

[20] Yamashita Y, Watanabe O, Miyazaki T, Yamamoto H, Harada M, Takahashi M. Cystic renal cell carcinoma. Imaging findings with pathologic correlation. Acta Radiol 1994, Jan;35(1):19-24.

[21] Pedrosa I, Sun MR, Spencer M, Genega EM, Olumi AF, Dewolf WC, Rofsky NM. MR imaging of renal masses: Correlation with findings at surgery and pathologic analysis. Radiographics 2008;28(4):985-1003.

[22] Roy C, Sauer B, Lindner V, Lang H, Saussine C, Jacqmin D. MR imaging of papillary renal neoplasms: Potential application for characterization of small renal masses. Eur Radiol 2007, Jan;17(1):193-200.

[23] Pedrosa I, Sun MR, Spencer M, Genega EM, Olumi AF, Dewolf WC, Rofsky NM. MR imaging of renal masses: Correlation with findings at surgery and pathologic analysis. Radiographics 2008;28(4):985-1003.

[24] Harmon WJ, King BF, Lieber MM. Renal oncocytoma: Magnetic resonance imaging characteristics. J Urol 1996, Mar;155(3):863-7.

[25] Taouli B, Thakur RK, Mannelli L, Babb JS, Kim S, Hecht EM, et al. Renal lesions: Characterization with diffusion-weighted imaging versus contrast-enhanced MR imaging. Radiology 2009, May;251(2):398-407.

[26] Sandrasegaran K, Sundaram CP, Ramaswamy R, Akisik FM, Rydberg MP, Lin C, Aisen AM. Usefulness of diffusion-weighted imaging in the evaluation of renal masses. AJR Am J Roentgenol 2010, Feb;194(2):438-45.

[27] Sohaib SA, Cook G, Allen SD, Hughes M, Eisen T, Gore M. Comparison of whole-body MRI and bone scintigraphy in the detection of bone metastases in renal cancer. Br J Radiol 2009, Aug;82(980):632-9.

[28] Ohno Y, Koyama H, Onishi Y, Takenaka D, Nogami M, Yoshikawa T, et al. Non-small cell lung cancer: Whole-body MR examination for m-stage assessment--utility for whole-body diffusion-weighted imaging compared with integrated FDG PET/CT. Radiology 2008, Aug;248(2):643-54.

[29] Smith AD, Lieber ML, Shah SN. Assessing tumor response and detecting recurrence in metastatic renal cell carcinoma on targeted therapy: Importance of size and attenuation on contrast-enhanced CT. AJR Am J Roentgenol 2010, Jan;194(1):157-65.

[30] Adiga GU, Dutcher JP, Larkin M, Garl S, Koo J. Characterization of bone metastases in patients with renal cell cancer. BJU Int 2004, Jun;93(9):1237-40.

[31] Staudenherz A, Steiner B, Puig S, Kainberger F, Leitha T. Is there a diagnostic role for bone scanning of patients with a high pretest probability for metastatic renal cell carcinoma? Cancer 1999, Jan 1;85(1):153-5.

[32] Hafez KS, Novick AC, Campbell SC. Patterns of tumor recurrence and guidelines for followup after nephron sparing surgery for sporadic renal cell carcinoma. J Urol 1997, Jun;157(6):2067-70.

[33] Levy DA, Slaton JW, Swanson DA, Dinney CP. Stage specific guidelines for surveillance after radical nephrectomy for local renal cell carcinoma. J Urol 1998, Apr;159(4): 1163-7.

[34] Koga S, Tsuda S, Nishikido M, Ogawa Y, Hayashi K, Hayashi T, Kanetake H. The diagnostic value of bone scan in patients with renal cell carcinoma. J Urol 2001, Dec; 166(6):2126-8.

[35] Blacher E, Johnson DE, Haynie TP. Value of routine radionuclide bone scans in renal cell carcinoma. Urology 1985, Nov;26(5):432-4.

[36] Ozülker T, Ozülker F, Ozbek E, Ozpaçaci T. A prospective diagnostic accuracy study of F-18 fluorodeoxyglucose-positron emission tomography/computed tomography in the evaluation of indeterminate renal masses. Nucl Med Commun 2011, Apr;32(4): 265-72.

[37] Divgi CR, Pandit-Taskar N, Jungbluth AA, Reuter VE, Gönen M, Ruan S, et al. Preoperative characterisation of clear-cell renal carcinoma using iodine-124-labelled antibody chimeric G250 (124i-cg250) and PET in patients with renal masses: A phase I trial. Lancet Oncol 2007, Apr;8(4):304-10.

[38] Mueller-Lisse UG, Mueller-Lisse UL. Imaging of advanced renal cell carcinoma. World J Urol 2010, Jun;28(3):253-61.

[39] Nakatani K, Nakamoto Y, Saga T, Higashi T, Togashi K. The potential clinical value of FDG-PET for recurrent renal cell carcinoma. Eur J Radiol 2011, Jul;79(1):29-35.

[40] Khandani AH, Rathmell WK. Positron emission tomography in renal cell carcinoma: An imaging biomarker in development. Semin Nucl Med 2012, Jul;42(4):221-30.

[41] Kayani I, Avril N, Bomanji J, Chowdhury S, Rockall A, Sahdev A, et al. Sequential FDG-PET/CT as a biomarker of response to sunitinib in metastatic clear cell renal cancer. Clin Cancer Res 2011, Sep 15;17(18):6021-8.

[42] Torigian DA, Huang SS, Houseni M, Alavi A. Functional imaging of cancer with emphasis on molecular techniques. CA Cancer J Clin 2007;57(4):206-24.

[43] Atri M. New technologies and directed agents for applications of cancer imaging. J Clin Oncol 2006, Jul;24(20):3299-308.

[44] Galbraith SM, Maxwell RJ, Lodge MA, Tozer GM, Wilson J, Taylor NJ, et al. Combretastatin A4 phosphate has tumor antivascular activity in rat and man as demonstrated by dynamic magnetic resonance imaging. J Clin Oncol 2003, Aug;21(15):2831-42.

[45] Jain RK. Normalization of tumor vasculature: An emerging concept in antiangiogenic therapy. Science 2005, Jan;307(5706):58-62.

[46] Desar IME, van Herpen CML, van Laarhoven HWM, Barentsz JO, Oyen WJG, van der Graaf WTA. Beyond RECIST: Molecular and functional imaging techniques for evaluation of response to targeted therapy. Cancer Treat Rev 2009, Jun;35(4):309-21.

[47] Jeswani T, Padhani AR. Imaging tumour angiogenesis. Cancer Imaging 2005;5:131-8.

[48] Cuenod CA, Fournier L, Balvay D, Guinebretière J-MM. Tumor angiogenesis: Pathophysiology and implications for contrast-enhanced MRI and CT assessment. Abdom Imaging 2006;31(2):188-93.

[49] Goh V, Padhani AR. Imaging tumor angiogenesis: Functional assessment using MDCT or MRI? Abdom Imaging 2006;31(2):194-9.

[50] Kambadakone AR, Sahani DV. Body perfusion CT: Technique, clinical applications, and advances. Radiol Clin North Am 2009, Jan;47(1):161-78.

[51] Ma S-HH, Le H-BB, Jia B-HH, Wang Z-XX, Xiao Z-WW, Cheng X-LL, et al. Peripheral pulmonary nodules: Relationship between multi-slice spiral CT perfusion imaging and tumor angiogenesis and VEGF expression. BMC Cancer 2008;8:186.

[52] Padhani AR. Diffusion magnetic resonance imaging in cancer patient management. Semin Radiat Oncol 2011, Apr;21(2):119-40.

[53] Li SP, Padhani AR. Tumor response assessments with diffusion and perfusion MRI. J Magn Reson Imaging 2012, Apr;35(4):745-63.

[54] Turkbey B, Kobayashi H, Ogawa M, Bernardo M, Choyke PL. Imaging of tumor angiogenesis: Functional or targeted? AJR Am J Roentgenol 2009, Aug;193(2):304-13.

[55] Gwyther SJ, Schwartz LH. How to assess anti-tumour efficacy by imaging techniques. Eur J Cancer 2008, Jan;44(1):39-45.

[56] van der Veldt AA, Meijerink MR, van den Eertwegh AJ, Boven E. Targeted therapies in renal cell cancer: Recent developments in imaging. Target Oncol 2010, Jun;5(2): 95-112.

[57] Figueiras RG, Padhani AR, Goh VJ, Vilanova JC, González SB, Martín CV, et al. Novel oncologic drugs: What they do and how they affect images. Radiographics 2011;31(7):2059-91.

[58] Garcia Figueiras R. CT perfusion techniques in oncologic imaging: A useful tool? AJR Am J Roentgenol 2013, Jan 1.

[59] Flaherty KT, Rosen MA, Heitjan DF, Gallagher ML, Schwartz B, Schnall MD, O'Dwyer PJ. Pilot study of DCE-MRI to predict progression-free survival with sorafenib therapy in renal cell carcinoma. Cancer Biol Ther 2008, Apr;7(4):496-501.

[60] Thiam R, Fournier LS, Trinquart L, Medioni J, Chatellier G, Balvay D, et al. Optimizing the size variation threshold for the CT evaluation of response in metastatic renal cell carcinoma treated with sunitinib. Ann Oncol 2010, May;21(5):936-41.

[61] van der Veldt AA, Meijerink MR, van den Eertwegh AJ, Haanen JB, Boven E. Choi response criteria for early prediction of clinical outcome in patients with metastatic renal cell cancer treated with sunitinib. Br J Cancer 2010, Mar 2;102(5):803-9.

[62] Nathan PD, Vinayan A, Stott D, Juttla J, Goh V. CT response assessment combining reduction in both size and arterial phase density correlates with time to progression in metastatic renal cancer patients treated with targeted therapies. Cancer Biol Ther 2010, Jan;9(1):15-9.

[63] Smith AD, Shah SN, Rini BI, Lieber ML, Remer EM. Morphology, attenuation, size, and structure (MASS) criteria: Assessing response and predicting clinical outcome in metastatic renal cell carcinoma on antiangiogenic targeted therapy. AJR Am J Roentgenol 2010, Jun;194(6):1470-8.

[64] Eisenhauer EA, Therasse P, Bogaerts J, Schwartz LH, Sargent D, Ford R, et al. New response evaluation criteria in solid tumours: Revised RECIST guideline (version 1.1). Eur J Cancer 2009, Jan;45(2):228-47.

[65] van Cruijsen H, van der Veldt A, Hoekman K. Tyrosine kinase inhibitors of VEGF receptors: Clinical issues and remaining questions. Front Biosci 2009;14:2248-68.

[66] Krajewski KM, Guo M, Van den Abbeele AD, Yap J, Ramaiya N, Jagannathan J, et al. Comparison of four early posttherapy imaging changes (EPTIC; RECIST 1.0, tumor shrinkage, computed tomography tumor density, choi criteria) in assessing outcome to vascular endothelial growth factor-targeted therapy in patients with advanced renal cell carcinoma. Eur Urol 2011, May;59(5):856-62.

[67] Nishino M, Jagannathan JP, Krajewski KM, O'Regan K, Hatabu H, Shapiro G, Ramaiya NH. Personalized tumor response assessment in the era of molecular medicine: Cancer-specific and therapy-specific response criteria to complement pitfalls of RECIST. AJR Am J Roentgenol 2012, Apr;198(4):737-45.

Section 2

Management of Localized Renal Tumor

Chapter 4

Renal Cell Carcinoma: Clinical Surgery

Carolin Eva Hach, Stefan Siemer and Stephan Buse

Additional information is available at the end of the chapter

http://dx.doi.org/10.5772/53778

1. Introduction

Renal cell cancer is the third most common genitourinary tumour and the seventh most common cancer. It accounts for about 3% of all malignancies. After prostate cancer and bladder cancer it is the third most common urological tumour. Among urological cancers it shows the highest mortality [1]. Its incidence has geographic, ethnic and age differences, however over the last two decades there has been a rising incidence of renal cell carcinoma particularly of early-stage tumours leading to a paradigm shift in the therapeutic management.

An increased risk of disease is described with a positive family history and the following diseases: Von Hippel-Lindau (VHL) syndrome, tuberous sclerosis, polycystic renal degeneration, chronic renal insufficiency, dialysis and condition after renal transplantation, arterial hypertension, adiposity and diabetes mellitus. Other risk factors are drugs (phenacetinabusus, diuretics) and a number of environmental factors such as asbestos, lead, arsenic, cadmium and aromatic hydrocarbon compounds. Previous described as typical triad of flank pain, hematuria and palpable flank tumour (Virchow`s triad) is nowadays rarely seen in far advanced tumour stages [2]. The same is true for B symptoms, which is usually a sign of metastasis already existing.

The increased availability and advances in diagnostic imaging (ultrasound, computed tomograhy and magnetic resonance imaging) (Fig.1) with an increase in the incidental diagnosis of renal tumours [3] and an improved understanding of the basic biology of renal cell carcinoma, led in recent years to an improvement in survival rates, however, in approximately one third of all patients when diagnosed there are metastasis [4] (mainly locoregional lymph nodes, lung, skeletal system, brain and liver) with a 5-year survival rate of less than 5%.

INTECH
open science | open minds

© 2013 Hach et al.; licensee InTech. This is a paper distributed under the terms of the Creative Commons Attribution License (http://creativecommons.org/licenses/by/3.0), which permits unrestricted use, distribution, and reproduction in any medium, provided the original work is properly cited.

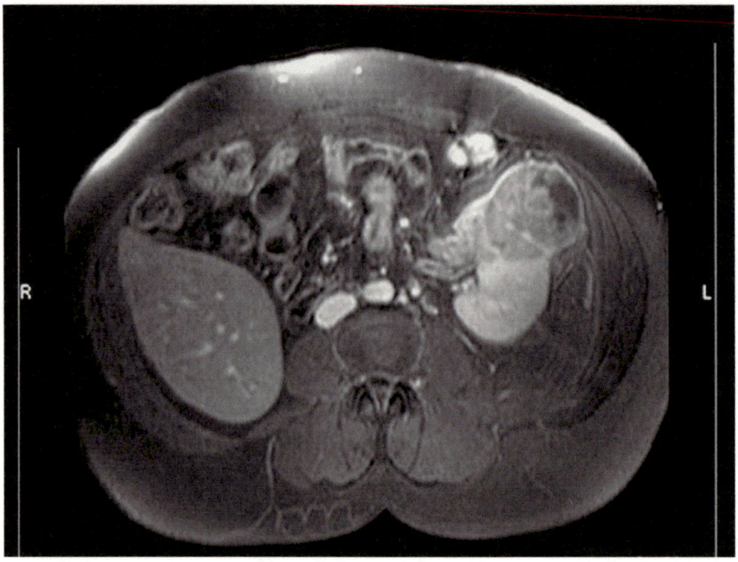

Figure 1. Abdominal magnetic resonance imaging (MRI): Renal tumour of the left upper pole: suspected renal cell carcinoma

Furthermore a third of patients that have been treated for a locally limited renal cell carcinoma (Fig. 2a,b,c) in the course show recurrence or metastasis. A tool to assess the risk of metastasis after a nephrectomy is the Mayo Scoring System (Tab.1).

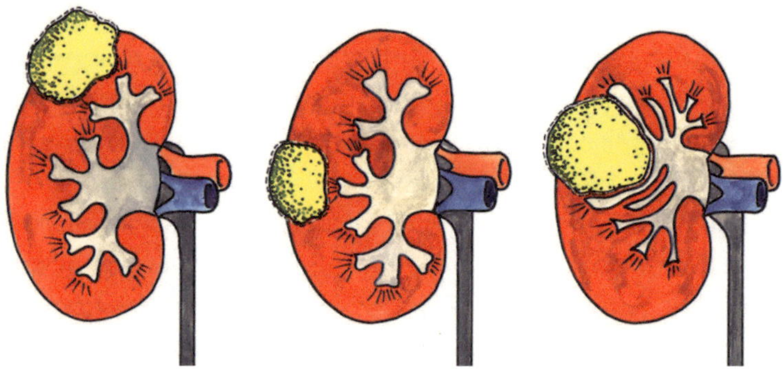

Figure 2. (a) Locally limited renal cell carcinoma of the upper pole; (b) Locally limited renal cell carcinoma in the lateral convexity; (c) Locally limited renal cell carcinoma with suppression of pelvicocaliceal system

Of crucial prognostic importance is therefore the question of the presence of a locally defined or metastatic renal cell carcinoma with a median survival of about 50% one year after the diagnosis of metastasis. This underlines the importance of early detection. Because of lack of radiosensitivity and chemosensitivity of renal cell carcinoma surgical treatment (nephrectomy or partial nephrectomy) remains the only curative treatment option for locally confined tumours. Partial nephrectomy/nephron-sparing nephrectomy, minimally invasive techniques, energy ablative techniques and active surveillance have been progressively used as an alternative option towards open radical nephrectomy which was the historical gold standard approach. Partial nephrectomy has demonstrated an equivalent oncologic outcome with an improved renal function and reduction of cardiovascular events. Over the past years laparoscopic and robot-assisted procedures gained in importance showing similar results in terms of oncologic control.

Feature	Score
Pathologic T stage[a]	
T1a	0
T1b	2
T2	3
T3-4	4
Regional lymph node status[a]	
pNx/pN0	0
pN1-2	2
Nuclear grading	
G1-2	0
G3	1
G4	3
Tumour size	
< 10cm	0
> 10cm	1
Histologic tumour necrosis	
No	0
Yes	1

[a] According to the 2002 American Joint Committee in Cancer staging system

Risk group	Score	Estimated metastasis-free survival after 3 years	Estimated metastasis-free survival after 10 years
Low risk	0-2	98%	92.5%
Intermediate risk	3-5	80%	64%
High risk	>6	37%	24%

Table 1. Mayo-Scoring-System (Leibovich BC, Blute ML, Cheville JC et al. Prediction of progression after radical nephrectomy for patients with clear cell carcinoma: a stratification tool for prospective clinical trials. Cancer 2003; 97:1663-1671)

In metastastic renal cell carcinoma the surgical removal of the primary tumour in the sense of reducing the tumour burden and metastasis respectively for palliative reasons or as part of a combined tumour therapy may be required. Through such combined therapy concepts in some cases significant extensions of survival times can be achieved. Integration of surgery and systemic therapy is essential in the treatment of metastatic renal cell carcinoma. The earliest possible diagnosis and careful selection of surgical procedure for each patient is the basis with the goal of curation and the best possible quality of life.

2. Therapy for localized renal cell carcinoma

For a long time radical nephrectomy was the standard treatment for normal contralateral renal function and absence of metastasis. The first successful nephrectomy took place on 2 August 1869 by the Heidelberg surgeon Gustav Simon. In the late 1960s the classic radical nephrectomy with the removal of kidney and adrenal gland within Gerota`s fascia, including removal of the perirenal adipose capsule, of the proximal ureter and the ipsilateral lymph nodes with a 5-year overall survival rate of 66% for organ-confined tumours was described by Robson [5], (Tab. 2 and 3).

TNM stage[a]	5-year cancer-specific survival rate
T1	83%
T2	57%
T3	42%
T4	28%

[a] According to the 1997 TNM system (AJCC)

Table 2. 5-year cancer-specific survival after nephrectomy/partial nephrectomy as a function of the 1997 TNM stage (AJCC) (Tsui KH, Shvarts O, Smith RB et al. Prognostic indicators for renal cell carcinoma: a multivariate analysis of 643 patients using the revised 1997 TNM staging criteria. J Urol 2000; 163:1090-1095)

Robson stage	5-year survival rate
I	75%
II	63%
III	38%
IV	11%

Table 3. 5-year survival rate after nephrectomy, depending on the Robson stage (Guinan PD, Vogelzang NJ, Fremgen AM et al. Renal cell carcinoma: tumour size, stage and survival. Members of the Cancer Incidence and End Results Committee. J Urol 1995; 153:901-903)

In the open surgical nephrectomy, the choice of the surgical approach should be taken depending on the location and size of the tumour as well as the experience of the surgeon. Basically the following methods are available: primary retroperitoneal approach to the lumbar by use of sub- or intercostal incision, transabdominal or thoracoabdominal. There seems to be no difference in terms of oncological results.

The laparoscopic nephrectomy (transperitoneal, retroperitoneal or "hand-assisted") is another method. This frequently surgical technique is especially used in T1 (up to 7cm tumour size) and T2 tumours (tumour larger 7cm, limited to the kidney). The surgical steps are basically those of the conventional open surgical approach. Comparable oncological results with open nephrectomy are seen in large tumours as well. [6].

The advantages of laparoscopic nephrectomy are reduction in postoperative pain symptoms with less pain medication and earlier mobilization. Furthermore faster recovery and better cosmetic results are mentioned. The frequently discussed risk of implantation metastasis in the abdominal puncture trocar has only been reported casuistic. A tumour cell spread by the applied pneumoperitoneum is not known.

The third and most recent method to be mentioned is the robotic-assisted laparoscopic nephrectomy. Major advantages of this method are the three-dimensional view for the surgeon, up to a 10-fold magnification of the surgical field, a suppression of tremor of the surgeon`s hands through a so-called tremor filter and the free movement of the instruments which are equivalent to those of the human wrist (so-called "endo wrist instruments"). Robot-assisted two approaches are possible: transperitoneal and retroperitoneal approach.

Specific complications of the nephrectomy, regardless of the surgical approach are mainly injuries to neighbouring organs in particular pleural lesions, spleen, pancreas and duodenal injuries and bleeding complications. Frequently occurring transient postoperative creatinine level elevation usually shows a rapid compensation with a healthy contralateral kidney.

As mentioned earlier, in recent years by increasing the availability and development of radiological examination techniques, there has been an increase of incidentally detected T1 renal tumours. After the first partial nephrectomy was done in 1887 by Vincenz Czerny at the University of Heidelberg, it is established today for tumours ≤ 4cm as the gold standard as well as for tumours up to 7cm in selected patients [7]. Becker et al. showed with the nephrectomy comparable oncologic results and low complication rates in tumours > 4cm [8] or ≥ 7cm [9] in selected patients. The 5- year tumour-free survival in this process is over 95%, the rate of local recurrence is < 1% [10], even though interestingly in section statistics up to 20% multifocal tumours are detected. A reason for this may lie in a different biological behaviour of tumours with a different aggressiveness. Whether the multifocal renal cell carcinoma is a primary multifocal tumour initiation or a secondary intrarenal metastasis is currently unknown. Careful preoperative imaging therefore is essential. Aim of the organ-preserving technique is a complete resection of the tumour with an optimal preserved renal function.

Tumour size	5-year cancer specific survival rate	10-year cancer specific survival rate
< 4cm (T1a)	96%	90%
> 4cm (T1b)	86%	66%

Table 4. 5-year and 10-year cancer-specific survival after partial nephrectomy depending on tumour size (Hafez KS, Fergany AF, Novick AC. Nephron sparing surgery for localized renal cell carcinoma: impact of tumour size on patient survival, tumour recurrence and TNM staging. J Urol 1999; 162:1930-1933)

Regarding the surgical procedure there is a distinction to be made, especially depending on tumour size and –localization between a number of techniques such as local tumour resection (Fig. 3 and 4) in which a safe distance of a few millimeters should be respected, the poleresection or segmentresection, the heminephrectomy up to nephrectomy with extracorporeal workbench tumour resection and subsequent autotransplantation of the kidney into the iliac fossa at very large central tumours and imperative implications.

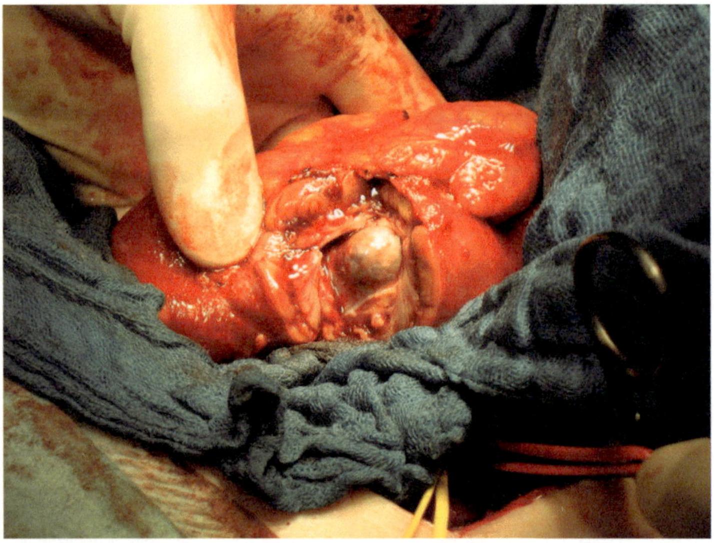

Figure 3. Local resection of a renal tumour

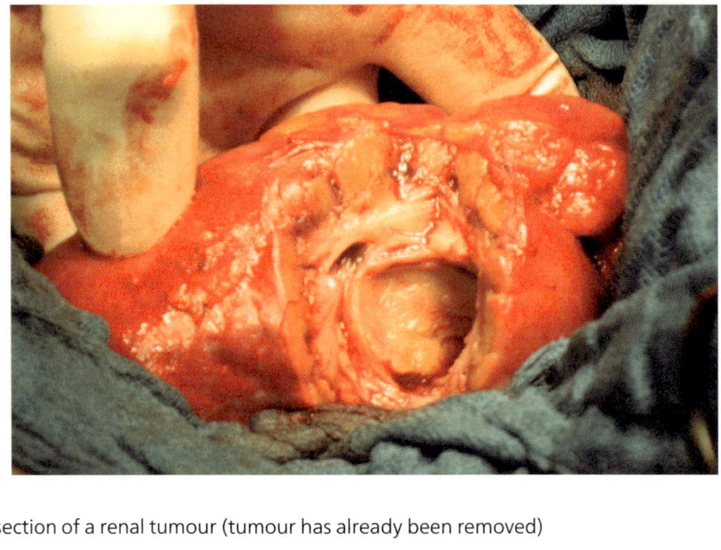

Figure 4. Local resection of a renal tumour (tumour has already been removed)

When doing a partial nephrectomy a differentiation is made between the most common existing elective indications for peripheral small unilateral tumours (≤ 4cm, equivalent to a tumour stage pT1a or in specialized centres tumours up to 7 cm diameter, equivalent to a tumour stage pT1b) in a healthy contralateral kidney, the relative indication in impaired renal function or pre-existing renal insufficiency, synchronous bilateral organ involvement and genetic predisposition for multiple tumours as well as the absolute/imperative indication of an existing solitary kidney (anatomic or functional). Furthermore with this surgical procedure a distinction is made between a partial nephrectomy without ischemia, in a warm ischemia in an anticipated ischemic time of < 20 minutes by disconnection of the renal artery and the renal vein at the renal hilum and partial nephrectomy in cold ischemia (cooling kidney down to 15-20°C) in an anticipated ischemic time of > 20 minutes by the application of 4°C cold perfusion solution through the renal artery or by surrounding the organ with ice. Additionally the implementation of so-called renoprotective measures can follow. These include intraoperative administration of an ACE inhibitor for the reduction of post-ischemic vascular resistance and of mannitol 5% 5-10 minutes before clamping and reopening of the renal artery, with the aim of reducing the intracellular edema and increasing the diuresis and as needed heparin for the prevention of renal artery thrombosis.

Retrospective studies have shown a benefit for partial nephrectomy compared to a nephrectomy with T1a tumours, which can be explained mainly by improved renal function with reduction of cardiovascular events [11]. Also Go et al. have demonstrated in a large prospective study that the loss of renal function is associated with an increase in cardiovascular mortality and shorter life expectancy [12].

Similar to the nephrectomy the partial nephrectomy is an established laparoscopic procedure performed for the fist time in 1993 by Winfield and Clayman. When performing a laparoscopic partial nephrectomy the preparation of the renal hilum takes place after colon mobilization, identification of the ureter as well as the vena cava. Subsequently the excision of the tumour with scissors usually in warm, rarely performed in cold ischemia takes place. After attending to the tumour bed with sutures and/or hemostyptics follows an adaptation of the remaining parenchyma by using a continuous suture. Last is the recovery of the surgical specimen in the extraction bag. Similar to the laparoscopic nephrectomy this method shows the advantages of a lower mean blood loss, lower analgetic requirements postoperatively as well as shorter convalescence and hospitalisation times however at a heightened risk of postoperative hemorrhage and usually prolonged ischemic times. Regarding the oncological and functional outcomes there are comparable results between open and laparoscopic partial nephrectomy [13].

Similar to the robot-assisted nephrectomy, the laparoscopic robot-assisted procedure also used with the nephron-sparing surgery represents another possibility of minimally invasive surgery. After the introduction of the method in 2004 at first primarily small peripherally located tumours were considered to be particularly suitable for this technique [14]. With increasing experience the indication was extended to more complex tumours. Excellent results of robot-assisted surgical technique in relation to more complex lesions, such as centrally located renal tumours or directly at the renal hilum neighbouring tumours are described [15].

The three-dimensional view and the magnification of the surgical field has the advantage of a more precise excision of the tumour. In addition, the robotic-assisted partial nephrectomy has a much shorter learning curve and shorter ischemic times than the conventional laparoscopic procedure. A special technique for the reduction of the ischemic time is the so-called "sliding clip renorrhaphy" during renal reconstruction. In this technique a continous absorbable suture with clips for securing both ends is used. These clips can then be moved along the sutures and this way the renal defect can be closed. With this the warm ischemic time could be reduced significantly [16]. Another method through which the warm ischemic time can be reduced is the early removal of the vascular clamps, so-called "early unclamping". Few sutures are used in order to avoid more bleeding before removal of the vascular clamps, to then care for the remaining still bleeding vessels without ischemia [17]. Also the selective disconnection of the tumour supplying segmental arteries can reduce the ischemic time, but at an increased risk of injury during preparation of the hilar vessels. While early experience with robotic partial nephrectomy have demonstrated no advantages of this surgical method compared to the conventional laparoscopic approach [14], recent work showed equivalent results in terms of oncologic outcomes for benefits such as a lower intraoperative blood loss and shorter warm ischemic times compared to those of conventional laparoscopy. A multicenter study showed comparable results in terms of the following parameters: duration of surgery (laparascopic partial nephrectomy 174 min vs. robotic-assisted partial nephrectomy 189 min), cavity opening (54 vs. 47%), R1-status (3.9 vs. 1%) and postoperative complications (10.2 vs. 8.6%) [18].

The criticism of the robot-assisted partial nephrectomy are essentially two:

1. Dependency of the surgeon on the assistant during surgery
2. High purchase and maintenance costs for the surgical robot

The surgeon sits at the console and does not stand at the operating table, therefore communication between him and his assistant surgeon is extremely important, especially during critical surgical steps such as the setting of vascular clamps and clips.

Comparative data on the ratio of the costs for an open, conventional laparoscopic and robotic partial nephrectomy are limited. Mir et al. compared the costs of open, laparoscopic and robotic partial nephrectomy in 33 patients. They showed laparoscopic partial nephrectomy to be more cost effective than open partial nephrectomy due to a shorter hospital stay. Moreover they demonstrated that the laparoscopic procedure is more cost effective compared the robotic approach because of lower instrumentation costs [19]. Studies on robotic-assisted cystectomy and prostatectomy however showed significantly higher costs of robotic surgeries [20, 21].

In summary it can be stated that the preservation of functioning renal parenchyma and therefore a reduction in renal dysfunction is a clear advantage of partial nephrectomy compared to nephrectomy. The laparoscopic as well as the robotic-assisted partial nephrectomy in studies with small numbers of patients (Fig. 5 and 6) represent a safe alternative with low morbidity for selected patients at appropriate centres with special expertise. Specific complications with a partial nephrectomy, regardless which type of surgical approach, most likely

http://dx.doi.org/10.5772/53778

are postoperative hemorrhage and extravasation of urine (urinoma) which can be treated by a transient ureter splint or nephrostomy. These complications occur more frequently in patients with imperative indications than in elective indications.

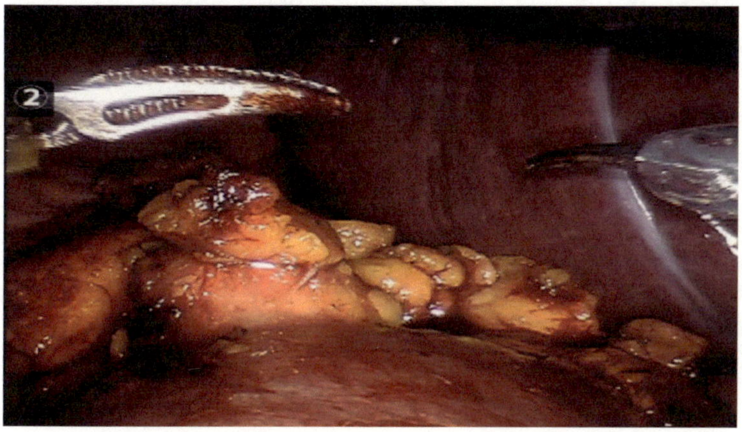

Figure 5. Robot-assisted laparoscopic partial nephrectomy

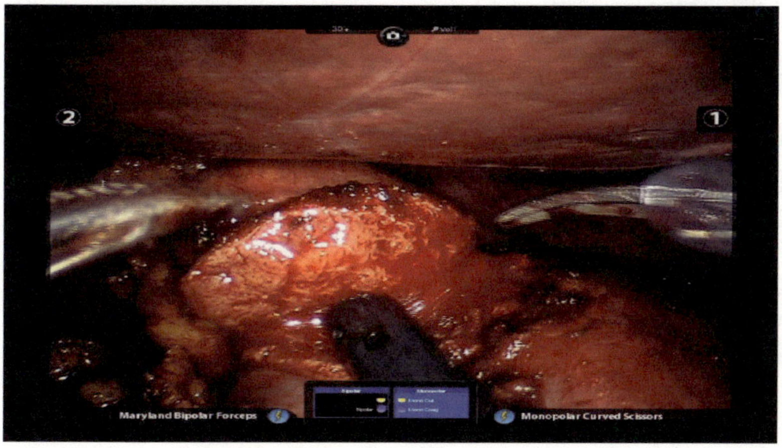

Figure 6. Robot-assisted laparoscopic partial nephrectomy (during enucleation of the tumour)

3. Surgical features

Adrenalectomy: After the ipsilateral adrenalectomy over a long period of time on the grounds of radicalism was seen regradless of size and extent of the renal tumour as essential, the indication for performing a routine adrenalectomy during a nephrectomy is not a standard these days. As an important aspect the fact is that an adrenal tumour rarely grows per continuitatem, but most likely it is a sign of haematogenous metastasis with poor prognosis. On the other side the safety of imaging by using CT is at 97%. The likelihood of adrenal metastasis in small T1 tumours is less than 1% [22]. After Robson in the 1960s described a survival benefit for patients that had a standard adrenalectomy [5], were not detected in subsequent studies [23]. The indication for removal of the adrenal gland is given in case of a very large renal tumour, an upper pole tumour and a suspected metastasis in the adrenal gland (preoperative imaging studies or intraoperative finding).

Lymphadenectomy: For a long time conducting a regional lymphadenectomy (paraaortic/paracaval) was an important part of the nephrectomy. The improved survival times when performing a lymphadenectomy were proven in part by the work of Robson. Especially in view of conversion of patients to small asymptomatic renal tumours, the removal of the ipsilateral lymph nodes is critical discussed similarly to the adrenalectomy. Though diagnostically useful, the value of the hilar ipsilateral lymphadenectomy due to few studies regarding their prognostic significance remains unclear. The therapeutic benefit has not been proven. Interestingly in autopsy studies it was proven that the result of lymph node metastasis usually shows an occult distant metastasis.

Renal vein thrombus and vena cava thrombus: A special feature of the renal cell carcinoma is the tendency of ingrowth into the venous system. A tumour thrombus in the vena cava is found in about 4-10% of all cases, a tumour thrombus with growth up into the right atrium in 0.4% of all cases. Surgical removal of the thrombus should be sought in principle. The surgical procedure must be scheduled in this case depending on the extent of the thrombus.

Level I:Infiltration of the renal vein

Level II:Infiltration of the infrahepatic vena cava

Level III:Infiltration of the intrahepatic vena cava

Level IV:Infiltration of the suprahepatic vena cava

Renal vein thrombi are removed by clamping the junction into the vena cava, thrombi of the vena cava below the diaphragm by a cavotomy. If there is an expansion beyond the hepatic hilum the use of a heart-lung machine is necessary. If there is an expansion to the right atrium the use of extracorporal circulation is required. An important aspect in the planning and implementation of these procedures is the interdisciplinary collaboration between urologists and cardiac surgeons. The prognosis of patients with a tumour thrombus after a successfully carried out surgery is not dependent on the size and extent of the thrombus, but the metastasis stage. After thrombectomy in a non-metastastic stage 5-year tumour specific survival rates up to nearly 70% can be achieved [24]. However almost half of all patients with an extensive vena cava thrombus at diagnosis show lymphatic or haematogenous metastasis.

Bilateral renal tumours: The incidence of synchronous bilateral renal tumours is at 1.6-6%. In principle a two-stage procedure is desirable, where initially the smaller and unifocal tumour can be treated in terms of a partial nephrectomy, with the aim to avoid dialysis in case a subsequent contralateral nephrectomy is required.

Local recurrence: The discovery of local recurrence in condition after partial nephrectomy without evidence of systemic metastasis is seen in <3% of all cases. In this case higher local recurrence rates are seen with imperative indications, which may be explained by a greater number of advanced tumours. In principal surgical removal should be made after exclusion of other metastasis.

4. Other techniques

Energy ablative therapy: The energy ablative method is based on tissue destruction by using cold or heat. Especially cryoablation (CA) and radiofrequency ablation (RFA) are to be mentioned. There are percutaneous and laparoscopic techniques available. Essentially the indication for performing the energy ablative method is limited to palliative situations or as an alternative for high-risk patients with small, conveniently located renal tumours. Potential benefits represent mainly the reduced morbidity and the possibility of treating multimorbid patients in an outpatient setting. The problem is, among other things, the increased risk of local recurrence [25].

LESS/NOTES: After establishing laparoscopic and robot-supported methods now further developments of the methodology in terms of a reduction of the required trocars (LESS = Laparoscopic Single Site Surgery) and the use of so-called "natural orifices" (NOTES = Natural Orifice Translumenal Endoscopic Surgery) take place. Concerning this matter so far however there are only casuistics and small case series available.

5. Surgical treatment of metastastic renal cell carcinoma

Given the fact that a third of patients who are suffering from a renal cell carcinoma have a synchronous and another third after curative intent therapy have a metachronous metastasis, the following shows the possibilities and the importance of surgical therapy for metastastic renal cell carcinoma.

Basically in metastatic renal cell carcinoma a distinction must be made between the sole palliative and the cytoreductive nephrectomy. Indication criterias for palliative nephrectomy for example are conservative uncontrolled pain or recurrent bleeding. In symptomatic multimorbid patients with a high surgical risk the possibility of a tumour embolization should be evaluated. Important here is a sufficient analgesic therapy after completion of the procedure, because severe pain is a common local complication. An impact on the survival rates cannot be seen with surgical procedure nor with tumour embolization. In the era of immunochemotherapy it was shown that cytoreductive nephrectomy followed by immunochemotherapy opposed to receiving only medical therapy shows significantly better survival rates (7.8 months for interferon vs. 13.6 months for nephrectomy plus interferon) [26]. Whether a nephrectomy in metastatic stage in the post-immunotherapy era is up-to date needs to be evaluated. Results of prospective randomized trials for example CARMENA study ("Clinical Trial to Assess the Importance of Nephrectomy") are still pending.

With regard to the surgical treatment of metastasis themselves this indication must be made primarily in response to the location, size and extent of metastasis findings, the symptoms and the overall situation of the affected patients.

Solitary pulmonary filiae should be checked for resectability. Are there only a few (up to three) localized metastasis, then a nephrectomy plus complete resection of metastasis can lead to a significant survival benefit. Basically patients with synchronous pulmonary metastasis have a significant worse prognosis than those with a metachronous metastasis. If it is a disseminated metastasis the initiation of a targeted therapy for (long-term) stabilization of the disease should be discussed with the patient. The basis for this inhibition of tumour growth is a modification of growth signaling inside the tumour cell and the (neo)angiogenesis. Currently seven substances (in different indications) are available: tyrosine kinase inhibitors such as sunitinib, sorafenib, pazopanib and axitinib, antibody-based therapies such as bevacizumab plus interferon-alpha and mTOR ("mamillian target of Rapamycin") inhibitors as temsirolimus and everolimus. The use of drugs in the adjuvant setting with advanced renal cell carcinoma with a high risk of disease progression is currently being evaluated in clinical trials.

In case of hepatic filiae with a median survival rate of 6-18 months the indication for resection in case of a solitary metastasis with a diameter <5 cm should be evaluated if liver function is intact. It is essential to inform the patient about this procedure`s high morbidity. For non-resectable liver metastasis it is possible to perform a CT-guided percutaneous radiofrequency induced thermal ablation (RITA).

In the detection of brain metastasis a surgical approach is to be discussed especially with the onset of neurological symptoms. The indication for resection of metastasis through stereotactic radiosurgery (GammaKnife, CyberKnife) or radiation therapy is to be weighed individually. When limited in size and number of brain metastasis very good results can be achieved in this case with regard to the local control of metastasis.

An indication for surgery in bone metastasis may present neurological deficits in a myelon compression, pain, and fracture risk in instability of the bone. However survival time extensions are described in an osseous metastasis only in individual cases.

Metachronous adrenal metastasis without evidence of further metastasis should be surgically removed.

6. Conclusion

Surgical therapy remains the only curative approach in the treatment of renal cell carcinoma being resistant opposite radiation and chemotherapy. (Radical) nephrectomy was the standard surgical procedure over a long period of time. The spread and further developments of imaging diagnostics resulted in an earlier diagnostic of incidentally detected small renal masses therefore an increase of the performance of nephron-sparing procedures. In the meantime partial nephrectomy represents the standard surgical technique in pT1a renal cell carcinomas (size of tumour ≤ 4cm). Over the past years laparoscopic procedures (laparoscopic nephrectomy and laparoscopic partial nephrectomy) showing similar results in consideration of the oncological outcome compared to open-surgical procedures gained in importance. Long-term results of the rather new technique of robotic nephrectomy and partial nephrectomy are encouraging but remain to be seen. LESS (Laparoscopic Single Site Surgery) and NOTES (Natural Orifice Translumenal Endoscopic Surgery) are first steps towards modifying established minimal invasive procedures.

Author details

Carolin Eva Hach*, Stefan Siemer and Stephan Buse

*Address all correspondence to: carolin.hach@krupp-krankenhaus.de

1 Department of Urology, Alfried Krupp Hospital, Essen, Germany

2 Department of Urology, Saarland University, Homburg/Saar, Germany

References

[1] Perez-Farinos, N, Lopez-Abente, G, & Pastor-Barriuso, R. (2006). Time trend and age-period-cohort effect on kidney cancer mortality in Europe, 1981-2000. *BMC Public Health*.

[2] Lee, C. T, Katz, J, Fearn, P. A, et al. (2002). Mode of presentation of renal cell carcinoma provides prognostic information. *Urol Oncol*, 7, 135-140.

[3] Pantuck, A. J, Zisman, A, & Belldegrun, A. S. (2001). The changing natural history of renal cell carcinoma. *J Urol*, 166, 1611-1623.

[4] Gupta, K., Miller, J. D., Li, J. Z., et al. (2008). Epidemiologic and socioeconomic burden of metastatic renal cell carcinoma (mRCC): a literature review. *Cancer Treat Rev*, 34, 193-205.

[5] Robson, C. J., Churchill, B. M., & Anderson, W. (1969). The results of radical nephrectomy for renal cell carcinoma. *J Urol*, 101, 297-301.

[6] Hemal, A. K., Kumar, A., Wadhwa, P., et al. (2007). Laparoscopic versus open radical nephrectomy for large tumours; a long-term prospective comparison. *J Urol*, 177, 862-866.

[7] Ljungberg, B., Cowan, N., Hanbury, D. C., et al. (2010). Guidelines on renal cell carcinoma. *EAU-Guidelines*.

[8] Becker, F., Siemer, S., Hack, M., et al. (2006). Excellent long-term cancer control with elective nephron-sparing surgery for selected renal cell carcinomas measuring more than 4 cm. *Eur Urol*, 49, 1058-1064.

[9] Becker, F., Roos, F. C., Janssen, M., et al. (2011). Short-term functional and oncologic outcomes of nephron-sparing surgery for renal tumours ≥ 7 cm. *Eur Urol*, 59, 931-937.

[10] Lau, W. K., Blute, M. L., Weaver, A. L., et al. (2000). Matched comparison of radical nephrectomy vs. nephron-sparing surgery in patients with unilateral renal cell carcinoma and a normal contralateral kidney. *Mayo Clin Proc*, 75, 1236-1242.

[11] Zini, L., Perrotte, P., Capitanio, U., et al. (2009). Radical versus partial nephrectomy: effect on overall and noncancer mortality. *Cancer*, 115, 1465-1471.

[12] Go, A. S., Chertow, G. M., Fan, D., et al. (2004). Chronic kidney disease and the risks of death, cardiovascular events, and hospitalization. *N Engl J Med*, 351, 1296-1305.

[13] Lane, B. R., & Gill, I. S. (2007). 5-year outcomes of laparoscopic partial nephrectomy. *J Urol*, 177, 70-74.

[14] Caruso, R. P., Phillips, C. K., Kau, E., et al. (2006). Robot assisted laparoscopic partial nephrectomy: initial experience. *J Urol*, 176, 36-39.

[15] Rogers, C. G., Singh, A., Blatt, A. M., et al. (2008). Robotic partial nephrectomy for complex renal tumours: surgical technique. *Eur Urol*, 53, 514-521.

[16] Benway, B. M., Wang, A. J., Cabello, J. M., et al. (2009). Robotic partial nephrectomy with sliding-clip renorrhaphy: technique and outcomes. *Eur Urol*, 55, 592-599.

[17] San Francisco, I. F., Sweeney, M. C., & Wagner, A. A. (2011). Robot-assisted partial nephrectomy: early unclamping technique. *J Endourol*, 25, 305-309.

[18] Benway, B. M., Bhayani, S. B., Rogers, C. G., et al. (2009). Robot assisted partial nephrectomy versus laparoscopic partial nephrectomy for renal tumours: a multi-institutional analysis of perioperative outcomes. *J Urol*, 182, 866-872.

[19] Mir, S. A., Cadeddu, J. A., Sleepner, J. P., et al. (2011). Cost comparison of robotic, laparoscopic, and open partial nephrectomy. *J Endourol*, 25, 447-453.

[20] Smith, A., Kurpad, R., Lal, A., et al. (2010). Cost analysis of robotic versus open radical cystectomy for bladder cancer. *J Urol*, 183, 505-509.

[21] Bolenz, C., Gupta, A., Hotze, T., et al. (2010). Cost comparison of robotic, laparoscopic, and open radical prostatectomy for prostate cancer. *Eur Urol*, 57, 453-458.

[22] Tsui, K., Shvarts, O., Barbaric, Z., et al. (2000). Is adrenalectomy a necessary component of radical nephrectomy? UCLA experience with 511 radical nephrectomies. *J Urol*, 163, 437-441.

[23] Leibovitch, I., Raviv, G., Mor, Y., et al. (1995). Reconsidering the necessity of ipsilateral adrenalectomy during radical nephrectomy for renal cell carcinoma. *Urology*, 46, 316-320.

[24] Zisman, A., Wieder, J. A., Pantuck, A. J., et al. (2003). Renal cell carcinoma with tumour thrombus extension: Biology, role of nephrectomy and response to immunotherapy. *J Urol*, 169, 909-916.

[25] Kunkle, D. A., Egleston, B. L., & Uzzo, R. G. (2008). Excise, aerlate or observe: the small renal mass dilemma- a meta-analysis and review. *J Urol*, 179, 1227-1233.

[26] Flanigan, R. C., Mickisch, G., Sylvester, R., et al. (2004). Cytoreductive nephrectomy in patients with metastatic renal cancer: a combined analysis. *J Urol*, 171, 1071-1076.

Chapter 5

Nephron-Sparing Surgery for the Treatment of Renal Cell Carcinoma 4 to 7 cm in Size

Ambrosi Pertia, Laurent Managadze and
Archil Chkhotua

Additional information is available at the end of the chapter

http://dx.doi.org/10.5772/53830

1. Introduction

The incidence of kidney cancer is gradually increasing over the past 2–3 decades [1]. 60 920 new cases of RCC have been diagnosed in the US in 2011 and 13 120 died of cancer [2]. The widespread use of modern radiological studies has substantially changed clinical presentation of the renal tumors. Currently, there is a trend towards more frequent diagnosis of asymptomatic, incidental, smaller lesions [1, 3]. Nephron sparing surgery (NSS) was initially used in the treatment of renal cell carcinoma (RCC) only for absolute and relative indications [4]. Excellent oncological outcome and reduced morbidity after NSS have led to more frequent use of organ preserving surgery in many centers [4-7]. Elective NSS is currently the treatment of choice for T1a tumors (<4 cm) in the patients with a normal contralateral kidney. Its safety and oncological results have been evaluated in numerous studies [3, 8-10].

The role of NSS in the tumors of 4–7 cm in size is less evaluated and controversial. It could be technically challenging as well [10]. The existing studies suggest that this policy might be feasible and safe. In this paper we present our single centre experience in using the NSS for RCC of 4–7 cm in size.

2. Technique of nephron-sparing surgery

All patients were operated through extraperitoneal, extrapleural incision above the 12th rib in 38 cases and above the 11th rib in 19 cases. The kidney was completely mobilized to exclude the presence of satellite tumors. Peritumoral fat was left in situ. Sharp incision of the

INTECH
open science | open minds

© 2013 Pertia et al.; licensee InTech. This is a paper distributed under the terms of the Creative Commons Attribution License (http://creativecommons.org/licenses/by/3.0), which permits unrestricted use, distribution, and reproduction in any medium, provided the original work is properly cited.

renal capsule was performed 2 to 3 mm away from the tumor margin. The renal pedicle was isolated completely and the renal artery was clamped just before beginning the incision on the renal capsule. The venous clamping was not used in any case. For diminishing the outcomes of renal ischemia vigorous hydration, infusion of Mannitol before the arterial clamping, and renal hypothermia was adopted in all cases. Tumors were enucleated without a layer of normal parenchyma in 17 cases and enucleoresection was performed in 40 cases. Tumor bed was inspected very carefully on the presense of residual tissue. Intraoperative frozen section of tumor bed was routinely performed. The results of frozen section were negative in all cases. The data of the patients who underwent nephrectomy due to positive margins on the frozen section were not included in the study. The visible bleeding vessels and opened calices were closed using running sutures. Finally, tumor bed was coagulated carefully for haemostatic and partly for oncological reasons. The coagulation was performed by means of diathermy. The parenchymal defect was closed using absorbable interrupted sutures. In case of large capsular defect it was covered with free peritoneal graft.

The stained slides from all tumor specimens were reviewed by urological pathologist. Shortly, the resected kidneys were evaluated macroscopically. The maximal tumor size was measured and 1.5 x 2cm tissue samples were taken for further assessment. Specimens were fixed, stained and evaluated by the same pathologist according to conventional technique. Pathological tumor staging was performed according to the 2002 TNM staging system [11] and nuclear grade was assigned according to the Furhman's grading system [12]. The removed tumor specimen was always inspected by pathologists and the surgical margins were inked.

Patients were followed with renal functional tests, chest X-ray, abdominal ultrasound or CT every 3 months during the first year, once in 6 months for the next two years and annually thereafter. In terms of statistical analysis the probability of cumulative and cancer-specific survival was estimated by the Kaplan-Meier method using the whole number of events.

3. Results

We retrospectively reviewed the records of 57 patients who underwent NSS at our institution from 1994 to 2011. The table 1 describes the clinical and pathological features of 57 patients operated at our institution. All patients were carefully evaluated to exclude the presence of distant metastases. Preoperative evaluation included: ultrasonography of the kidney, CT of the abdomen and chest X-ray in all patients. Renal function was assessed by measuring serum creatinine level and creatinine clearance.

The mean follow-up was 70.1 months (range: 10-157 months). Out of the 57 patients 35 (61.4%) were male and 22 (38.6%) were female. The median patient age was 53.1 years (range: 37-68 years). Left side tumor was detected in 34 (59.6%) cases and right side in 23 (40.4 %) cases. The tumor was located in the upper pole in 21 (36.8 %), in the mid kidney in 7 (12.2 %) and in the lower pole in 29 (51%) patients. Tumors were located peripherally in 46 (80.7%) cases and the central tumor location was detected in 11 (19.3%) cases. The peripheral location was defined as: peripherally located and enveloped by cortical parenchyma tumor, without extension into the renal sinus. At the diagnosis 53 (92.9 %) tumors were detected incidentally and 4 (7.1%) were associated with microscopic haematuria. The NSS was performed for absolute indications in 5 (8.7%) and for relative indications in 11 (19.9%) cases. 41 (71.9%) patients underwent NSS for elective indications.

Age at surgery (years)	53.1 (37-68)
Gender	
Male	35 (61.4 %)
Female	22 (38.6 %)
Tumor location	
Left	34 (59.6%)
Right	23 (40.4 %)
Upper pole	21 (36.8 %)
Mid kidney	7 (12.2 %)
Lower pole	29 (51%)
Central	11 (19.3%)
Peripheral	46 (80.7%)
Clinical presentation	
Incidental	53 (93%)
Presented by haematuria, pain etc.	4 (7%)
Tumor size (mm.)	48.1 (41-70)
Stage	
pT1b	53 (93%)
pT3a	4 (7%)
Fuhrman grade	
G1	22 (38.6 %)
G2	27 (47.4 %)
G3	8 (14 %)
Histological subtype (%)	
Clear cell	49 (85.9 %)
Pappilary	5 (8.7 %)
Chromophobe	2 (3.7 %)
Cystic RCC	1 (1.75 %)
Surgical complications	
Bleeding	1(1.75 %)
Urinary leakage	4 (7%)
Disease Recurrence	
Local recurrence	2 (3.5 %)
Distant metastases	4 (7%)

Table 1. Clinico-pathological characteristics of 57 patients operated with NSS.

The mean tumour size was 48.1 mm. (range: 41-70 mm.). The mean tumor size in the patients who underwent NSS for elective indications was 44.7 mm. and in the patients who underwent NSS for absolute and relative indications was 65.8 mm ($p<0.04$). The difference between the later two groups was not significant. Fifty three out of 57 tumors were pT1b (92.9 %) and 4 (7.1%) were pT3a. Pathological T3a stage was confirmed by tumor microinvasion into the perirenal fat. The final pathological evaluation did not reveal any case of tumor extension out of the inked area of the surgical specimens. Grade I tumor was diagnosed in 22 (38.6%), Grade 2 in 27 (47,4%) and Grade 3 in 8 (14%) cases. Morphological evaluation revealed 49 (85.9%) clear cell, 5 papillary (8.7%), 2 chromophobe (3.7%) and 1 cystic (1.75%) RCCs.

The mean duration of renal ischemia was 22 minutes (range: 18-35 mm.). No perioperative mortality and/or serious general complications (myocardial infarction, deep venous thrombosis etc.) have been observed. Postoperative complications occurred in 5 (8.8%) patients including: one (1.7%) postoperative bleeding and 4 (7%) urinary fistulas. The bleeding was observed in peripherally located, large (6 cm. in size) tumor operated for absolute indication. Urinary leakage occurred in two patients operated for centrally located (18.1%) and in two (4.2%) peripherially located tumors. This difference was statistically significant in favor of peripherially located tumors ($p<0.0001$). All patients required a double "J" stenting. Perirenal hematoma was observed in 2 (3.5%) cases but did not need any intervention and resolved spontaneously. Renal functions were stable in all patients during the follow-up period with a median postoperative creatinine level of 0.9 mg/dl (range: 0.7–1.4 mg/dl). The median hospital stay was 6 days (range: 4-15 days).

The tumor has recurred in 6 (10.5%) patients. Of them, local recurrence was detected in 2 (3.5%) and systemic recurrence in 4 (7%) patients. At the end of the follow-up overall survival was 85.8%, the disease-free survivals was 88.2 %. Both disease-free and overall survival were significantly better in groups of relative and elective indications as compared with absolute indication ($p=0.014$ and $p=0.023$, respectively) (Figure 1).

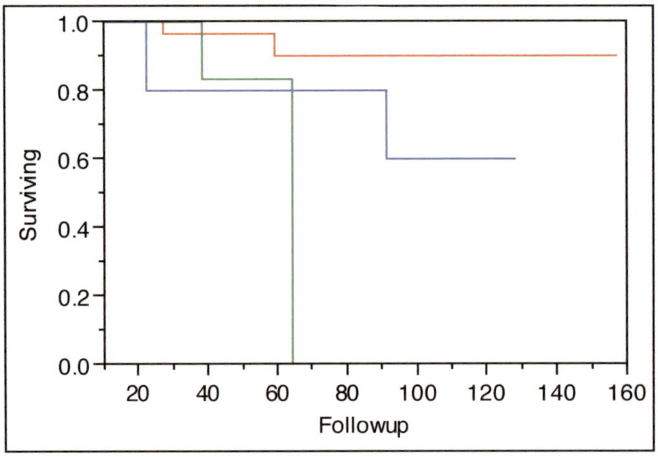

Figure 1. Cancer-specific survival in the patients with elective, relative and absolute indications for NSS. ——— Elective; ——— Relative; ——— Absolute

4. Discussion

The widespread use of modern radiological modalities substantially changed clinical presentation of renal tumors in recent decades. Currently, there is a trend towards the diagnosis of asymptomatic, incidental, smaller lesions at lower stages [1, 3, 10]. The local disease recurrence is the major drawback of NSS mostly due to the incomplete resection of the primary tumor. In this due radical nephrectomy still remains the gold standard for the treatment of RCC [4, 10].

Improved diagnostic and surgical techniques have led to wider use of NSS. Uzzo RG. and Novick AC. in their review of the results of more than 1800 cases of NSS have showed that the true biological significance of multicentric renal tumors and its implications for NSS remains to be elucidated [3]. In a prospective, randomized EORTC (European Organisation for Research and Treatment of Cancer) phase 3 study comparing open partial nephrectomy (OPN) with open radical nephrectomy (ORN) in small renal tumors (< 5 cm.) found comparable oncological results in the both arms [8, 9]. Moreover, excellent 5 and 10 year disease-free survival rates of 98.5% and 96.7% have been reported after NSS in non-randomized studies [5-7]. These data are now widely accepted. Finally, the recent evidence favoring the NSS over radical nephrectomy in the prevention of chronic kidney disease and possibly linking it to a better overall survival will constitute a strong argument for wider use of NSS. On the other hand, NSS is technically more demanding than RN even for small renal tumors [13]. The previous report of the EORTC 30904 trial revealed that complication rate in NSS was slightly higher than in radical nephrectomy [8].

Based on the success of NSS in the tumors of ≤ 4 cm, it has been increasingly used for the treatment of 4-7 cm. tumors in case of a normal contralateral kidney. Leibovich BC. *Et al.* retrospectively compared the results of NSS and radical nephrectomy in the tumors of 4 to 7 cm in size. There were no statistically significant differences in cancer-specific survival and distant metastases-free survival after adjusting for important pathological features. Thus, the authors concluded that the NSS has excellent results for the treatment of 4 to 7 cm renal tumors in appropriately selected patients [14].

Dash A. *et al.* compared the outcomes of the patients who had an elective partial or radical nephrectomy for clear cell renal cell carcinoma of 4–7 cm. in size. With the median follow-up of 21 months the authors failed to show that radical nephrectomy was associated with a better cancer control than the NSS. In terms of functional results the authors found that the serum creatinine level 3 months after surgery was significantly lower in the patients who had NSS [15].

Becker F. *et al.* reported the excellent results of NSS performed for elective indications. 69 patients with the tumor size of more than 4 cm. underwent NSS. After a mean follow-up of 6.2 years seven patients (10.1%) have died, none of them due to the tumor-related causes. Tumor recurrence was detected in four patients (5.8%). The 5-year overall survival was 94.9%. The 10-year and 15-year overall survival was 86.7%. Cancer-specific survival was 100% at 5, 10, and 15 years. The authors concluded that the selected patients with localized

RCC of > 4 cm. can be treated with elective NSS providing optimal long-term outcome. The surgeon's decision for organ-preserving surgery should depend on the tumor location and technical feasibility rather than on the tumor size [16].

Pahernick S. *et al.* compared the results of NSS for the tumors of less and more than 4 cm. in size. Out of 474 treated patients 102 had the tumor of more than 4 cm. The mean follow-up was 4.7 years. The 5 and 10-year cancer-specific survival for small and large tumors were: 97.9% and 95.8%, 94.9% and 95.8%, respectively. In contrast to the tumor size, stage pT3a was associated with a significantly higher risk of tumor related death. The authors advocated that the surgeon's decision with regard to the organ preservation should consider the tumor location and safe surgical resectability, rather than the tumor size [17]. This conclusion has been later supported by Antonelli A. *et al.* [18].

Joniau S. *et al.* presented their results of NSS for the patients with bigger than 4 cm renal tumors. The following data have been collected and analyzed: surgical indication, tumor characteristics, complications, serum creatinine level, time to recurrence and time to the patient death. Local cancer control has been achieved in the vast majority of patients. The renal function was preserved in the patients with elective indications. NSS for absolute indications was significantly correlated with the loss of renal function but not with a cancer-specific survival [19].

In our study the local disease recurrence was detected in 2 (3.5%) and the systemic recurrence in 4 (7%) patients. We could not reveal any changes in the serum creatinine level pre- and postoperatively in the both groups, despite cold ischemia which was used in all patients. Both, the cancer-specific and overall survival was significantly better in the groups of relative and elective indications as compared with the absolute indication ($p<0.014$ and $p<0.023$, respectively). These data are similar to the results of the eight-institution multicentre review of 1048 NSS procedures [13].

It has been shown by Badalato GM. *et al.* in their recent publication that the oncological efficacy of NSS for pT1b renal tumors was comparable to that of radical nephrectomy [20]. The authors compared the NSS with radical nephrectomy in the patients with T1b RCC using a propensity scoring approach. 11 256 cases of 4-7 cm. tumors that underwent partial or radical nephrectomy have been evaluated. The propensity score analysis was used to adjust for the potential differences in the baseline characteristics of the patients between the two groups. Overall and disease-free survival of the patients was compared in stratified and adjusted analysis, controlling for propensity scores. For the entire patient cohort, no difference in the survivals was found in the NSS and radical nephrectomy groups. The survival difference between the groups in a propensity-adjusted cohort of patients could not be confirmed even when stratified by the tumor size and patient age.

We've observed that the NSS for centrally located tumors was associated with a higher complication rate. This goes in accordance with the data of Ficarra V. *et al.* who recently proposed a new tumor scoring system [21]. According to the authors this system can better predict the complications after NSS than linear tumor size.

The weak points of our study are retrospective nature and absence of control group consisting of RN patients. However, the prospective randomized study is very difficult to conduct especially in the era of minimally invasive approaches for the treatment of RCC.

5. Conclusion

In conclusion, the NSS is a feasible procedure for RCCs of 4-7 cm in size. The local cancer control can be achieved in most patients. Oncological outcome of the treatment is negatively related with the tumor size. Long-term prospective studies on the higher number of patients are required to prove the similar oncological efficacy of NSS and radical nephrectomy in the RCCs of 4-7 cm. in size.

Author details

Ambrosi Pertia, Laurent Managadze and Archil Chkhotua

National Centre of Urology, Tbilisi, Georgia

References

[1] Hollingsworth JM, Miller DC, Daignault S, Hollenbeck BK. Rising incidence of small renal masses: a need to reassess treatment effect. J Natl Cancer Inst 2006; 98: 1331–1334.

[2] Siegel R, Ward E, Brawley O, Jemal, A. Cancer Statistics, 2011. CA Cancer J Clin 2011; 61(4): 212–236.

[3] Uzzo RG, Novick AC. Nephron sparing surgery for renal tumors: indications, techniques and outcomes. J Urol. 2001; 166(1): 6-18.

[4] Herr HW. A history of partial nephrectomy for renal tumors. J Urol. 2005; 173: 705-708.

[5] Lerner SE, Hawkins CA, Blute ML. Disease outcome in patients with low stage renal cell carcinoma treated with nephron sparing or radical surgery J Urol. 1996; 155: 1868-1873.

[6] Herr HW. Partial nephrectomy for unilateral renal carcinoma and a normal contralateral kidney: 10-year follow-up J Urol. 1999; 161: 33-34.

[7] Fergany AF, Hafez KS, Novick AC. Long-term results of nephron sparing surgery for localized renal cell carcinoma: 10-year followup. J Urol. 2000; 163: 442–445.

[8] Van Poppel H, Da Pozzo L, AlbrechtW, et al. A prospective randomized EORTC intergroup phase 3study comparing the complications of elective nephron-sparing surgery and radical nephrectomy for lowstage renal cell carcinoma. Eur Urol 2007; 51: 1606–1615.

[9] Van Poppel H, Da Pozzo L, AlbrechtW, et al. A prospective, randomized EORTC intergroup phase 3 study comparing the oncologic outcome of elective nephron-sparing surgery and radical nephrectomy for low-stage renal cell carcinoma. Eur Urol 2011; 59: 543–552.

[10] Van Poppel H, Becker F, Cadeddu J, et al. Treatment of localized Renal cell Carcinoma Eur. Urol 2011; 60: 662-672.

[11] Sobin L, Wittekind Ch. TNM Classification of Malignant Tumours. New York, John Wiley & Sons. 2002; vol. 6. p. 193.

[12] Fuhrman SA, Lasky LC, Limas C. Prognostic significance of morphologic parameters in renal cell carcinoma. Am J Surg Pathol. 1982; 6: 655-663.

[13] Patard J-J, Pantuck AJ, Crepel M, et al. Morbidity and clinical outcome of nephron-sparing surgery in relation to tumour size and indication. Eur Urol 2007; 52: 148–154.

[14] Leibovich BC, Blute ML, Cheville JC, Lohse CM, Weaver AL, Zincke H. Nephron sparing surgery for appropriately selected renal cell carcinoma between 4 and 7 cm results in outcome similar to radical nephrectomy. J Urol 2004; 171: 1066–1070.

[15] Dash A, Vickers AJ, Schachter LR, Bach AM, Snyder ME, Russo P. Comparison of outcomes in elective partial vs radical nephrectomy for clear cell renal cell carcinoma of 4-7 cm. BJU Int 2006; 97: 939–945.

[16] Becker F, Siemer S, Hack M, Humke U, Ziegler M, Stockle M. Excellent long-term cancer control with elective nephron-sparing surgery for selected renal cell carcinomas measuring more than 4 cm. Eur Urol 2006; 49: 1058–64.

[17] Pahernik S, Roos F, Röhrig B, et al. Elective nephron sparing surgery for renal cell carcinoma larger than 4 cm. J Urol 2008; 179: 71–74.

[18] Antonelli A, Cozzoli A, Nicolai M, et al. Nephron-sparing surgery versus radical nephrectomy in the treatment of intracapsular renal cell carcinoma up to 7 cm. Eur Urol 2008; 53: 803–809.

[19] Joniau S, Vander Eeckt K, Srirangam SJ, Van Poppel H. Outcome of nephron-sparing surgery for T1b renal cell carcinoma. BJU Int 2009; 103: 1344–1348.

[20] Badalato GM, Kates M, Wisnivesky JP, Choudhury AR, McKiernan JM. Survival after partial and radical nephrectomy for the treatment of stage T1bN0M0 renal cell carcinoma (RCC) in the USA: a propensity scoring approach. BJU Int 2012; 109: 1457-1462.

[21] Ficarra V, Novara G, Secco S, et al. Preoperative aspects and dimensions used for an anatomical (PADUA) classification of renal tumours in patients who are candidates for nephron-sparingsurgery. Eur Urol 2009; 56: 786–793.

Chapter 6

Renal Artery Embolization in Treatment of Renal Cancer with Emphasis on Response of Immune System

H. Zielinski, T. Syrylo and S. Szmigielski

Additional information is available at the end of the chapter

http://dx.doi.org/10.5772/54116

1. Introduction

Role of renal artery embolization (RAE) in strategy of treatment of renal carcinoma (RC) has a multiyear history in scientific literature and in personal experience. In view of personal experience we have a strong feeling that RAE is beneficial both in operable and advanced RC, partially because of longer survival and stimulation of certain immune reactions [1].

RAE was introduced to clinical practice in the 70's of last century. The pioneers who developed the technique of surgery were Lalli et al, in 1973 while Almgard et al. presented their own experience with the application of RAE in renal cancer in humans [2,3]. At that time arteriography was the basic diagnostic methods and identification of renal tumors was made during the embolization. Today, vascular embolization procedures are becoming widely used in the treatment of persistent bleeding, vascular defects and cancer.

In urology RAE is well established in the treatment of bleeding observed after jatrogennie complications of NSS (nephron sparing surgery), PCN (percutaneous nephrostomy), ESWL (extracorporeal shock wave lithotripsy), PCNL (percutaneous nephrolithotrypsy), closing arteriovenous fistulas and the need to rempve kidney in the case of severe nephrotic syndrome or secondary arterial hypertension [4, 7, 22].

Basic form of treatment of locoregional RC is surgical resection of kidney containing the tumor (optionally with adrenal gland and extraperitoneal lymph nodules). Recently it is adviced to introduce new, less invasive surgical techniques (laparoscopy and use of robots), as well as NSS (nephron sparing surgery). These techniques are used mostly in less advanced RC (T1) [25, 28, 29, 30].

In the strategy of treatment of more advanced RC frequently there is adviced application of RAE [2,3]. RAE is a procedure based on introduction, with use of an angiographic catheter,

INTECH
open science | open minds

© 2013 Zielinski et al.; licensee InTech. This is a paper distributed under the terms of the Creative Commons Attribution License (http://creativecommons.org/licenses/by/3.0), which permits unrestricted use, distribution, and reproduction in any medium, provided the original work is properly cited.

into blood vessel an obstruction material aimed to interrupt blood supply to an organ or to its particular region. At present different coils, haemostatic spongues, cyanoacrylic glues and alcohols are applied as materials for RAE [2, 11, 19]. This leads to acute necrosis of tissues where blood flow has been amputeed, which in turn results in development of acute phase reaction in the organism.

RAE is applied in treatment of RC for about 40 years [3]. It may be evoked prior to surgery, considered as a technique succouring the surgery, or used as palliative embolization in large, inoperable RC, mostly with intensive bleedings and/or pains. RAE which preceedes nephrectomy provides better conditions for the surgery and allows to shorten time of the intervention [1,4]. There exist informations that RAE may lead to stabilization and/or regression of distal metastases. These effects may be due to immunomodulating effects of RAE suggested by some authors [1,5]. However, knowledge on influence of RAE on immune status and response of immunocompetent cells is still scarce and fragmentaric. Systematic studies of this issue are needed.

In view of multiple limitations in efficacy and safety of RAE the present indications for application of this procedure include mostly [6, 7, 18]:

- Palliative RAE in advanced RC which results in relief of life-treatening haematuria and lumbar pains;
- Embolization of large, highly vascularized neoplasms prior to surgery (effective RAE results in contraction of vascular collaterals, facilitates dissection of the tumour, and allows to change the sequence of affixing renal vascular pedicle, ie first artery and the renal vein later);
- Embolization of highly vascularized RC metastases (e.g. vertebral metastases).

Opinions on the role of preoperative RAE in the management of patients with RC are controversial. Although a significant number of studies on RAE are reported in RC patients, there is no consensus on the benefits and morbidity associated with the procedure [7, 22]. Moreover, many large studies on the use of RAE both prior to nephrectomy and in advanced RC were conducted in the 1980s, before the development of improved techniques and imaging. Most proponents of preoperative RAE report the facilitation of nephrectomy through decreased operative blood loss, ease of dissection secondary to the development of oedema in tissue planes, and decreased operative time [8,9]. For those patients with significant tumour thrombus there might be a beneficial effect of decreasing the size or extent of tumour thrombus before surgery [10]. Interestingly, there might also be an advantage in the form of immunomodulation, whereby RAE-induced tumour necrosis stimulates a tumour-specific response from the immune system of the host [11-13].

Own experience [1] includes 474 patients with RC of which 118 had RAE before nephrectomy. It was reported that RAE significantly prolonged survival time in T2 and T3 RC. Additionally, it was found preliminarly that RAE exerted immunotropic effects and enhanced immune status of the patients. This diminished risks of the surgery. Recently we continued these investigations and performed series of studies on response of immune system in patients with RC undergoing RAE [14]. We analyzed 50 patients with RC exceeding diameter of 7 cm (T≥2) and tested immune status of persons with less and more advanced RC. 30 patients underwent palliative RAE and assessment of immune status at different times after embolization. The complex assessment of immune status included large battery of microculture tests of peripheral blood mononuclear cells (PBMC), estimation of levels of certain cytokines and cytometric measurement of lymphocyte subpopulations in peripheral blood. It was found that RAE lowers the suppressive action of neoplastic cells on the immune system, results in normalization of disordered proportion of lymphocyte subpopulations (CD4, CD8) and enhances the antiinflamatory response (increases levels of certain cytokines- IL-10 and IL-1ra). All together, the result reveal stimulation of certain functions of immunocompetent cells isolated from blood of RAE-treated RC patients. Clinical relevance of these findings and concluding whether or not RAE improved immune status of patients needs further studies.

2. Techniques of renal artery embolization

The initial indications developed in the 1970s for RAE were limited to symptomatic haematuria and palliation for metastatic renal cancer [2,3]. With technical advances and growing experience the indications have broadened to include conditions such as vascular malformations, medical renal disease, angiomyolipomas (AMLs), and preoperative infarction. The introduction of smaller delivery catheters and more precise embolic agents has drastically improved the morbidity associated with this technique [4]. RAE has continued to gain popularity as a minimally invasive approach for various urological conditions.

The technique of embolising hypervascular renal carcinomas dates back to 1969 when first reported by Lalli et al [2]. Since then, various techniques and embolic materials have been described. RAE has been used pre-operatively to facilitate nephrectomy [8], or to stimulate a possible systemic response in patients with metastases [5]. Renal embolisation has been established as a palliative treatment for unresectable renal carcinoma and in patients with less advanced disease (stage I–III) who, for whatever reason, are unsuitable or unwilling to undergo surgery [18, 22, 24]. In this group of patients the technique reduces tumour bulk and relieves local symptoms such as pain or intractable haematuria.

However, opinions on the role of preoperative RAE in the management of patients with RC are controversial. Although a significant number of studies on RAE are reported in these patients, there is no consensus on the benefits and morbidity associated with the procedure [7-9].

Effective embolization induces acute ischemic necrosis zone to form infarct of the organ tissues, which results in the onset of symptoms called postembolization syndrome, which usually occurs within the first few days after RAE [8]. Greater risk of developing the postembolization syndrome occurs in patients with small tumors, developing peripherally, when still remains a large part of the normal, not embolized part of the kidney [9]. The side effects which occur after RAE include: pain in the lumbar region, nausea and vomiting, hyperthermia, and fluctuations of blood pressure. These symptoms are usually temporary and transient, and their severity depends on the extent of ischemia in the kidney area. In a small percentage RAE may also lead to serious complications that are associated primarily with the movement (migration) or embolic material backflow [12, 22]. The consequence of this may be embolization of contralateral artery, mesenteric arteries, arteries of the lower limbs, and ischemic spinal cord injury. The risk of serious complications is low, if RAE is performed well and professionally. In our clinic material including hundreds of treatments was observed and serious complications developed, except of various symptoms of postembolization syndrome [1].

If there is a real benefit to be gained, most proponents of preoperative RAE cite the facilitation of nephrectomy through decreased operative blood loss, ease of dissection secondary to the development of oedema in tissue planes, and decreased operative time [10, 11, 26]. For those patients with significant tumour thrombus there might be a beneficial effect of decreasing the size or extent of tumour thrombus before surgery [12]. Interestingly, there might also be an advantage in the form of immunomodulation, whereby RAE-induced tumour necrosis stimulates a tumour-specific response [1,5,13]. It is likely that RAE is underutilized, perhaps because of a lack of prospective randomized studies demonstrating these potential benefits.

In our Departament of Clinical Urology the treatment of REA is performed under local anesthesia wit 1% xylocaine after puncturing the femoral artery under fluoroscopic control [1,14]. Vascular catheter is inserted into the abdominal aorta (Seldinger method). Aortonephrography is performed as the first step of the procedure (Fig.1 - A). This is followed by selective catheterisation of renal arteries and contrast agent (usually Omnipac) is applied using an automatic syringe (Fig. 1 - B). Image of arterial and venous intermediate is obtained with angiographic confirmation of following RC characteristics:

- Increased flow through the renal artery and the resulting expansion of the arteries,
- Presence of pathological vascularization in arterial phase (numerous, tortuous vessels with impaired angioarchitectonics)
- Nephrograms with the image of tumorous discoloration occuring due to retention of contrast in blood vessels,
- Loss of saturable renal parenchyma.

This is followed by injecting the embolizing material through a vascular catheter. Most frequently used is Spongostan which is fragmented and placed at the end of a syringe filled with 0.9% NaCl, and then injected into renal artery. Spongostan embolization often supplemented with different coils. In case of confirmation in renal arteriography of tumor vascularization by more than one artery, respectively all the supplying vessels are embolized, as above.

The whole procedure of RAE (Fig. 1 A – D) lasts about 30 – 60 minutes and its effectiveness (lack of blood flow in renal vessels) is confirmed in angiography after re-injection of contrast medium through the catheter withdrawn to the aorta.

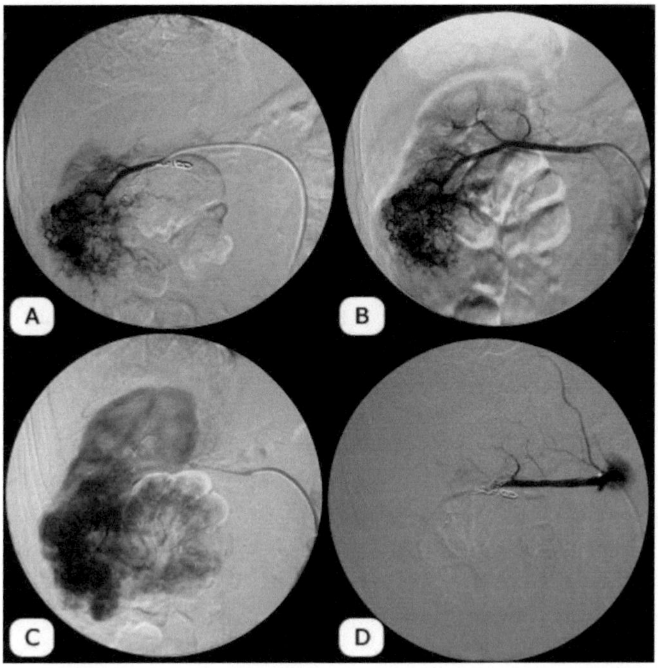

Figure 1. Stages of vascular embolization of renal artery. A. arteriography; B. vascularization of renal tumour; C. material for embolization injected to renal artery; D. closed renal artery.

After completing the RAE procedure the femoral artery puncture site is deemed temporary with pressure dressing. Few hours after RAE standard blood tests, monitoring of urine output and assessment of severity of postembolization symptoms (lumbar pain - a symptom that occurs in nearly all patients after effective RAE, nausea, vomiting, fever, transient renal failure and symptoms of gastrointestinal paralytic ileus). Medication (analgesic, antispasmodic, prokinetic agents, anticoagulants drugs and antibiotics) are prescribed appropriately to symptoms and depending on the clinical situation. In the study group of 474 patients there were no clinically significant complications (death, femoral hematoma, migration of embolizing material or ischemic spinal cord injury) [1,14].

Time schedules of RAE and nephrectomy are not established precisely, usually RAE is made few – several days before nephrectomy. In some cases RAE is made one only day before surgery to avoid acute postembolization syndrome.

3. Survival of renal cancer patients treated with renal artery embolization

Up to 30% of patients diagnosed with RC have metastatic disease at presentation [27]. Despite its sometimes favourable course, patients with metastatic RC generally die within 2 years of diagnosis. DeKernion et al [20] found that cumulative survival in 86 patients with metastatic RCC was 53% at 6 months, 43% at 1 year, 26% at 2 years and 13% at 5 years. The treatment of patients with metastatic RC has not improved over the years and continues to pose a problem for clinicians. Surgery is not curative in this group; however, recent advances in immunotherapy have rekindled interest in cytoreductive nephrectomy. A combined analysis [21] of two prospective randomized trials, [15, 16], found a small survival advantage (5.8 months) in patients who underwent nephrectomy followed by interferon-alpha based immunotherapy compared with immunotherapy alone. This survival benefit relates to patients with a good performance status whose primary tumour has been assessed to be surgically operable and who are good candidates for subsequent immunotherapy. Unfortunately, many elderly patients with disseminated RC do not fit these criteria and have significant comorbidity. Radical nephrectomy may cause significant morbidity post-surgery, particularly in elderly patients, and in some cases precludes the use of systemic therapy. It is in this situation that renal artery embolisation appears to have a role.

Previous studies had reported that delayed nephrectomy following embolisation of RC may be of clinical benefit to high risk patients with reduction in the size and vascularity of the primary tumour prior to surgery [9]. Subsequent studies have, however, found no survival benefit for patients with metastatic disease undergoing embolisation and nephrectomy [23]. The survey also indicated that a significant proportion of respondents (35%) still believed that the technique had a role in palliation of haematuria or pain in unfit or inoperable cases, or as the sole treatment modality in patients with metastatic disease.

Park et al [19] investigated the effectiveness of RAE with a mixture of ethanol and lipiodol in 27 patients with unresectable RC. 10 of the patients had stage III disease with 15 of the 27 patients having stage IV disease. Overall the median survival of the 27 patients was 8.5 months. The median survival was 23 months in the 10 patients with stage III disease and 7 months in 15 patients with stage IV disease. A similar study by Onishi et al [24] compared two groups of patients with unresectable RC with stage IV disease. 24 patients underwent renal embolisation with ethanol while 30 patients did not have any intervention. The median survival for the renal embolisation group was 229 days and for the control group 116 days. Those undergoing renal embolisation had a significantly better prognosis than those who did not (p=0.019). Other authors [18, 25, 26] have reported median survival times for patients treated with renal embolisation ranging from 4 months to 8.4 months. This equates to a 1 year survival rate of 36.8% and a 2 year survival rate of 15.8%. Ridley et al. [28] support the view that embolisation is not a curative treatment and probably only minimally alters the natural course of the disease, but it gives palliation of local symptoms related to advanced renal malignancy and is a safe alternative to radical nephrectomy, with low morbidity and complication rate and shorter hospital stay.

In own studies [1] a series of 474 patients with RC, who had radical nephrectomy during a period of 15 years, was studied to assess the prognostic significance of various pathologic parameters (tumor stage [pT], lymph node status, metastasis, tumor grade, venous involvement) and value of preoperative RAE. There were: 20 (4%) pT1, 204 (43%) pT2, 245 (52%) pT3, and 5 (1%) pT4 patients. All 474 patients underwent nephrectomy including a group of 118 (25%) patients (24 pT2, 90 pT3, and 4 pT4) who underwent preoperative embolization of the renal artery. To compare treatment outcomes in embolized patients with RC, a group of 116 (24%) nonembolized patients with RC was selected. This group was matched for sex, age, stage, tumor size, and tumor grade, with the embolized patients ($p < 0.01$). All important prognostic factors were studied as to their influence on survival by the treatment group. The overall 5- and 10-year survival was 62% and 47%, respectively (Figure 2). The 5- and 10-year survival rates were significantly better ($p < 0.01$) for patients with pT2 than for those with pT3 tumors (79% vs. 50% and 59% vs. 35%, respectively) (Figure 2). Involvement of regional lymph nodes (N+) was an important prognostic factor for survival in patients with pT3 tumors. The 5-year survival for pT3 N+ was 39%, compared with 66% in those with pT3N0 ($p < 0.01$). Preoperative embolization was also an important factor influencing survival (Figure 3).

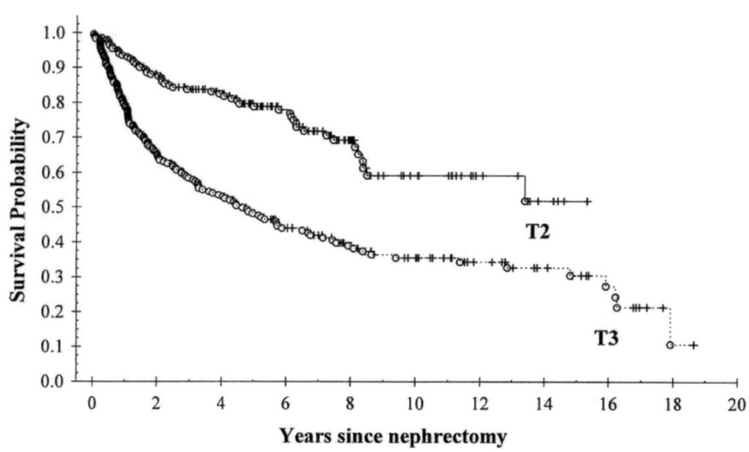

Figure 2. Estimated probability of survival from all causes of death by pathologic stage, pT2 vs. pT3. Open circles represent death of a patient. Tick marks represent a patient who was alive at last follow-up.

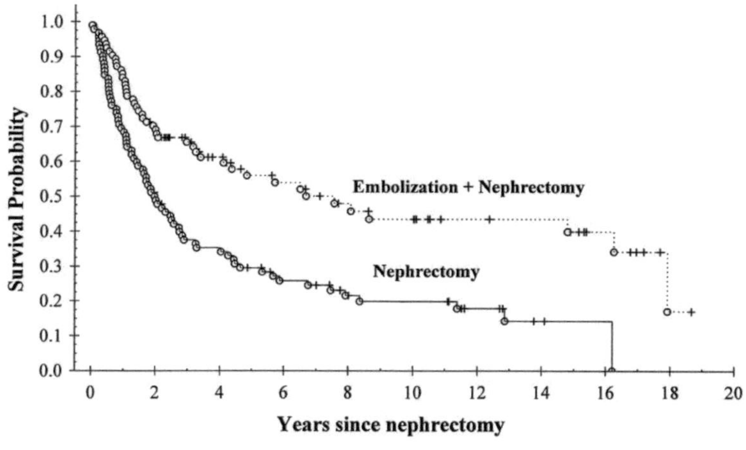

Figure 3. Estimated probability of survival in the 118 patients treated with preoperative embolization as compared to the 116 patients in radical nephrectomy alone group (matched patients).

The overall 5- and 10-year survival for 118 patients embolized before nephrectomy was 62% and 47%, respectively, and it was 35% and 23%, respectively, for the matched group of 116 patients treated with surgery alone ($p = 0.01$). The most important finding of this study was an apparent importance of preoperative embolization in improving patients' survival. This finding needs to be interpreted with caution and confirmed in a prospective randomized trial.

In conclusion, the available data suggest that RAE is a convenient, relatively tolerable management option in patients with unresectable renal tumours and in patients unfit or unwilling to undergo surgery as a means of palliation of local symptoms and improving clinical status. We believe there is also a role for this procedure in asymptomatic patients who have potentially resectable disease who are unfit or unwilling to undergo surgery, and in asymptomatic patients with inoperable metastatic disease.

4. Reaction of immune system to renal artery embolization

RC, with the tumor growth, and then the spread of tumor tissue beyond the original location, begins to affect the activity of the immune system [14]. Nakano et al [5] indicate the importance of cell proliferation inhibitory factor present in the serum of patients with RC. Lymphocytes in RC patients without any therapy, stimulated in vitro with PHA (phytohemagglutinin) in the presence of own serum responded very weakly to this mitogen. After RAE the impact of this inhibiting factor enhanced and proliferation of PHA-stimulated lymphocyte was still lowered [5]. Nephrectomy in patients not treated with RAE before surgery did not influence the ability of cells to stimulation by PHA. In contrary, patients who had RAE prior to nephrectomy the proliferation inhibitory factor quickly disappeared and proliferative response to PHA was normal already 2 months after surgery [5]. Catalona et al [34] reported that cell response to Con A (concanavalin A) is impaired in case of urological cancers, including RC, and the cells have a high immuno-suppressor activity. The abolition of the high suppressor activity may be necessary for effective treatment of RC [34]. Osada et al [35] in their study of 50 patients with RC confirmed a significant increase of helper and cytotoxic NK lymphocytes 10-12 months after RAE. This was very impressive, when compared to lowered values of these cells prior to RAE, suggesting that RAE enhanced the immune status [35]. Similar results were obtained by Bakke et al [13], who conducted a study of NK cell activity in patients with RC after RAE. Blood samples of 30 patients were taken before RAE and 24, 48, 72 and 96 hours after surgery. Surgery was performed to remove the kidney from 5 to 7 days after RAE. RAE resulted in increase in NK cells, with peak values observed after 48 hours [13]. RAE in patients with RC is performed in presence of potential existence of immune deficiency caused by cancer itself. Therefore, in this case, the immune responses (still poorly understood and inconsistent) observed at different times after embolization (usually few-several days after RAE) will be the result of the two, often different operating mechanisms: 1. response to ischemia and tissue necrosis and inflammation in the area of embolization of a probable stimulation of the macrophage-monocyte system; 2. release from tumor tissues of various factors affecting the immune system, at least some of which appear to have an immunosuppressive effect. The main task of the immune system is to maintain homeostasis. The basic unit, often defined as "immune orchestra conductor" is thymus-dependent T lymphocyte, which, based on the phenomenon of restriction major histocompatibility complex I and II expresses the phenomenon of violence against its own unnormal or changed antigens, and the phenomenon of tolerance to its own antigens [32, 33]. Embolization may lead to stimulation of the immune system in the following mechanism: close off blood supply to the tumor leads to necrosis which gives a chance to enhance antigenicity of cancer cells and evoke the potential amplification of the immune system [14]. This leads in turn to destruction of tumor tissue by infiltration with cytolytic immunocompetent cells.

Recent studies in patients with metastatic RC have shown a small survival advantage in patients undergoing radical nephrectomy followed by immunotherapy; however, these studies are biased towards patients with good performance status aqccording to ECOG (Eastern Cooperative Oncology Group) scale status 0 or status 1. This small survival benefit should also be viewed in light of the morbidity and mortality associated with a large surgical procedure. The increased morbidity associated with radical nephrectomy may preclude or delay the administration of systemic immunotherapy, which has demonstrated reproducible response rates of 10–20% [15].

In two randomized trials with identical design, patients who underwent nephrectomy followed by interferon alpha (IFN-α) therapy had improved survival (median 13.6 months) compared with those treated with IFN-α alone (median 7.8 months) [15, 16]. The antivascular endothelial growth factor (VEGF) antibody; the multityrosine kinase inhibitors, sorafenib, sunitinib, and pazopanib; and the mammalian target of rapamycin (mTOR) inhibitors, temsirolimus and everolimus, have become the mainstay of therapy for the vast majority of patients with metastatic renal cell carcinoma (mRCC). Large randomized controlled clinical trials have shown improved progression-free survival with these agents and improved survival in selected populations, but the majority of these study patients had prior nephrectomy and good performance status [16, 17, 20, 21].

In own studies [14] we examined functional status of immunocompetent cells isolated from peripheral blood of patients with advanced RC treated with RAE. Blood samples were collected by vein puncture and peripheral blood mononuclear cells (PBMC) were isolated on Ficol-Paque gradient, and after determination of cell viability (usually no less than 80% viable cells), the microcultures were set up in triplicates (10^5 cells/0.2 ml RPMI + 15% autologous inactivated serum) in Nuncoln microplates. Respective triplicates were left without stimulation or stimulated with phytohemagglutinin (PHA, HA16, Murex Biotech Ltd Dartford U.K., 0.4 μg/cult.) or with concanavalin A (Con A, Sigma, 8 μg/cult.). The plates were placed inside the anechoic chamber in the ASSAB incubator at 37° C and 5% CO_2. An identical plate of control cultures was also set up and placed in the ASSAB incubator beyond the chamber. At 24h of incubation, rearrangements of the cultures were performed as described elsewhere [32,33].

As a result of rearrangements of cultures performed at 24 h, the following parameters of T cell and monocyte activities were measured at the end of cultures: T lymphocyte response to PHA and to Con A, saturation of IL-2 receptors, T cell suppressive activity (SAT index), and the index of monocyte immunogenic activity (LM) related to the ratio of produced monokines (IL-1β versus IL-1ra) [32]. For the last 18h of incubation, 3H-thymidine (3HTdR, Amersham, U.K., spec act. 5Ci/mM) was added into the cultures in a dose of 0.4 μCi/cult.

At 72h the cultures were harvested and incorporation of 3HTdR was measured in Packard Tri carb 2100 TR scintillation counter. The results were calculated as a mean value of dpm (desintegrations per minute) per triplicate of cultures ± SD. The experiments were repeated 10 times, and the results observed in the exposed cultures were compared with those obtained in the control cultures. The data were analyzed with STATGRAPHICS PLUS 6.0 version. The differences between the mean values were assumed statistically significant if the p values, calculated withthe use of U Mann-Whitney's test, were lower than 0.05.

The results obtained in this study are summarized in Table 1 and described in detail elsewhere [14].

In the analysis of 50 patients with RC treated with RAE, we selected 30 patients where RAE was the only form of treatment. In this group of patients the immune response was studied at different times after the palliative RAE (output test, the test after 2-6 weeks and at 12 weeks after RAE) successive assessment of significant differences in the magnitude and direction of change of parameters characterizing the efficiency of the immune system. It was found that RAE performed in patients with advanced RC exerts immunomodulatory effect on the immune response manifested by the increase of the proliferative response to PHA and the percentage of CD4 + cells, and significant increase in the value of saturation of the receptors, IL-2, a cytokine with protrophic properties (Table 1). After RAE significant increase was observed in inflammatory response manifested by the increase of T regulatory cells, which can be a potential source of IL-10, cytokine inhibition of the function of the inflammatory response (Table 1).

It was found that RAE lowers the suppressive action of neoplastic cells on the immune system, results in normalization of disordered proportion of lymphocyte subpopulations (CD4, CD8) and enhances the antiinflamatory response (increases levels of certain cytokines- IL-10 and IL-1ra). All together, the result reveal stimulation of certain functions of immunocompetent cells isolated from blood of RAE-treated RC patients. Clinical relevance of these findings and concluding whether or not RAE improved immune status of patients needs further studies [1, 14].

The changes in the immune system may, however be heterogeneous and multidirectional and individually changebale. This would indicate that the systemic inflammatory response is not only associated with the release of cytokines from a kidney tumor, and it rather results from the defective immune response in patients with advanced cancer [14].

http://dx.doi.org/10.5772/54116

Investigated parameter	RAE-treated RC patients (T 3 and 4) N=30
PHA	Lowering after 2-6 weeks * Increase after 12 weeks
ConA	Lowering after 2-6 weeks * Lowering after 12 weeks
IL-2	Lowering after 2-6 weeks Increase after 12 weeks
LM	No significant differences after 2-6 weeks Lowering after 12 weeks
SAT	Increase after 2-6 weeks No significant differences after 12 weeks
$CD3^+$	Increase after 2-6 weks No significant differences after 12 weeks
$CD4^+$	Increase after 2-6 weeks Increase after 12 weeks
$CD8^+$	Lowering after 2-6 weeks * Lowering after 12 weeks
$CD4^+/CD25^{high}$	Increase after 2-6 weeks Increase after 12 weeks
NK	No significant differences after 2-6 weeks No significant differences after 12 weeks
IL-1β	Increase after 2-6 weeks Lowering after 12 weeks
IL-6	Increase after 2-6 weeks Lowering after 12 weeks
TGF-β	Lowering after 2-6 weeks * Increase after 12 weeks
IL-1ra	Lowering after 2-6 weeks * Increase after 12 weeks
IL-10	Lowering after 2-6 weeks * Increase after 12 weeks

Table 1. Summary of changes in investigated functional parameters of immune system in a group of 30 patients with advanced RC treated with RAE ($p<0.05$).

5. Summary and conclusions

In summary, the present authors conclude that patients with advanced RC benefit from RAE with longer survival. RAE applied prior to nephrectomy facilitates surgery and additionally prolongs survival. Additionally, RAE appears to be a potent immunostimulatory agent. It is our strong feeling that in specialistic urologic centers RAE is a safe procedure which succours the complex therapeutic process in patients with RC.

Author details

H. Zielinski[1], T. Syrylo[1*] and S. Szmigielski[2]

*Address all correspondence to: tsyrylo@wp.pl

1 Department of Clinical Urology, Military Institute of Medicine, Warsaw, Poland

2 Military Institute of Hygiene and Epidemiology, Warsaw, Poland

References

[1] Zielinski H, Szmigielski S, Petrovich Z. Comparison of preoperative embolization followed by radical nephrectomy with radical nephrectomy alone for renal cell carcinoma. *Am J Clin Oncol* 2000; 23: 6–12

[2] Lalli AF, Peterson N, Bookstein JJ. Roentgen-guided infarctions of kidney and lungs: a potential therapeutic technique. *Radiology* 1969;93:434–5.

[3] Almgard LE, Fernström I, Haverling M, Ljungqvist A. Treatment of renal adenocarcinoma by embolic occlusion of the renal circulation. *Br J Urol* 1973; 45: 474-9

[4] Kadir S, Marshall FF, White RI Jr, Kaufman SL, Barth KH. Therapeutic embolization of the kidney with detachable silicone balloons. *J Urol* 1983; 129: 11–3

[5] Nakano H, Nihira H, Toge T. Treatment of renal cancer patients by transcatheter embolization and its effects on lymphocyte proliferative responses. *J Urol* 1983; 130: 24–7

[6] Keller FS. Interventional radiology: new paradigms for the new millennium. *J Vasc Interv Radiol* 2000; 11: 677–81

[7] Teasdale C, Kirk D, Jeans WD, Penry JB, Tribe CT, Slade N. Arterial embolization in renal carcinoma: a useful procedure? *Br J Urol* 1982; 54: 616–9

[8] Kaisary AV, Williams G, Riddle PR. The role of preoperative embolization in renal cell carcinoma. *J Urol* 1984; 131: 641–6

[9] Christensen K, Dyreborg U, Andersen JF, Nissen HM. The value of transvascular embolization in the treatment of renal carcinoma. *J Urol* 1985; 133: 191–3

[10] Bakal CW, Cynamon J, Lakritz PS, Sprayregen S. Value of preoperative renal artery embolization in reducing blood transfusion requirements during nephrectomy for renal cell carcinoma. *J Vasc Interv Radiol* 1993; 4: 727–31

[11] Klimberg I, Hunter P, Hawkins IF, Drylie DM, Wajsman Z. Preoperative angioinfarction of localized renal cell carcinoma using absolute ethanol. *J Urol* 1985; 133: 21–4

[12] Blute ML, Leibovich BC, Lohse CM, Cheville JC, Zincke H. The Mayo Clinic experience with surgical management, complications and outcome for patients with renal cell carcinoma and venous tumour thrombus. *BJU Int* 2004; 94: 33–41

[13] Bakke A, Gothlin JH, Haukaas SA, Kalland T. Augmentation of natural killer cell activity after arterial embolization of renal carcinomas. *Cancer Res* 1982; 42: 3880–3

[14] Syrylo T. Influence of renal artery embolization on efficacy of immune system in patients with renal cancer [In Polish]. D.M.Sc. thesis. Military Institute of Medicine, Warsaw, Poland, 2012; 1 – 90.

[15] Mickisch GH, Garin A, van Poppel H, de Prijck L, Sylvester R. European Organisation for Research and Treatment of Cancer (EORTC). Radical nephrectomy plus interferon-alfa-based immunotherapy compared with interferon alfa alone in metastatic renal cell carcinoma: a randomized trial. *Lancet* 2001;358:966–70.

[16] Flanigan RC, Salmon SE, Blumenstein BA, Bearman SI, Roy V, McGrath PC, et al. Nephrectomy followed by interferon alfa-2b compared with interferon alfa-2b alone for metastatic renal cell cancer. *N Engl J Med* 2001;345:1655–9.

[17] Motzer RJ, Russo P. Systemic therapy for renal cell carcinoma. J Urol 2000;163:408–17.

[18] Nurmi M, Satokari K, Puntala P. Renal artery embolization in the palliative treatment of renal adencarcinoma. *Scand J Urol Nephrol* 1987;21:93–6.

[19] Park JH, Kim SH, Han JK, Chung JW, Han MC. Transcatheter arterial embolization of unresectable renal cell carcinoma with a mixture of ethanol and iodised oil. *Cardiovasc Intervent Radiol* 1994;17:323–7.

[20] deKernion JB, Ramming KP, Smith RB. The natural history of metastatic renal cell carcinoma: a computer analysis. *J Urol* 1978;120:148–52.

[21] Flanigan RC, Mickisch G, Sylvester R, Tangan C, van Poppel H, Crawford ED. Cytoreductive nephrectomy in patients with metastatic renal cancer: A combined analysis. *J Urol* 2004;171:1071–6.

[22] Lanigan D, Jurriaans E, Hammonds JC, Wells IP, Choa RG. The current status of embolization in renal cell carcinoma – a survey of local and national practice. *Clin Radiol* 1992;46:176–8.

[23] Flanigan RC. The failure of infarction and/or nephrectomy in stage IV renal cell cancer to influence survival or metastatic regression. *Urol Clin North Am* 1987;14:757–62.

[24] Onishi T, Oishi Y, Suzuki Y, Asano K. Prognostic evaluation of transcatheter arterial embolization for unresectable renal cell carcinoma with distant metastases. *BJU Int* 2001;87:312–5.

[25] Tigrani VS, Reese DM, Small EJ, Presti JC, Carroll PR. Potential role of nephrectomy in the treatment of metastatic renal cell carcinoma: A retrospective analysis. *Urology* 2000;55:36–40.

[26] Bono AV, Caresano A. The role of embolization in the treatment of kidney carcinoma. *Eur Urol* 1983;9:334–7.

[27] Parker S, Tong T, Bolden S, Wingo PA. Cancer statistics, 1996. *Cancer J Clin* 1996;46:5–27.

[28] Ridley SL, Culp SH, Jonascg F et al. Outcome of patients with metastatic renal cell carcinoma treated with targeted therapy without cytoreductive nephrectomy. *Ann Oncol* 2011; 22: 1048-53

[29] Mahnken AH, Rohde D, Brkovic D, Gunther RW, Tacke JA. Percutaneous radiofrequency ablation of renal cell carcinoma – preliminary results. *Acta Radiol* 2005;46:208–14.

[30] Marberger M, Schatzl G, Cranston D, Kennedy JE. Extracorporeal ablation of renal tumours with high-intensity focused ultrasound. *BJU Int* 2005;95(Suppl. 2):52–5.

[31] Stenzel A, deKernion JB. Pathology, biology, and clinical staging of renal cell carcinoma. *Sem Oncol (Suppl.)* 1989;16:3–11.

[32] Dąbrowski MP, Stankiewicz W, Płusa T, Chciałowski A, Szmigielski S. Competition of IL-1 and IL-1 ra determines lymphocyte response to delayed stimulation with PHA. *Mediators of Inflammation*. 2001; 10, 101-7.

[33] Dąbrowski MP, Stankiewicz W. Desirable and undesirable immunotropic effects of antibiotics: immunomodulating properties of cefaclor. *J Chemotherapy*, 2001, 13, 1-6.

[34] Catalona WJ, Ratliff TL, McCool RE. Concanavalin A-activated suppressor cell activity in peripheral blood lymphocytes of urologic cancer patients. *J Natl Cancer Inst.* 1980; 65: 553-7.

[35] Osada J, Pietruczuk M, Dabrowska M, Kordecki K, Janica J, Walecki J. An assessment of lymphocytic population in peripheral blood of patients with renal cell carcinoma before and after embolization [In Polish]. *Rocz Akad Med* Bialystok. 2000; 45: 228-39.

Chapter 7

Paraneoplastic Glomerulopathy Associated with Renal Cell Carcinoma

Akihiro Tojo

Additional information is available at the end of the chapter

http://dx.doi.org/10.5772/53534

1. Introduction

Renal cell carcinoma is often associated with paraneoplastic syndromes caused by the secretion of tumor cell products such as hormones, cytokines, growth factors and tumor antigens, which show manifestations including impaired glucose metabolism, hypercalcemia, hypertension, Cushing syndrome, polycythemia, thrombosis, eosinophilia, leukemoid reactions and amyloidosis [1]. It has been reported that 10-40% of patients with renal cell carcinoma present paraneoplastic symptoms [1]. However, paraneoplastic glomerulonephritis associated with renal cell carcinoma has often been overlooked, for the urinary abnormalities including proteinuria and hematuria are often interpreted as clinical manifestations of the tumor itself, especially when the proteinuria is non-nephrotic.

The term of paraneoplastic glomerulopathy was first described by Galloway in 1922 in a case of nephrotic syndrome associated with Hodgkin's disease [2]. Hodgkin's lymphoma is associated with minimal change nephrotic syndrome, while solid carcinomas including lung cancer and carcinomas of the gastrointestinal tract frequently develop membranous nephropathy, which is the most common paraneoplastic glomerulopathy [3,4]. Although renal cell carcinoma is not a frequent cause of paraneoplastic glomerulopathy, recent advances in the study of the molecular mechanism of renal cell carcinoma as a cytokine producing tumor have promoted a better understanding of the mechanism of paraneoplastic nephropathy associated with renal cell carcinoma. In this chapter, I will discuss the mechanisms of paraneoplastic nephropathies associated with renal cell carcinoma.

INTECH
open science | open minds

© 2013 Tojo; licensee InTech. This is a paper distributed under the terms of the Creative Commons Attribution License (http://creativecommons.org/licenses/by/3.0), which permits unrestricted use, distribution, and reproduction in any medium, provided the original work is properly cited.

1.1. Pathological types of renal cell carcinoma and molecular mechanisms of paraneoplastic syndrome

Renal cell carcinoma accounts for 85 % of renal neoplasms, and 25% of patients with renal cell carcinoma show advanced disease with local invasion or metastasis at the time of diagnosis [5]. Renal cell carcinoma is classified pathologically into five types: clear cell (75%), papillary (12%), chromophobe (4%), oncocytoma (4%), collecting duct carcinoma (<1%), and unclassified (3-5%) [5]. The most common type, clear cell renal cell carcinoma, shows hypervascularity. About 60% of sporadic clear cell renal cell carcinoma have mutations in the von Hippel-Lindau tumor suppressor gene (*VHL*) [6], which is a causative gene for von Hippel-Lindau disease, an autosomal dominant familial cancer syndrome consisting retinal angioma, hemangioblastoma of the central nervous system, pheochromocytomas, and clear cell renal cell carcinoma. VHL protein normally suppresses hypoxia-inducible genes by inhibiting HIF-1α [7] (Figure 1). However, when VHL protein is lost in clear cell renal cell carcinoma, various cytokines and growth factors induced by HIF-1α are enhanced; vascular endothelial growth factor (VEGF) which stimulates angiogenesis of carcinoma, platelet-derived growth factor (PDGF) and transforming growth factor alpha (TGF- α), which lead to tumor growth, glucose transporter (GLUT-1) and carbonic anhydrase IX (CA IX), which leads to tumor cell survival in an acidic environment [8-10]. NF-kB activity is also regulated by VHL protein, and cytokine-inducible transcription factors including NF-kB and STAT3 are activated in renal cell carcinoma [11-15]. Renal cell carcinoma tissue and cell lines of the tumor express mRNA of IL-6 and IL-6 receptor [16, 17], which may play a role in cancer cell growth in an autocrine or paracrine manner.

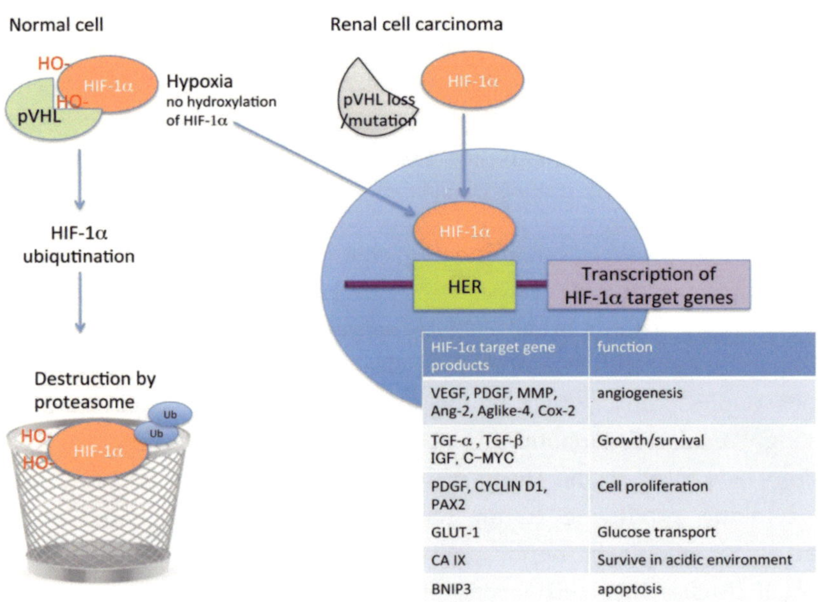

Figure 1. Molecular mechanisms of renal cell carcinoma as a cytokine-producing tumor.

The von Hippel-Lindau protein (pVHL) binds with hypoxia inducible factor 1α (HIF-1α) transcription factor and promotes the ubiqutination of HIF-1α, resulting in degradation by the proteasome under normoxic conditions. In renal cell carcinoma, the absence of wild type pVHL stimulates the accumulation of HIF-1α and activates transcription at hypoxia-response elements (HREs) in genes including vascular endothelial growth factor (VEGF), platelet-derived growth factor (PDGF), transforming growth factor α (TGF-α) and TGF-β, glucose transporter (GLUT-1) and carbonic anhydrase IX (CA IX).

MMP: matrix metalloproteinase; Ang-2: angiopoietin-2; Aglike-4: angiopoietin-like 4; COX-2: cyclooxygenase-2; BNIP3: BCL2/adenovirus E1B 19 kD interacting protein 3; PAX2: paired box gene 2.

The serum levels of VEGF and IL-6 are increased according to the stage of renal cell carcinoma, whereas TNF-α and IL-1β showed a slight increase as they are probably produced by infiltrating monocytes or macrophages (Figure 2) [18,19]. This indicates that clear cell renal cell carcinoma is a cytokine-producing tumor, whose functions are linked to the development of the various features of the paraneoplastic syndrome [9,20].

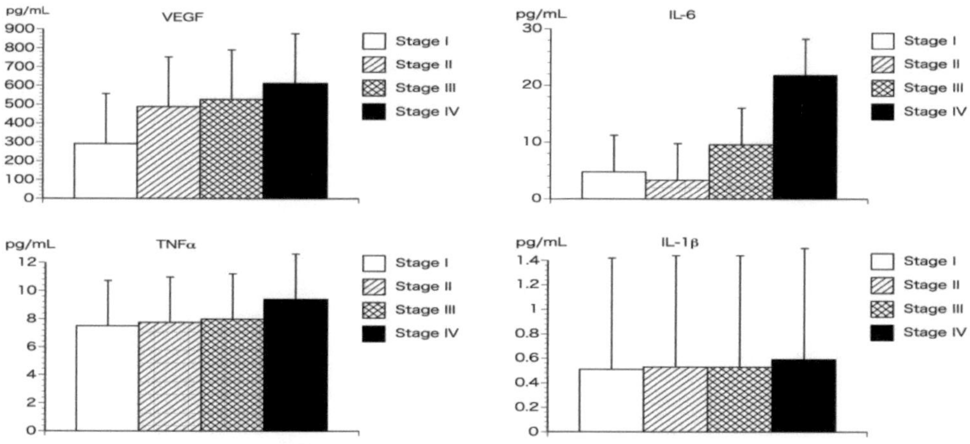

Figure 2. Serum vascular endothelial growth factor (VEGF), interleukin-6 (IL-6), tumor necrosis factor α (TNF-α) and interleukin-1β (IL-1β) in various stages of renal cell carcinoma. Adapted from [18] and [19].

2. Incidence of paraneoplastic syndrome and glomerulopathy in renal cell carcinoma

The most frequent features of the paraneoplastic syndrome in renal cell carcinoma are hypercalcemia, hypertension and polycythemia. Their prevalence and their causative hormones and cytokines are listed in Table1 [1].

Phenomenon	Prevalence %	Hormones and cytokines
Hypercalcemia	13-20%	Non-bone metastatic disease 50%, PTH, PTHrP, TGF-α, β, OAF, IL-1, TNF
Hypertension	40%	Renin
Polycythemia	1-8%	Erythropoietin
Nonmetastatic hepatic dysfunction (Stauffer's syndrome)	3-20%	Hepatotoxines, lysosomal enzymes stimulating hepatic cathepsins or phosphatases, IL-6
Constitutional syndrome (fever, weight loss, fatigue)	20-30%	TNF-α, IL-6. IL-1, prostaglandins
	6%	β-HCG
Cushing's syndrome	2%	ACTH
Abnormal glucose metabolism		Insulin, glucagon
Galactorrhea		Prolactin
Amyloidosis	3-8%	SAA protein
Neuromyopathies	rare	unknown
Nephropathy		
Vasculopathy		
Coagulopathy		

PTHrP: parathyroid hormone-related peptide, OAF: osteoclast activating factor, TNF: tumor necrosis factor, HCG: human chorionic gonadotropin, ACTH: adrenocorticotropin, SAA: serum amyloid A.

Table 1. Prevalence and features of paraneoplastic syndromes in renal cell carcinoma.

Paraneoplastic glomerulopathy is believed to be a rare manifestation of the paraneoplastic syndrome. However, immunohistochemical analysis of resected kidneys from 60 patients of renal cell carcinoma revealed 27% of them had immune complex nephropathy including 11 patients (18%) with IgA nephropathy and 5 patients (8%) with focal segmental glomerulosclerosis [21]. Another immunofluorescence study revealed a positive staining for C3, IgM, or IgA in the mesangial deposits in 35% (14/40) of patients with renal cell carcinoma versus 5.4% in the control subjects [22] (Table 2). Thus, the occurrence of glomerular diseases is not so rare in renal cell carcinoma.

	Prevalence %	Outcomes after resection of renal carcinoma	Reference
IgA nephropathy	11/60 (18%)	Remission 6, Azotemia 2	Magyarlaki [21]
FSGS	5/60 (8%)	Azotemia 3	
Diabetic nephropathy	3/60 (5%)	Nephrotic /Azotemia 2	
Nephrosclerosis	4/60 (7%)	Nephrotic /Azotemia 2	
Tubulointerstitial nephritis	16/60 (27)	-	
IgA/C3 deposition	1/40 (2.5%)	N.D.	Beaufils [22]
C3/IgM deposition	13/40 (33%)		
CEA deposition	2/9 (22%)		
HBs Ag/Ab deposition	6/29(21%)		

Table 2. Evaluation of glomerulopathy in resected kidneys of renal cell carcinoma patients.

3. Diagnosis and mechanism of paraneoplastic glomerulopathy associated with renal cell carcinoma

Recent development or worsening of diabetes mellitus, increased platelet or C-reactive protein (CRP), and hypercalcemia also suggests the existence of paraneoplastic syndrome. Glomerulonephritis is considered when urinalysis shows dysmorphic red blood cells and red blood cell casts, as hematuria caused by renal cell carcinoma usually shows isomorphic red blood cells. When proteinuria exceeds 1g per day, it is also better to speculate overlapping glomerulonephritis and examine serological tests including immunoglobulins (IgG, IgA, IgM), complements (CH50, C3, C4), anti-nuclear antibody, and anti-dsDNA antibody. A final diagnosis of glomerulonephritis can only be given by a renal biopsy. Renal cysts or masses identified by renal ultrasonography at the time of renal biopsy should be further investigated with CT and MRI. Renal cancer will progress rapidly after steroid therapy for glomerulonephritis.

The diagnosis of paraneoplastic glomerulopathy will be suggested following the criteria; 1) existence of a time relationship between the diagnosis of the glomerulopathy and cancer, 2) no obvious etiology for glomerular diseases, 3) clinical or histological remission of glomerulopathy after complete remission by surgical removal of carcinoma, 4) recurrence of the carcinoma associated with deterioration of glomerular diseases [3,23].

As mentioned above, inactivation of the *VHL* gene by frame-shift mutation is observed in about 60% of sporadic RCC [5]. Activated HIF-1α without VHL protein stimulates hypoxia-related proteins such as vascular endothelial growth factor (VEGF) and platelet-derived growth factor (PDGF), which lead to tumor growth and trigger angiogenesis (Figure 1) [8,10]. The increased VEGF accelerates glomerular permeability and causes proteinuria, and

PDGF and IL-6 stimulates mesangial cell proliferation, and TGF-β increases the mesangial matrix, contributing to the development of glomerulonephritis.

It is interesting that IgA nephropathy showed a higher prevalence than membranous nephropathy in renal cell carcinoma, whereas about 50% of glomerulopathies associated with gastrointestinal neoplasias and lung cancers were membranous nephropathy (Table 3). The mechanisms of paraneoplastic nephropathy may be different in renal cell carcinoma compared with gastrointestinal neoplasias and lung cancers. The paraneoplastic nephropathy of renal cell carcinoma may depend more upon overproduction of cytokines rather than cross-reaction with tumor antigen and production of autoantibodies.

	Renal cell carcinoma N=49	**Gastrointestinal neoplasia N=48**	**Lung cancer N=41**
Membranous nephropathy	10 (20%)	26 (54%)	20 (49%)
IgA nephropathy	15 (31%)	1 (2%)	2 (5%)
Minimal change disease	6 (12%)	9 (19%)	9 (22%)
Focal segmental glomerulonephritis	5 (10%)	2 (4%)	1 (2%)
Membranoproliferative glomerulonephritis	3 (6%)	2 (4%)	5 (12%)
Crescentic glomerulonephritis	10 (20%)	8 (17%)	4 (10%)

Table 3. Type of glomerulopathy in renal cell carcinoma compared with gastrointestinal neoplasia and lung cancer. Modified from [3].

4. Types of paraneoplastic nephropathy

4.1. IgA nephropathy and renal cell carcinoma

Although IgA nephropathy is more common in younger patients, when it occurs in patients older than 60 years, a high prevalence of malignancy (23%) is observed [24]. Solid tumors that invade mucosal tissue like the respiratory tract, the buccal cavity, and the nasopharynx increase circulating IgA levels and show deposition of IgA in the mesangium [24]. Several cases of IgA nephropathy associated with renal cell carcinoma have been reported previously [21,25-28]. In Figure 3, a 66 year-old male diagnosed IgA nephropathy with mesangial IgA deposition but weak C3 staining showed a rapid increase in renal cyst during steroid treatment, and a clear cell renal cell carcinoma was found in the resected kidney (Figure 3). The infiltrating plasma cells around the renal cell carcinoma produced IL-6 and IgA (Figure 3). Elevated levels of IL-6 have been reported in 18 (25%) of 71 patients with renal cell carcinoma [29], and IL-6 increased in more than 50% of patients with metastatic renal cell carcinoma, playing a role as a prognostic marker [19,20,30,31]. IL-6 stimulates IgA production

[32], thus, the elevated IL-6 in renal cell carcinoma may increase circulating IgA, which deposits in the mesangial area causing IgA nephropathy.

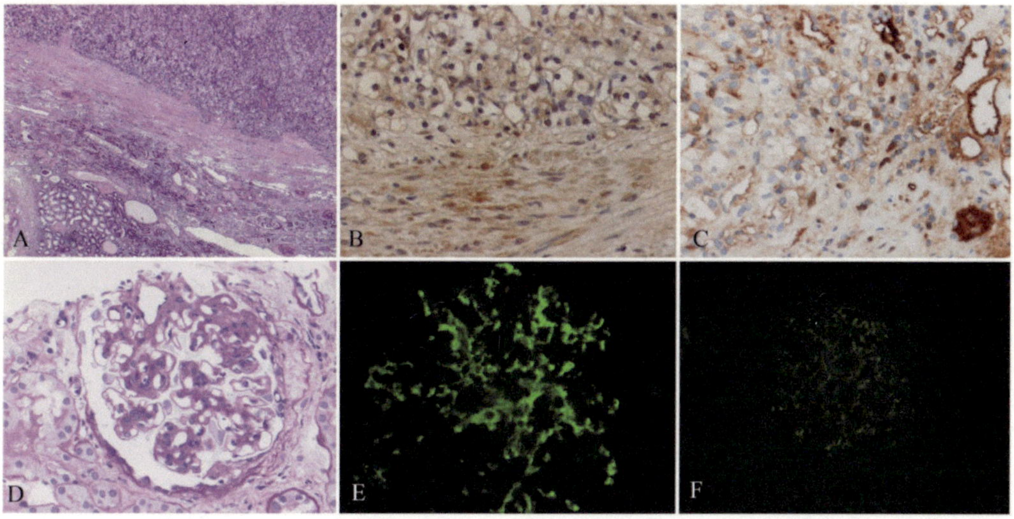

Figure 3. Clear cell renal cell carcinoma in association with IgA nephropathy. (A) PAS staining of clear cell carcinoma with a capsule. (B) immunostaining for IL-6 showing positive immunoreactivity in the infiltrating lymphocytes and plasma cells around the clear cell carcinoma and capsule. (C) IgA immunoreactivity positive in the plasma cells around renal cell carcinoma. (D) Renal biopsy sample showing segmental mesangial cell proliferation. (E) Immunofluorescence showed positive staining of IgA in the mesangial area, and weak staining of C3 (F).

4.2. Membranous nephropathy and renal cell carcinoma

The most frequent paraneoplastic glomerulopathy associated with solid tumors is membranous nephropathy and it is easy to detect because most of the cases manifest the nephrotic syndrome (paraneoplastic nephrotic syndrome) [3,23,33]. Since membranous nephropathy associated with malignancy has been attributed to tumor antigen-antibody immune complex formation, the cancer related antigens have been identified in immune complex in some cases including PSA in prostate cancer, CEA in gastrointestinal cancer [34]. Renal cell carcinoma has been reported to be associated with membranous nephropathy [35-43], but its prevalence is lower compared with gastrointestinal cancer and lung cancer (Table 3). As antibodies against phospholipase A2 receptor antibody have been identified in 70 % of patients with primary membranous nephropathy [44], a diagnosis of secondary membranous nephropathy should be considered when it is negative. IgG subclass immunofluorescence is useful to distinguish the primary membranous nephropathy in which IgG4 is stained predominately. In a case of secondary membranous nephropathy associated with renal cell carcinoma, showed predominantly IgG1 and IgG3 staining compared to IgG4 (Figure 4). The renal tubular epithelial antigen (RTE) has been identified in one case of renal cell carcinoma [45], but in most cases the tumor antigen-antibody complex were not identified in the serum and elutes of glomeruli in patients with membranous nephropathy associated with renal cell carcinoma [35,40].

Even though tumor antigen-antibodies have not been identified yet, renal tumors may have some contribution to the pathogenesis of membranous nephropathy because nephrotic syndrome is transiently ameliorated after tumor excision [40-43].

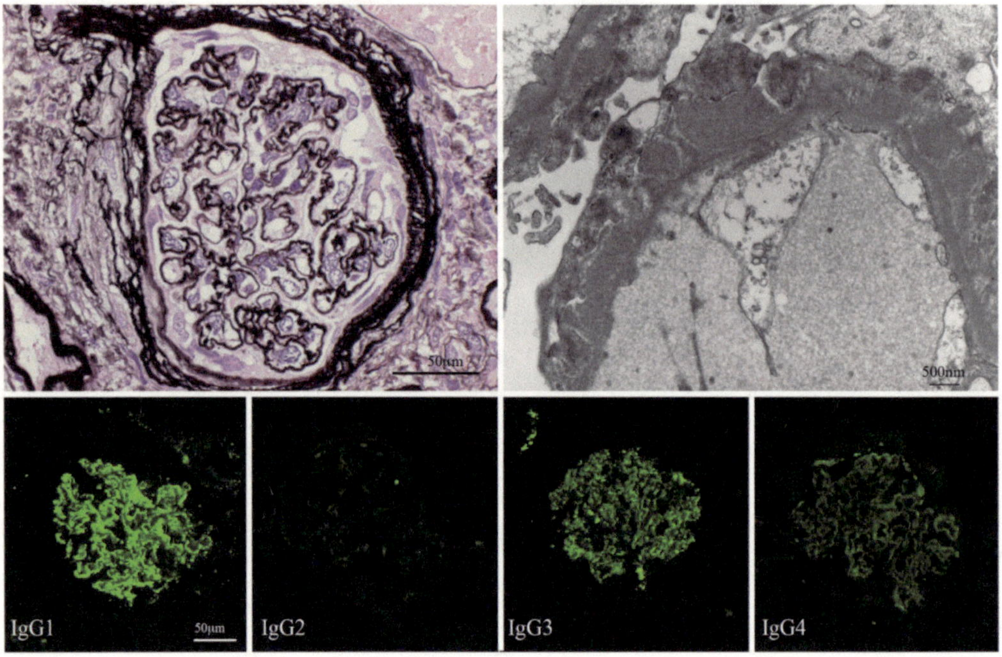

Figure 4. Secondary membranous nephropathy associated with clear cell renal cell carcinoma.

Light microscopy of PAM staining demonstrated thickening of the glomerular basement membrane, and electron microscopy revealed subepithelial electron dense deposits with spike formation. IgG1 and IgG3 were more strongly stained along the capillary wall than IgG4, suggesting secondary membranous nephropathy.

4.3. Minimal change disease and focal segmental glomerulosclerosis with renal cell carcinoma

In contrast to Hodgkin's disease, renal cell carcinoma associated with minimal change nephrotic syndrome is rare [46,47]. The onset of nephrotic syndrome is simultaneous [48,49] or precedes the diagnosis of renal tumor by 3-4 weeks [47,50], and there was a case in which complete remission was achieved after nephrectomy without steroids [49]. These lines of evidence suggest that occurrence of minimal change nephrotic syndrome may be a paraneoplastic syndrome associated with renal cell carcinoma. Renal oncocytoma, characterized by increased cytoplasmic volume containing abundant fine eosinophilic granules and mitochondria, also show the paraneoplastic minimal change nephrotic syndrome [51]. The pathogenesis of minimal change nephrotic syndrome in not clear, but T cell-mediated immune response has been postulated. The increased secretion of VEGF from renal cell carcinoma may alter glomerular permeability and induce minimal change nephrotic syndrome.

Magyarlaki et al [21] reported 5 cases (8%) of focal segmental glomerulosclerosis in 60 autopsy cases of renal cell carcinoma, however, there are only a few reports of focal segmental glomerulosclerosis with renal cell carcinoma [52] and Wilms' tumor [53]. Glomerulosclerotic lesions are often observed in the renal parenchyma adjacent to a tumor, so parenchymal compression and urinary outflow obstruction by renal tumor may be involved in the development of focal segmental glomerulosclerosis.

4.4. Crescentic rapidly progressive glomerulonephritis and vasculitis with renal cell carcinoma

Crescentic glomerulonephritis with rapid progressive renal failure in conjunction with renal cell carcinoma has been reported previously [54-57]. The prevalence of renal cell carcinoma is significantly higher in patients with ANCA-positive Wegener's granulomatosis (7 in 477 patients) than in those with rheumatoid arthritis (1 in 479 patients) with an odds-ratio for development of renal cell carcinoma of 8.73 ($p=0.0464$, 95% CI 1.04-73.69) [58]. In most of the 7 cases, Wegener's granulomatosis was developed shortly after or simultaneously with the diagnosis of renal cell carcinoma [58]. There are many infiltrating cells around the clear cell renal cell carcinoma (Figure 5), and the chronic inflammation observed in renal cell carcinoma may induce anti-neutrophil cytoplasmic antibodies (ANCA) or the renal cancer cells may serve as an antigen source [59]. The renal prognosis in crescentic glomerulonephritis with renal cell carcinoma becomes poor when an anti-GBM antibody exists, and a rapid progression to end-stage renal failure with need of hemodialysis has been reported [54].

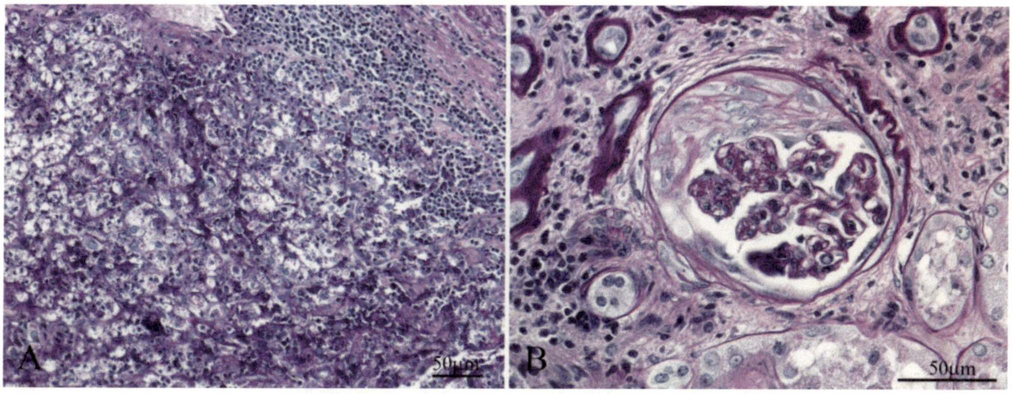

Figure 5. ANCA-related crescentic nephritis associated with renal cell carcinoma. A) The clear cell renal cell carcinoma was surrounded by many infiltrating inflammatory cells including lymphocytes, plasma cells and some neutrophils. B) Some glomeruli around the renal cell carcinoma demonstrated crescents, and the MPO-ANCA level was decreased from 217 EU to 99 EU after nephrectomy.

Membranoproliferative glomerulonephritis with crescents has been reported in patients with renal cell carcinoma, and elective nephrectomy improved both proteinuria and renal function after seven months [60]. Henoch-Schönlein purpura with leukocytoclastic vasculitis was also observed in a 25-year-old man with a small size (0.9x0.8cm) clear cell renal cell carcinoma [61]. Vasculitis associated with cancer is common in lymphoma and leukemia, but only 37 cases associated with solid tumor malignancies have been reported [62], including lung cancer, prostate cancer, colon cancer, renal cell carcinoma, breast cancer and squamous cell carcinoma [63]. Cytokine production by malignant cells, like renal cell carcinoma, may contribute to the development of vasculitis.

4.5. Scleroderma and lupus erythematosus with renal cell carcinoma

Renal cell carcinoma has an immunogenic feature. An interesting case was reported recently where clinical manifestations of scleroderma and proteinuria associated with renal cell carcinoma and membranous nephropathy in a 55-year-old man improved after heminephrectomy of the renal cell carcinoma [43]. Similarly, lupus nephritis developed in a 64 year-old male with clear cell renal carcinoma with para-aortic lymph node metastasis. After one year of partial nephrectomy, the renal cell carcinoma recurred with nephrotic syndrome and pericarditis, and laboratory examination showed an increase in IgG (3449 mg/dL), IgA (371 mg/dL), IgM (715 mg/dL), anti-nuclear antibody (x320) and anti-double strand DNA antibody (41 IU/mL) with low complement levels (CH50 10 U/mL, C3 60, C4 10 mg/dL). Immunohistochemical examination of the resected kidney and para-aortic lymph nodes revealed increased infiltration of plasma cells producing IgG, IgM and IgA around the tumor (Figure 6), suggesting that renal cell carcinoma may have some role in the development of lupus erythematosus.

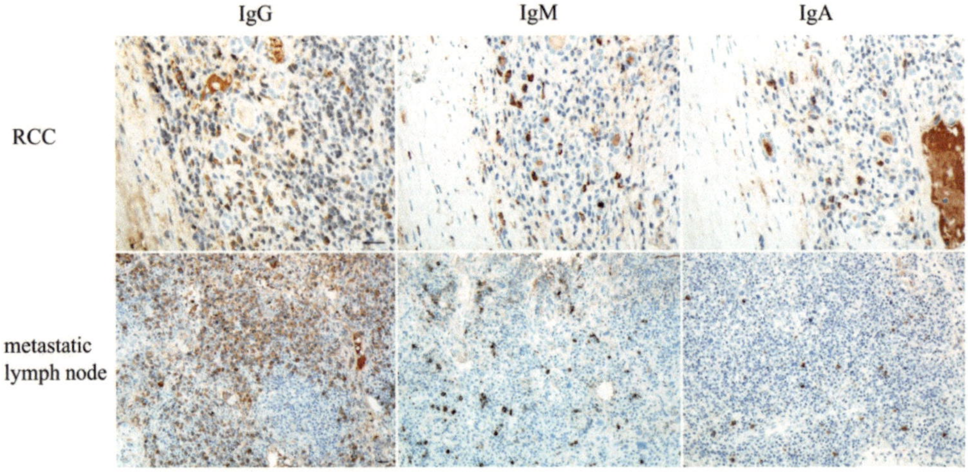

Figure 6. Immunohistochemistry for IgG, IgM, and IgA in the resected kidney of renal cell carcinoma and its para-aortic lymph node metastasis. The patient developed lupus erythematosus and nephrotic syndrome when renal cell carcinoma recurred and progressed.

4.6. Amyloidosis associated with renal cell carcinoma

About 3% of patients with renal cell carcinoma develop systemic amyloidosis [64], and the amyloid is composed of AA protein [65,66]. The renal cell carcinoma may be involved in the stimulation of hepatic production of acute phase reaction proteins including serum amyloid A protein, and the modification of amyloidogenic proteins by the monocyte-macrophage system in the chronic inflammatory lesion of renal cell carcinoma, causing the secondary amyloidosis. Remission of amyloidosis and nephrotic syndrome has been reported after nephrectomy [65,67,68].

4.7. Tubulointerstitial nephritis

Tubulointerstitial nephritis is often difficult to identify because it does not show obvious abnormalities in urine. However, 27% of patients with renal cell carcinoma showed tubulointerstitial nephritis in resected kidney (Table 2) [21]. Recently, as a mechanism of tubulointerstitial nephritis, the antibody against carbonic anhydrase II (CAII) was identified in Sjögren syndrome with renal tubular acidosis [69] and IgG4 related tubulointerstitial nephritis [70]. Carbonic anhydrase is a zinc metalloenzyme that catalyzes the hydration of carbon dioxide and the dehydration of bicarbonate in the proximal tubules and the distal nephron including the intercalated cells of the collecting duct. CA has 15 isoforms and CAII accounts for more than 95 % of CA activity in the kidney and exists in the cytosol, and the remaining 5% renal CA is membrane associated CAIV and CAXII [71]. CAIX is not expressed in the normal kidney, however, in renal cell carcinoma CAIX is induced by hypoxia as a tumor-associated antigen [72,73]. Inactivation of the VHL gene complex leads to the stabilization of hypoxia inducible factor-1α which activates CAIX gene expression [74]. CAIX may promote tumor growth and survival in hypoxic and acidic environments [73]. Serum levels of CAIX are higher in clear cell renal cell carcinoma than non-clear cell renal cell carcinoma and it is a useful marker for the differential diagnosis of renal cell carcinoma and also as a maker of tumor size [75]. It could be possible that an autoantibody against CAIX could be induced and cause tubulointerstitial nephritis in renal cell carcinoma.

5. Treatment of paraneoplastic glomerulopathy associated with renal cell carcinoma

The primary treatment for renal cell carcinoma is surgical excision including radical nephrectomy, nephron-sparing partial nephrectomy, laparoscopic nephrectomy and percutaneous ablation by radiofrequency heat or cryoablation [5]. Most cases of nephrotic syndrome associated with renal cell carcinoma showed remission or transient reduction of proteinuria just after nephrectomy as summarized in Table 4. It is interesting that only nephrectomy can achieve remission of nephropathy with amyloidosis [65,67,68], which is usually refractory to treatment. Some cases of IgA nephropathy, membranous nephropathy, crescentic glomerulonephritis and focal segmental nephrosclerosis associated with renal cell carcinoma progressed to end stage renal failure. In addition to nephrectomy, treatment with prednisolone was attempted in some cases, especially in minimal change nephrotic syndrome, and showed reduction of proteinuria. However, it is noteworthy to recognize that the cyst at the time of biopsy rapidly enlarged after treatment with prednisolone for IgA nephropathy, and a diagnosis of renal cell carcinoma was made later [28]. Thus, the first line of treatment of paraneoplastic glomerulopathy associated with renal cell carcinoma is nephrectomy, and the use of steroids should be limited only to cases of controlled renal cell carcinoma.

Glomerulopathy	Age, sex	Treatment	Outcomes	References
IgAN	61 M	nephrectomy	Remission	Tanaka [26]
IgAN	8 cases	nephrectomy	Remission (6/8)	Magyarlaki [21]
IgAN	58 M 66 M 59 M	Steroid, nephrectomy Steroid 30mg, nephrectomy nephrectomy	Remission ESRD Remission	Mimura [28]
MN	76 F	nephrectomy	Died (33 days)	Stein [37]
MN	69 M	steroid 50mg	Died (6 months)	Nishihara [38]
MN	62 M	Partial nephrectomy	PR	Fujita [39]
MN	57 M	nephrectomy	TR/relapse	Togawa [40]
MN	72M	nephrectomy	TR/ESRD	Kapolas [41]
MN	77 F	nephrectomy	remission	Kuroda [42]
MN	55 M	nephrectomy	remission	Nunez [43]
MCNS	49 M	Nephrectomy, steroid	PR	Forland [51]
MCNS	70 M	nephrectomy	Remission after biopsy	Lee [49]
MCNS	69 M	Steroid 80mg, CPM150mg	Died of infection	Abouchacra [48]
MCNS	64 F	Nephrectomy, steroid 60mg	PR	Woodrow [50]
MCNS	78 M	nephrectomy, steroid 1mg/kg	Complete remission	Auguet [47]
FSGS	48 M	nephrectomy	Worsened sCr	Ejaz [52]
CresGN /GBM-Ab	74 M	nephrectomy	ESRD	Hatakeyama [54]
CresGN/MPO-ANCA	68 F	nephrectomy, steroid	Remission	Karim [56]
CresGN	35 F	HD	ESRD died on HD	Jain [57]
MPGN	26 F	nephrectomy	remission	Tydings [76]
MPGN	65 M	nephrectomy	remission	Ahmed [60]
amyloidosis	66 F	diuretics	NS, Died (respiratory failure)	Pras [66]
amyloidosis	58 F	Nephrectomy, splenectomy	Remission (7months)	Vanatta [65]
amyloidosis	62 M	nephrectomy	Remission (3years)	Karsenty [67]
amyloidosis	54 F	nephrectomy	Remission (5years) died of relapse	Tang [68]

IgAN: IgA nephropathy, MN: membranous nephropathy, MCNS: minimal change nephrotic syndrome, FSGS: focal segmental glomerulosclerosis, cresGN: crescentic glomerulonephritis, MPGN: Membranoproliferative glomerulonephritis, PR: partial remission, ESRD: end-stage renal disease, TR transient remission, CPM cyclophosphamide, HD: hemodialysis, NS: nephrotic syndrome.

Table 4. Treatment and outcomes of glomerulopathy with renal cell carcinoma

http://dx.doi.org/10.5772/53534

6. Molecular-target therapy related nephropathy in renal cell carcinoma

About 30% patients will have distant metastasis at the time of diagnosis, and medical therapies including interleukin-2, interferons, and molecular-target therapy are generally offered for advanced renal cancer as listed in Table 5. Interleukin-2 showed transient proteinuria and renal dysfunction, but these changes are reversible and did not cause long-term intrinsic renal damage [77-79]. Interferons are well known to show proteinuria in 15-20% of patients [80]. The nephrotic syndrome and acute renal failure induced by interferon therapy are histologically due to minimal change disease and acute tubulointerstitial nephritis [80-82].

Bevacizumab, a humanized monoclonal anti-vascular endothelial growth factor antibody, is used for the treatment of metastatic renal cell carcinoma, but adverse effects such as hypertension, anorexia and proteinuria are increased with combination therapy of bevacizumab and interferon α compared with interferon α monotherapy [83,84]. High-dose bevacizumab therapy showed proteinuria of more than 1+ in 64% of patients with renal cell carcinoma and nephrotic range proteinuria of more than 3.5 g/day in 7.7% patients [85]. Renal biopsy revealed thrombotic microangiopathy in two patients treated with Bevacizumab and interferon-α [86]. As VEGF is expressed in the podocyte and its receptors are found in glomerular endothelial cells, blocking VEGF may disturb the function of VEGF to maintain the glomerular capillary permeability barrier, causing thrombotic microangiopathy [87,88].

Treatment of renal cell carcinoma with sunitinib or sorafenib, which inhibit the VEGF receptor and multi-tyrosine kinases, induced severe nephrotic syndrome with acute renal failure, and renal biopsy revealed minimal change disease and thrombotic microangiopathy with acute tubular necrosis [89,90]. Sunitinib also develops other pathological forms of renal diseases including acute interstitial nephritis [91], acute nephritic syndrome with subendothelial C3 deposition [92], FSGS [93], and sorafenib is also associated with IgA nephropathy [94], and interstitial nephritis [95]. Withdrawal of sunitinib or sorafenib with or without use of steroids ameliorated increased serum creatinine and proteinuria as well as hypertension and edema [91,93-95], but in some advanced cases hemodialysis was needed [89, 92] or proteinuria persisted [90]. Thus, early detection of renal adverse effects of these drugs is necessary.

Temsirolimus is a highly specific inhibitor of the mammalian target of rapamycin, which is a central regulator of intracellular signaling pathways and an inhibitor of angiogenesis. Temsirolimus has prolonged overall survival in patients with advanced renal cell carcinoma compared to interferon-α [96]. However, temsirolimus reduced synaptopodin and nephrin expression in podocytes and induced nephrotic syndrome caused by focal segmental glomerulosclerosis [97]. The amount of proteinuria decreased after withdrawal of temsirolimus, so it is necessary to notice the nephrotic adverse effects of this drug.

Medical therapy	Mechanism	Renal diseases	References
Interleukin-2	immunomodulatory cytokine	Proteinuria, transient increase in sCr	Belldegrun [77]
			Shalmi [78]
			Guleria [79]
Interferon α, γ	immunomodulatory cytokine	proteinuria, MCNS, IN, ARF	INF-α: Quesada [80]
			IFN-γ: Nair [81], Tashiro [82]
Bevacizumab	Humanized VEGF-neutralizing antibody	Proteinuria, TMA	Rini [83], Summers [84],
			Roncone [86]
Sunitinib	VEGF receptor and multiple tyrosine kinase inhibitor	MCNS, iATN	Chen [89]
		AIN	Winn [91]
		AGN	Rolleman [92]
		FSGS, TMA	Costero [93]
Sorafenib	VEGF receptor and multiple tyrosine kinase inhibitor	TMA, MCNS	Overkleeft [90]
		IgAN	Jonkers [94]
		AIN	Izzedine [95]
Temsirolimus	Inhibitor of the mammalian target of rapamycin	FSGS	Izzedine [97]

MCNS: minimal change nephrotic syndrome, IN: interstitial nephritis, ARF: acute renal failure, TMA: thrombotic microangiopathy, iATN: ischemic acute tubular necrosis, AGN:acute glomerulonephritis.

Table 5. Interleukin, interferon and molecular-target drugs related nephropathy in the renal cell carcinoma

7. Summary

Recent advances in the molecular understanding of renal cell carcinoma have shed light on the mechanism of paraneoplastic glomerulopathy. Clear cell renal cell carcinoma with a VHL gene mutation stimulates HIF-1α transcription, and produces various cytokines and growth factors including VEGF, PDGF, TGF–α/β, IL-6, CAIX and EPO. Renal cell carcinoma has a feature of cytokine disease or immunogenic disease, and enhanced cytokines and growth factors stimulate lymphocytes and plasma cells, and the latter works as a causative factor for various forms of paraneoplastic glomerulopathies. The precise mechanism of glomerulonephritis has not been completely elucidated, and further investigation of renal cell carcinoma related glomerulopathies will open a new perspective in the understanding of glomerular diseases.

http://dx.doi.org/10.5772/53534

Acknowledgements

I thank Dr. Maristela L. Onozato, MD, PhD in Department of Pathology, Massachusetts General Hospital, Boston, MA and Dr. Satoshi Kinugasa, MD, PhD in Division of Nephrology and Endocrinology, The University of Tokyo for critical review of this manuscript.

Author details

Akihiro Tojo

Address all correspondence to: akitojo-tky@umin.ac.jp

Division of Nephrology and Endocrinology, The University of Tokyo, Tokyo, Japan

References

[1] Palapattu GS, Kristo B, Rajfer J. Paraneoplastic syndromes in urologic malignancy: the many faces of renal cell carcinoma. Rev Urol. 2002 Fall;4(4):163-170.

[2] Galloway J. Remarks ON HODGKIN'S DISEASE. Br Med J. 1922 Dec 23;2(3234): 1201-1208 1202.

[3] Bacchetta J, Juillard L, Cochat P, Droz JP. Paraneoplastic glomerular diseases and malignancies. Crit Rev Oncol Hematol. 2009 Apr;70(1):39-58.

[4] Lien YH, Lai LW. Pathogenesis, diagnosis and management of paraneoplastic glomerulonephritis. Nat Rev Nephrol. [Research Support, N.I.H., Extramural Review]. 2011 Feb;7(2):85-95.

[5] Cohen HT, McGovern FJ. Renal-cell carcinoma. N Engl J Med. 2005 Dec 8;353(23): 2477-2490.

[6] Kim WY, Kaelin WG. Role of VHL gene mutation in human cancer. J Clin Oncol. 2004 Dec 15;22(24):4991-5004.

[7] Iliopoulos O, Levy AP, Jiang C, Kaelin WG, Jr., Goldberg MA. Negative regulation of hypoxia-inducible genes by the von Hippel-Lindau protein. Proc Natl Acad Sci U S A. 1996 Oct 1;93(20):10595-10599.

[8] Kaelin WG, Jr. The von Hippel-Lindau gene, kidney cancer, and oxygen sensing. J Am Soc Nephrol. 2003 Nov;14(11):2703-2711.

[9] Oya M. Renal cell carcinoma: biological features and rationale for molecular-targeted therapy. Keio J Med. 2009 Mar;58(1):1-11.

[10] Baldewijns MM, van Vlodrop IJ, Vermeulen PB, Soetekouw PM, van Engeland M, de Bruine AP. VHL and HIF signalling in renal cell carcinogenesis. J Pathol. Jun;221(2): 125-138.

[11] Horiguchi A, Oya M, Marumo K, Murai M. STAT3, but not ERKs, mediates the IL-6-induced proliferation of renal cancer cells, ACHN and 769P. Kidney Int. 2002 Mar; 61(3):926-938.

[12] An J, Rettig MB. Mechanism of von Hippel-Lindau protein-mediated suppression of nuclear factor kappa B activity. Mol Cell Biol. 2005 Sep;25(17):7546-7556.

[13] Yang H, Minamishima YA, Yan Q, Schlisio S, Ebert BL, Zhang X, Zhang L, Kim WY, Olumi AF, Kaelin WG, Jr. pVHL acts as an adaptor to promote the inhibitory phosphorylation of the NF-kappaB agonist Card9 by CK2. Mol Cell. 2007 Oct 12;28(1): 15-27.

[14] Anglesio MS, George J, Kulbe H, Friedlander M, Rischin D, Lemech C, Power J, Coward J, Cowin PA, House CM, Chakravarty P, Gorringe KL, Campbell IG, Okamoto A, Birrer MJ, Huntsman DG, de Fazio A, Kalloger SE, Balkwill F, Gilks CB, Bowtell DD. IL6-STAT3-HIF signaling and therapeutic response to the angiogenesis inhibitor sunitinib in ovarian clear cell cancer. Clin Cancer Res. Apr 15;17(8):2538-2548.

[15] Pantuck AJ, An J, Liu H, Rettig MB. NF-kappaB-dependent plasticity of the epithelial to mesenchymal transition induced by Von Hippel-Lindau inactivation in renal cell carcinomas. Cancer Res. Jan 15;70(2):752-761.

[16] Takenawa J, Kaneko Y, Fukumoto M, Fukatsu A, Hirano T, Fukuyama H, Nakayama H, Fujita J, Yoshida O. Enhanced expression of interleukin-6 in primary human renal cell carcinomas. J Natl Cancer Inst. 1991 Nov 20;83(22):1668-1672.

[17] Miki S, Iwano M, Miki Y, Yamamoto M, Tang B, Yokokawa K, Sonoda T, Hirano T, Kishimoto T. Interleukin-6 (IL-6) functions as an in vitro autocrine growth factor in renal cell carcinomas. FEBS Lett. 1989 Jul 3;250(2):607-610.

[18] Jacobsen J, Rasmuson T, Grankvist K, Ljungberg B. Vascular endothelial growth factor as prognostic factor in renal cell carcinoma. J Urol. 2000 Jan;163(1):343-347.

[19] Yoshida N, Ikemoto S, Narita K, Sugimura K, Wada S, Yasumoto R, Kishimoto T, Nakatani T. Interleukin-6, tumour necrosis factor alpha and interleukin-1beta in patients with renal cell carcinoma. Br J Cancer. 2002 May 6;86(9):1396-1400.

[20] Blay JY, Rossi JF, Wijdenes J, Menetrier-Caux C, Schemann S, Negrier S, Philip T, Favrot M. Role of interleukin-6 in the paraneoplastic inflammatory syndrome associated with renal-cell carcinoma. Int J Cancer. 1997 Jul 29;72(3):424-430.

[21] Magyarlaki T, Kiss B, Buzogany I, Fazekas A, Sukosd F, Nagy J. Renal cell carcinoma and paraneoplastic IgA nephropathy. Nephron. 1999 Jun;82(2):127-130.

[22] Beaufils H, Patte R, Aubert P, Camey M, Kuss R, Barbagelatta M, Chomette G. Renal immunopathology in renal cell carcinoma. Virchows Arch A Pathol Anat Histopathol. 1984;404(1):87-97.

[23] Ronco PM. Paraneoplastic glomerulopathies: new insights into an old entity. Kidney Int. 1999 Jul;56(1):355-377.

[24] Mustonen J, Pasternack A, Helin H. IgA mesangial nephropathy in neoplastic diseases. Contrib Nephrol. 1984;40:283-291.

[25] Abu-Romeh SH, al-Adnani MS, Asfar S. Renal cell carcinoma presenting with acute renal failure and IgA glomerulonephritis. Nephron. 1988;50(2):169-170.

[26] Tanaka K, Kanzaki H, Taguchi T. IgA glomerulonephritis in a patient with renal cell carcinoma. Nihon Jinzo Gakkai Shi. 1991 Jan;33(1):87-90.

[27] Sessa A, Volpi A, Tetta C, Meroni M, Torri Tarelli L, Battini G, Camussi G, Conte F, Ferrario G, Giordano F, et al. IgA mesangial nephropathy associated with renal cell carcinoma. Appl Pathol. 1989;7(3):188-191.

[28] Mimura I, Tojo A, Kinugasa S, Uozaki H, Fujita T. Renal cell carcinoma in association with IgA nephropathy in the elderly. Am J Med Sci. 2009 Nov;338(5):431-432.

[29] Tsukamoto T, Kumamoto Y, Miyao N, Masumori N, Takahashi A, Yanase M. Interleukin-6 in renal cell carcinoma. J Urol. 1992 Dec;148(6):1778-1781; discussion 1781-1772.

[30] Blay JY, Negrier S, Combaret V, Attali S, Goillot E, Merrouche Y, Mercatello A, Ravault A, Tourani JM, Moskovtchenko JF, et al. Serum level of interleukin 6 as a prognosis factor in metastatic renal cell carcinoma. Cancer Res. 1992 Jun 15;52(12):3317-3322.

[31] Negrier S, Perol D, Menetrier-Caux C, Escudier B, Pallardy M, Ravaud A, Douillard JY, Chevreau C, Lasset C, Blay JY. Interleukin-6, interleukin-10, and vascular endothelial growth factor in metastatic renal cell carcinoma: prognostic value of interleukin-6--from the Groupe Francais d'Immunotherapie. J Clin Oncol. 2004 Jun 15;22(12):2371-2378.

[32] Beagley KW, Eldridge JH, Lee F, Kiyono H, Everson MP, Koopman WJ, Hirano T, Kishimoto T, McGhee JR. Interleukins and IgA synthesis. Human and murine interleukin 6 induce high rate IgA secretion in IgA-committed B cells. J Exp Med. 1989 Jun 1;169(6):2133-2148.

[33] Lefaucheur C, Stengel B, Nochy D, Martel P, Hill GS, Jacquot C, Rossert J. Membranous nephropathy and cancer: Epidemiologic evidence and determinants of high-risk cancer association. Kidney Int. 2006 Oct;70(8):1510-1517.

[34] Ronco P, Debiec H. Molecular pathomechanisms of membranous nephropathy: from Heymann nephritis to alloimmunization. J Am Soc Nephrol. 2005 May;16(5):1205-1213.

[35] Kerpen HO, Bhat JG, Feiner HD, Baldwin DS. Membranes nephropathy associated with renal cell carcinoma. Evidence against a role of renal tubular or tumor antibodies in pathogenesis. Am J Med. 1978 May;64(5):863-867.

[36] Cudkowicz ME, Sayegh MH, Rennke HG. Membranous nephropathy in a patient with renal cell carcinoma. Am J Kidney Dis. 1991 Mar;17(3):349-351.

[37] Stein HD, Yudis M, Sirota RA, Snipes ER, Gronich JH. Membranous nephropathy associated with renal cell carcinoma. Am J Kidney Dis. 1993 Aug;22(2):352.

[38] Nishibara G, Sukemi T, Ikeda Y, Tomiyoshi Y. Nephrotic syndrome due to membranous nephropathy associated with renal cell carcinoma. Clin Nephrol. 1996 Jun;45(6):424.

[39] Fujita Y, Kashiwagi T, Takei H, Takada D, Kitamura H, Iino Y, Katayama Y. Membranous nephropathy complicated by renal cell carcinoma. Clin Exp Nephrol. 2004 Mar;8(1):59-62.

[40] Togawa A, Yamamoto T, Suzuki H, Watanabe K, Matsui K, Nagase M, Hishida A. Membranous glomerulonephritis associated with renal cell carcinoma: failure to detect a nephritogenic tumor antigen. Nephron. 2002 Feb;90(2):219-221.

[41] Kapoulas S, Liakos S, Karkavelas G, Grekas D, Giannoulis E. Membranous glomerulonephritis associated with renal cell carcinoma. Clin Nephrol. 2004 Dec;62(6): 476-477.

[42] Kuroda I, Ueno M, Okada H, Shimada S, Akita M, Tsukamoto T, Deguchi N. Nephrotic syndrome as a result of membranous nephropathy caused by renal cell carcinoma. Int J Urol. 2004 Apr;11(4):235-238.

[43] Nunez S, Konstantinov KN, Servilla KS, Hartshorne MF, Williams WL, Gibel LJ, Tzamaloukas AH. Association between scleroderma, renal cell carcinoma and membranous nephropathy. Clin Nephrol. 2009 Jan;71(1):63-68.

[44] Beck LH, Jr., Bonegio RG, Lambeau G, Beck DM, Powell DW, Cummins TD, Klein JB, Salant DJ. M-type phospholipase A2 receptor as target antigen in idiopathic membranous nephropathy. N Engl J Med. 2009 Jul 2;361(1):11-21.

[45] Ozawa T, Pluss R, Lacher J, Boedecker E, Guggenheim S, Hammond W, McIntosh R. Endogenous immune complex nephropathy associated with malignancy I. Studies on the nature and immunopathogenic significance of glomerular bound antigen and antibody, isolation and characterization of tumor specific antigen and antibody and circulating immune complexes. Q J Med. 1975 Oct;44(176):523-541.

[46] Martinez-Vea A, Panisello JM, Garcia C, Cases A, Torras A, Mayayo E, Carrera M, Richart C, Oliver JA. Minimal-change glomerulopathy and carcinoma. Report of two cases and review of the literature. Am J Nephrol. 1993;13(1):69-72.

[47] Auguet T, Lorenzo A, Colomer E, Zamora A, Garcia C, Martinez-Vea A, Richart C, Oliver JA. Recovery of minimal change nephrotic syndrome and acute renal failure in a patient withRenal cell carcinoma. Am J Nephrol. 1998;18(5):433-435.

[48] Abouchacra S, Duguid WP, Somerville PJ. Renal cell carcinoma presenting as nephrotic syndrome complicated by acute renal failure. Clin Nephrol. 1993 Jun;39(6): 340-342.

[49] Lee SJ, Richards NT. Nephrotic syndrome cured by renal biopsy. Nephrol Dial Transplant. 1992;7(3):265-266.

[50] Woodrow G, Innes A, Ansell ID, Burden RP. Renal cell carcinoma presenting as nephrotic syndrome. Nephron. 1995;69(2):166-169.

[51] Forland M, Bannayan GA. Minimal-change lesion nephrotic syndrome with renal oncocytoma. Am J Med. 1983 Oct;75(4):715-720.

[52] Ejaz AA, Geiger XJ, Wasiluk A. Focal segmental glomerulosclerosis in kidney resected for renal cell carcinoma. Int Urol Nephrol. 2005;37(2):345-349.

[53] Thorner P, McGraw M, Weitzman S, Balfe JW, Klein M, Baumal R. Wilms' tumor and glomerular disease. Occurrence with features of membranoproliferative glomerulonephritis and secondary focal, segmental glomerulosclerosis. Arch Pathol Lab Med. 1984 Feb;108(2):141-146.

[54] Hatakeyama S, Kawano M, Konosita T, Nomura H, Iwainaka Y, Koni I, Tofuku Y, Takeda R, Nisino A, Tokunaga S, et al. [A case of renal cell carcinoma associated with rapidly progressive glomerulonephritis]. Nihon Jinzo Gakkai Shi. 1990 Oct; 32(10):1125-1132.

[55] Kagan A, Sinay-Trieman L, Czernobilsky B, Barzilai N, Bar-Khayim Y. Is the association between crescentic glomerulonephritis and renal cell carcinoma coincidental? Nephron. 1993;65(4):642-643.

[56] Karim MY, Frankel A, Paradinas FJ, Moss J. Anti-neutrophil cytoplasmic antibody-positive crescentic nephritis occurring together with renal cell carcinoma. Nephron. 2000 Aug;85(4):368-370.

[57] Jain S, Kakkar N, Joshi K, Varma S. Crescentic glomerulonephritis associated with renal cell carcinoma. Ren Fail. 2001 Mar;23(2):287-290.

[58] Tatsis E, Reinhold-Keller E, Steindorf K, Feller AC, Gross WL. Wegener's granulomatosis associated with renal cell carcinoma. Arthritis Rheum. 1999 Apr;42(4):751-756.

[59] Mayet WJ, Hermann E, Csernok E, Knuth A, Poralla T, Gross WL, Meyer zum Buschenfelde KH. A human renal cancer line as a new antigen source for the detection of antibodies to cytoplasmic and nuclear antigens in sera of patients with Wegener's granulomatosis. J Immunol Methods. 1991 Sep 20;143(1):57-68.

[60] Ahmed M, Solangi K, Abbi R, Adler S. Nephrotic syndrome, renal failure, and renal malignancy: an unusual tumor-associated glomerulonephritis. J Am Soc Nephrol. 1997 May;8(5):848-852.

[61] Hong YH. Renal cell carcinoma presenting as Henoch-Schonlein purpura with leukocytoclastic vasculitis, hematuria, proteinuria and abdominal pain. Rheumatol Int. Aug;30(10):1373-1376.

[62] Naschitz JE, Yeshurun D, Eldar S, Lev LM. Diagnosis of cancer-associated vascular disorders. Cancer. 1996 May 1;77(9):1759-1767.

[63] Kurzrock R, Cohen PR, Markowitz A. Clinical manifestations of vasculitis in patients with solid tumors. A case report and review of the literature. Arch Intern Med. 1994 Feb 14;154(3):334-340.

[64] Azzopardi JG, Lehner T. Systemic amyloidosis and malignant disease. J Clin Pathol. 1966 Nov;19(6):539-548.

[65] Vanatta PR, Silva FG, Taylor WE, Costa JC. Renal cell carcinoma and systemic amyloidosis: demonstration of AA protein and review of the literature. Hum Pathol. 1983 Mar;14(3):195-201.

[66] Pras M, Franklin EC, Shibolet S, Frangione B. Amyloidosis associated with renal cell carcinoma of the AA type. Am J Med. 1982 Sep;73(3):426-428.

[67] Karsenty G, Ulmann A, Droz D, Carnot F, Grunfeld JP. Clinical and histological resolution of systemic amyloidosis after renal cell carcinoma removal. Nephron. 1985;40(2):232-234.

[68] Tang AL, Davies DR, Wing AJ. Remission of nephrotic syndrome in amyloidosis associated with a hypernephroma. Clin Nephrol. 1989 Nov;32(5):225-228.

[69] Takemoto F, Hoshino J, Sawa N, Tamura Y, Tagami T, Yokota M, Katori H, Yokoyama K, Ubara Y, Hara S, Takaichi K, Yamada A, Uchida S. Autoantibodies against carbonic anhydrase II are increased in renal tubular acidosis associated with Sjogren syndrome. Am J Med. 2005 Feb;118(2):181-184.

[70] Nishi H, Tojo A, Onozato ML, Jimbo R, Nangaku M, Uozaki H, Hirano K, Isayama H, Omata M, Kaname S, Fujita T. Anti-carbonic anhydrase II antibody in autoimmune pancreatitis and tubulointerstitial nephritis. Nephrol Dial Transplant. 2007 Apr;22(4):1273-1275.

[71] Purkerson JM, Schwartz GJ. The role of carbonic anhydrases in renal physiology. Kidney Int. 2007 Jan;71(2):103-115.

[72] Ivanov SV, Kuzmin I, Wei MH, Pack S, Geil L, Johnson BE, Stanbridge EJ, Lerman MI. Down-regulation of transmembrane carbonic anhydrases in renal cell carcinoma cell lines by wild-type von Hippel-Lindau transgenes. Proc Natl Acad Sci U S A. 1998 Oct 13;95(21):12596-12601.

[73] Ivanov S, Liao SY, Ivanova A, Danilkovitch-Miagkova A, Tarasova N, Weirich G, Merrill MJ, Proescholdt MA, Oldfield EH, Lee J, Zavada J, Waheed A, Sly W, Lerman MI, Stanbridge EJ. Expression of hypoxia-inducible cell-surface transmembrane carbonic anhydrases in human cancer. Am J Pathol. 2001 Mar;158(3):905-919.

[74] Sufan RI, Jewett MA, Ohh M. The role of von Hippel-Lindau tumor suppressor protein and hypoxia in renal clear cell carcinoma. Am J Physiol Renal Physiol. 2004 Jul; 287(1):F1-6.

[75] Zhou GX, Ireland J, Rayman P, Finke J, Zhou M. Quantification of carbonic anhydrase IX expression in serum and tissue of renal cell carcinoma patients using enzyme-linked immunosorbent assay: prognostic and diagnostic potentials. Urology. Feb;75(2):257-261.

[76] Tydings A, Weiss RR, Lin JH, Bennett J, Tejani N. Renal-cell carcinoma and mesangiocapillary glomerulonephritis presenting as severe pre-eclampsia. N Y State J Med. 1978 Oct;78(12):1950-1954.

[77] Belldegrun A, Webb DE, Austin HA, 3rd, Steinberg SM, Linehan WM, Rosenberg SA. Renal toxicity of interleukin-2 administration in patients with metastatic renal cell cancer: effect of pre-therapy nephrectomy. J Urol. 1989 Mar;141(3):499-503.

[78] Shalmi CL, Dutcher JP, Feinfeld DA, Chun KJ, Saleemi KR, Freeman LM, Lynn RI, Wiernik PH. Acute renal dysfunction during interleukin-2 treatment: suggestion of an intrinsic renal lesion. J Clin Oncol. 1990 Nov;8(11):1839-1846.

[79] Guleria AS, Yang JC, Topalian SL, Weber JS, Parkinson DR, MacFarlane MP, White RL, Steinberg SM, White DE, Einhorn JH, et al. Renal dysfunction associated with the administration of high-dose interleukin-2 in 199 consecutive patients with metastatic melanoma or renal carcinoma. J Clin Oncol. 1994 Dec;12(12):2714-2722.

[80] Quesada JR, Talpaz M, Rios A, Kurzrock R, Gutterman JU. Clinical toxicity of interferons in cancer patients: a review. J Clin Oncol. 1986 Feb;4(2):234-243.

[81] Nair S, Ernstoff MS, Bahnson RR, Arthur S, Johnston J, Downs MA, Neuhart J, Kirkwood JM. Interferon-induced reversible acute renal failure with nephrotic syndrome. Urology. 1992 Feb;39(2):169-172.

[82] Tashiro M, Yokoyama K, Nakayama M, Yamada A, Ogura Y, Kawaguchi Y, Sakai O. A case of nephrotic syndrome developing during postoperative gamma interferon therapy for renal cell carcinoma. Nephron. 1996;73(4):685-688.

[83] Rini BI, Halabi S, Rosenberg JE, Stadler WM, Vaena DA, Archer L, Atkins JN, Picus J, Czaykowski P, Dutcher J, Small EJ. Phase III trial of bevacizumab plus interferon alfa versus interferon alfa monotherapy in patients with metastatic renal cell carcinoma: final results of CALGB 90206. J Clin Oncol. May 1;28(13):2137-2143.

[84] Summers J, Cohen MH, Keegan P, Pazdur R. FDA drug approval summary: bevacizumab plus interferon for advanced renal cell carcinoma. Oncologist.15(1):104-111.

[85] Yang JC, Haworth L, Sherry RM, Hwu P, Schwartzentruber DJ, Topalian SL, Steinberg SM, Chen HX, Rosenberg SA. A randomized trial of bevacizumab, an anti-vascular endothelial growth factor antibody, for metastatic renal cancer. N Engl J Med. 2003 Jul 31;349(5):427-434.

[86] Roncone D, Satoskar A, Nadasdy T, Monk JP, Rovin BH. Proteinuria in a patient receiving anti-VEGF therapy for metastatic renal cell carcinoma. Nat Clin Pract Nephrol. 2007 May;3(5):287-293.

[87] Schrijvers BF, Flyvbjerg A, De Vriese AS. The role of vascular endothelial growth factor (VEGF) in renal pathophysiology. Kidney Int. 2004 Jun;65(6):2003-2017.

[88] Eremina V, Jefferson JA, Kowalewska J, Hochster H, Haas M, Weisstuch J, Richardson C, Kopp JB, Kabir MG, Backx PH, Gerber HP, Ferrara N, Barisoni L, Alpers CE, Quaggin SE. VEGF inhibition and renal thrombotic microangiopathy. N Engl J Med. 2008 Mar 13;358(11):1129-1136.

[89] Chen YS, Chen CL, Wang JS. Nephrotic Syndrome and Acute Renal Failure Apparently Induced by Sunitinib. Case Rep Oncol. 2009;2(3):172-176.

[90] Overkleeft EN, Goldschmeding R, van Reekum F, Voest EE, Verheul HM. Nephrotic syndrome caused by the angiogenesis inhibitor sorafenib. Ann Oncol. Jan;21(1): 184-185.

[91] Winn SK, Ellis S, Savage P, Sampson S, Marsh JE. Biopsy-proven acute interstitial nephritis associated with the tyrosine kinase inhibitor sunitinib: a class effect? Nephrol Dial Transplant. 2009 Feb;24(2):673-675.

[92] Rolleman EJ, Weening J, Betjes MG. Acute nephritic syndrome after anti-VEGF therapy for renal cell carcinoma. Nephrol Dial Transplant. 2009 Jun;24(6):2002-2003.

[93] Costero O, Picazo ML, Zamora P, Romero S, Martinez-Ara J, Selgas R. Inhibition of tyrosine kinases by sunitinib associated with focal segmental glomerulosclerosis lesion in addition to thrombotic microangiopathy. Nephrol Dial Transplant. Mar;25(3): 1001-1003.

[94] Jonkers IJ, van Buren M. Nephrotic-range proteinuria in a patient with a renal allograft treated with sorafenib for metastatic renal-cell carcinoma. Clin Exp Nephrol. 2009 Aug;13(4):397-401.

[95] Izzedine H, Brocheriou I, Rixe O, Deray G. Interstitial nephritis in a patient taking sorafenib. Nephrol Dial Transplant. 2007 Aug;22(8):2411.

[96] Hudes G, Carducci M, Tomczak P, Dutcher J, Figlin R, Kapoor A, Staroslawska E, Sosman J, McDermott D, Bodrogi I, Kovacevic Z, Lesovoy V, Schmidt-Wolf IG, Barbarash O, Gokmen E, O'Toole T, Lustgarten S, Moore L, Motzer RJ. Temsirolimus, interferon alfa, or both for advanced renal-cell carcinoma. N Engl J Med. 2007 May 31;356(22):2271-2281.

[97] Izzedine H, Boostandoot E, Spano JP, Bardier A, Khayat D. Temsirolimus-induced glomerulopathy. Oncology. 2009;76(3):170-172.

Section 3

Management of Metastatic/Advanced Renal Tumor

Chapter 8

Surgical and Oncological Results of Treatment of Metastases of Renal Cell Carcinoma to the Contralateral Adrenal Gland

Archil Chkhotua, Laurent Managadze and
Ambrosi Pertia

Additional information is available at the end of the chapter

http://dx.doi.org/10.5772/53745

1. Introduction

Urooncological diseases account about 40% of all oncological pathologies in men and more than 10% in women. Renal cell carcinoma (RCC) accounts for about 4% of all adult malignancies and is the most lethal urological cancer. 60 920 new cases of RCC have been diagnosed in the US in 2011 and 13 120 died of cancer [1]. The patient death rate from RCC has decreased in the last 15 years due to the improvements in early diagnosis and surgical treatment of the disease [1]. However, it is estimated that 1/3 of the patients with localized cancer will develop distant metastasis after radical treatment [2]. Therefore, early identification of metastatic disease, timely and proper treatment is the main goal in the management of RCC.

The most common sites of metastases of RCC are: lymph nodes, lungs, liver, bones and brain [3]. It is known that the disease can metastasize to almost every organ. Adrenal metastasis of RCC is relatively rare. It can be: synchronous or metachronous; ipsilateral, contralateral or bilateral; solitary or part of a massive metastatic spread. Malignant involvement of the ipsilateral adrenal gland has been detected in up to 10% of the radical nephrectomy specimens [4-8]. Contralateral adrenal metastasis however, is uncommon. In the autopsy study of more than 400 patients who had undergone nephrectomy for RCC, the solitary contralateral adrenal metastasis has been detected in only 2.5% of cases [9].

The predisposing factors for the disease spread and the optimal treatment of this rare complication are not fully understood. It is well-known that some patients with isolated metastasis may benefit from surgical treatment. However, the optimal diagnosis and treatment of the contralateral adrenal metastasis from RCC is not yet well defined. The available infor-

INTECH
open science | open minds

© 2013 Chkhotua et al.; licensee InTech. This is a paper distributed under the terms of the Creative Commons Attribution License (http://creativecommons.org/licenses/by/3.0), which permits unrestricted use, distribution, and reproduction in any medium, provided the original work is properly cited.

mation on the outcomes of various treatment options of this complication is limited and mainly based on a sporadic case reports.

In this chapter we analyze all 65 cases of the contralateral adrenal metastases of RCC reported in the literature [10-32]. Our single center experience of treatment of four patients with this complication is also presented. The chapter describes the current view on the pathogenesis, diagnosis and management as well as the surgical, pathological and oncological results of treatment of this rare complication.

The natural course of the RCC is unpredictable. The disease can metastasize to any organ, any time even many years after the operation [33, 10]. Metastasis from the RCC has been discovered as late as 23 and 31 years after radical nephrectomy [33, 34]. The contralateral adrenal metastasis from RCC is extremely rare. Only 69 cases (including our series) can be found in the literature.

The exact reasons of late development of the adrenal metastasis are not completely clear. One of the possible explanations could be that some metastases, especially those of low grade, can grow very slowly. Besides, improper patient follow-up i.e. not using a routine imaging studies for a long time might explain the late detection of some metastasis.

Adrenal metastasis from renal tumors is more common to the ipsilateral adrenal gland. The pathological mechanisms for secondary involvement of the contralateral adrenal gland are unknown. It is thought that the disease spreads via hematogenous route as in case of other organ metastases. However, the autopsy studies illustrate that contralateral adrenal metastases occur far more often than should be expected on the basis of organ size [18]. Explanation of this fact can be a rich blood supply of the adrenal gland and its high blood volume-to-unit weight ratio [35]. It has been speculated that as far as the contralateral adrenal metastasis has occurred the adrenal gland will have a higher affinity to the RCC cells than other organ tissues [4]. In another words, if the tumor cell reaches the adrenal gland the later acts as a fertile soil and stimulates raise of these cells [18]. In consistent with this theory some studies are showing that the adrenal metastases from the contralateral primary RCC grew to a considerable size without metastasing to other organs. Utsumi T, et al. describe a huge (85X90mm) contralateral adrenal metastasis that had invaded the kidney, renal vein, and inferior vena cava but without any involevement of other organs [32].

The risk-factors for development of the adrenal metastasis have been analyzed by some of the studies. Importance of the several clinicopathological features of the primary RCC has been reported. These are: tumor size, left sided tumor, advanced T-stage, and upper-pole tumor location [4, 36].

Adrenal metastases are usually anatomically and functionally silent and patients rarely have symptoms or signs of adrenal insufficiency. Therefore, abdominal imaging is not routinely used for follow-up and the isolated contralateral adrenal metastasis from RCC is rarely diagnosed during a lifetime. This should contribute to the late disease diagnosis, treatment and the worse prognosis.

Due to rare occurrence, the optimal diagnostic approach to a solitary contralateral adrenal metastasis in the patients with a history of RCC is controversial. It can be different from the adrenal incidentalomas. Imaging studies usually cannot verify with certainty the adrenal masses detected in the patients previously operated due to the RCC. It is always difficult to determine whether the mass is: primary adrenal tumor (carcinoma), benign tumor (i.e. an adrenal cortical adenoma) or metastasis. Preoperative diagnosis of synchronous adrenal metastases is relatively easy and is mainly based on radiological findings from abdominal CT and/or MRI. The finding of solitary adrenal mass without elevated serum adrenocortical hormones is strongly suggestive of a metastatic lesion. Metastatic adrenal tumors are usually well-vascularized as compared with the adrenal cortical adenoma or primary adrenal carcinoma. The later ones are more hypovascular [30].

CT is a highly specific in diagnosing adrenal metastases. In 82% of cases reported in the literature, contralateral adrenal metastases have been diagnosed by abdominal CT. Antonelli et al. reviewed clinical records of 1179 surgically treated RCC patients and found that 15 had suspicious findings in the contralateral adrenal glands on CT. Only one of the 15 surgically removed adrenals was found to be free of tumor. The authors reported positive and negative predictive value of CT as 73% and 96% in detecting the adrenal metastases. Remarkably, the positive predictive value of CT in diagnosing the contralateral adrenal metastases was higher [32]. It should be noted that accuracy of CT for distinguishing between benign and malignant contralateral adrenal nodules has improved recently using CT protocols to evaluate the wash-out of contrast media [37].

We've analyzed the records of six hundred twenty nine patients who underwent radical nephrectomy for RCC in our center between 1991 and 2005. The mean patient age was 55.7±11.3 years (range: 12-85 years). 422 (67.2%) were man and 207 (32.8%) were women. The mean follow-up is 60.5±1.7 months (range: 1-187 months). The pathological stage distribution of the tumor was the following: T1 –132 (21%); T2 – 229 (36.4%); T3 – 256 (40.7%); T4 - 12 (1.9%) patients. 123 (19.4%) cancers were G1, 277 (44.1%) - G2 and 229 (36.5 %) - G3. Morphological evaluation revealed clear cell RCC in 475 patients (75.6%). 38 (6.1%) patients had lymph node and 28 (4.5%) patient had distant metastases at the time of surgery. 170 (27%) tumors were discovered incidentally, 332 (52.8%) were locally symptomatic and 127 patients (20.2%) had a systemic disease symptoms.

Four cases (0.6%) of isolated contralateral adrenal metastasis have been diagnosed with the mean follow-up of 83.3 months (range: 23-196 months). In accordance with the existing data from the literature all four metastases have been detected by CT. The metastases have been diagnosed synchronously in one (0.1%) and metachronously in three (0.5%) cases. Mean age of the patients was 56 years (range: 47-68 years). All the patients underwent adrenalectomy through flank incision above the 11th rib. No patient received any form of adjuvant systemic therapy.

All four patients had undergone contralateral radical nephrectomy due to the conventional RCC. All removed kidneys and adrenal were sent to the department of pathology of the same institution (National Centre of Urology). The same team of personnel according to the single protocol has technically processed all the tissue specimens. The surgical margins of the primary nephrectomy specimens were recorded as positive or negative based on the gross and microscopic examination of the specimen. The adrenal gland was examined macroscopically, sliced in 2- to 3-mm cross sections and processed for further microscopical evaluation.

Morphological parameters assessed for both the primary and metastatic tumors included: stage, histological subtype, nuclear grade and presence of tumor necrosis. The stained slides from all tumor and metastases specimens were reviewed by urological pathologist, as described previously [38]. Shortly, the resected kidneys and adrenals were evaluated macroscopically. The maximal tumor size was measured and 1.5 x 2cm tissue samples were taken for further assessment. Specimens were fixed, stained and evaluated by the same pathologist according to conventional technique. The tumors were staged according to the AJCC classification system and graded according to Fuhrman's grading system.

The mean (range) diameter of the primary renal tumor was 76±27.9 mm (12-200 mm) and the mean diameter of the adrenal metastases was 6.4 cm (range: 3–9 cm). The clinical and pathological features of the primary tumors for the 4 patients with contralateral adrenal metastasis are summarized in Table 1. The pathological stage of the adrenal metastasis was pT_2N0 and pT3aN0 in two patients each. Grade 2 tumor was detected in one and grade 3 in three cases.

N	Age	Sex	Time from surgery to metastasis (months)	Side of metastasis	Stage	Grade	Follow-up	Patient status
1	47	M	18	Right	T3a	3	31	Dead
2	58	M	64	Right	T2	3	78	Dead
3	57	F	24	Right	T3a	3	165	Alive
4	73	F	156	Left	T2	2	180	Alive

Table 1. The characteristics of four patients with contralateral adrenal metastasis.

One patient had synchronous contralateral adrenal metastasis. The mean time from the primary nephrectomy to contralateral adrenal metastasis for the remaining three patients was 65.5 months (range: 18–156 months).

Adrenal biopsy can be advocated in some cases. The biopsies of RCC has been lately abandoned due to the following reasons: a) the predictive value of the imaging findings usually is so high that a negative biopsy result would not alter the management strategy; b) 10-20% of biopsies are reported to be non-conclusive; c) high risk of complications associated with the biopsy [39].

Early diagnosis and treatment of metachronous adrenal metastases is more challenging as it can occur many years after the operation. This depends on the mode of follow-up, diagnostic techniques used and early referral of the patient to the specialized clinic. In our study the adrenal metastases have been detected at the mean 65.5 months after radical nephrectomy. A wide variability of latency in diagnosis of the metastases has been reported by others as well. These data indicate on the necessity of prolonged surveillance, especially in the high risk patients i.e. with advanced disease stage [31, 40].

The survival of patients with RCC mainly depends on the disease spread. Widely metastatic RCC usually have a poor prognosis with a mean survival of 11 months. On the contrary, in the patients with solitary or limited metastases resection of the metastases can be associated with prolonged survival (30% survival at 5 years) [39]. Reports of successful outcomes and subsequent long-term survival after treatment of solitary metastases of the RCC justify an aggressive surgical approach [10]. In light of the existing data, complete resection of the primary renal and metastatic adrenal tumors should be the main clinical strategy in these patients. Thus, in case of adrenal metastases whether it is synchronous or metachronous, ipsilateral or contralateral, complete removal of adrenal gland is a treatment of choice providing the best results [30].

Adrenalectomy can be performed either laparoscopically, retroperitoneoscopically or by robotic surgery, decreasing the surgery-associated morbidity and hospital stay [20]. We've performed open adrenalectomy in all our patients. The operation was uneventful in all of them. The mean operation time was 136 minutes (range: 110-160 minutes). All metastases were clear cell RCC tumors. The mean blood loss was 175 ml (range: 50-350 ml). The mean hospital stay was 6 days (range: 4-10 days). No patient had positive surgical margins from the adrenalectomy. There are no data on the efficacy of any form of systemic therapy in the treatment of solitary adrenal metastasis.

The available data on the outcome of the surgical treatment of the contralateral adrenal metastases form RCC are limited and biased. Table 2 summarizes the data of 65 patients with contralateral adrenal metastasis reported in the literature [10-32]. Characteristics of the patients (age, sex), interval between the primary surgery and diagnosis of the adrenal metastasis, and clinical outcome of the patients are described.

These are mainly the case reports of 1-2 cases. The biggest series of 11 cases has been reported by Lau WK, et al. from the Mayo clinic in 2003. In this report 82% of the metastases were metachronous, diagnosed at the mean 4.2 years (0-9.2 years) after the nephrectomy. Other relatively big series of 7 and 8 patients have been reported by Plawner J. and Antonelli A. in 1991 and 2006, respectively.

57% of all metastases reported up to now have been detected synchronously and 43% were discovered metachronously at the mean 2.8 years (0-23 years) after the radical nephrectomy. 58% of the patients were male and 42% were female. The majority (62%) of metastases developed on the left side. Abdominal CT was the preferred method of diagnosis in the vast majority of cases (82%) followed-up by arteriography (6%) and IVP (2%).

At the mean follow-up of 6.8 years (0.3-14.3 years) 29 patients (55%) were alive without evidence of disease and 18 patients (34%) were dead of disease. Surgical removal of the adrenal gland was the only treatment used in these patients. None of the patients received any form of adjuvant systemic therapy.

Reference	N of cases	Chronicity	Age (years)	Sex	Time from nephrectomy (years)	Side	Method of diagnosis	Follow-up (years)	Patient status
10	1	s	NS	NS	0	NS	NS	0.6	NED
12	2	s, s	58, 80	M, M	0, 0	L, R	NS, IVP	1.5, 1.8	DOD, NED
13	2	s, s	54, 57	M, F	0, 0	R, L	Art, Art	3, NS	NED, NS
14	2	s, s	54, 55	F, F	0, 0	L, R	CT, Art	1.7, 2	NED, NED
15	2	m, m	57, 46	M, F	0.5, 1	R, L	CT, CT	2.2, 1.8	NED, NED
16	2	s, m	67, 68	M, M	0, 15	R, L	CT, CT	0.4, 1	NED, NED
17	2	m, m	46, 69	M, M	2, 4	L, R	CT, CT	2.5, 4	DOD, NED
18	1	s	60	F	0	R	CT	0.8	NED
19	7	s, s, m, s, m, m, s	63, 55, 55, 48, 70, 57, 71	All M	0, 0, 3.6, 0, 7, 6.8, 0	L, R/L, R, R, L, L, L	NS	14.3, 4.8, 0.8, 0.6, 5, 2.7, 6.7	DOD, DOD, DOD, DOD, NED, NED DOD
20	2	m, m	49, 82	M, M	5, 5	R, R	CT, CT	0.3, 1.3	NED, NED
21	5	All m	47, 59, 69, 57, 72	F, F, F, M, M	1.5, 1.5, 5.3, 2, 17.8	NS	All CT	2, 0.7, 3.7, 5.3, 3.5	DOD, DOD, NED, NED, NED
22	2	s, m	63, 64	M, F	0, 4	L, L	CT, CT	1, 5	NED, NED
23	1	s	52	M	0	R	CT	7	NED
24	1	m	52	M	0.8	R	CT	7.3	NED
25	1	m	NS	M	23	NS	NS	1	NED
26	1	s	NS	NS	0	NS	CT	NS	NS
27	4	s, s, s, m	All NS	All NS	0, 0, 0, NS	NS	NS	9, 5.4, NS, NS	DOD, AWD, NS, NS
28	1	m	63	M	22	L	CT	5.6	NED
29	1	m	50	F	7.5	R	CT	2.5	NED
30	11	m, m, m, m, s, m, m, m, s, m, m	69, 43, 49, 64,54, 54, 67, 53,68, 70, 79,	M, M, M, M, M, M, F, M, M, F, M	6.1, 7.3, 9.2, 9.1, 0, 1, 6.7, 5.8, 0, 0.8, 1	L, L, R, R, R, L, L, L, R, R, L	All CT	1.7, 0.9, 1.9, 0.5, 6.6, 9.9, 3.4, 3.7, 9.2, 4.4, 1.2	DU, DOD, DOD, NED, DOD, DOD, DOC, DOD, NED, DOD, DOD,
31	8	s-6, m-2	NS	NS	NS	NS	All CT	NS	NS
32	1	s	64	M	0	R	CT	0.5	NED

Art, arteriography; AWD, alive with disease; DOC, dead of other causes; DOD, dead of disease; DU, dead of unknown cause; F, female; IVP, intravenous pyelogram; L, left; m, metachronous; M, male; NED, no evidence of disease; NS, not stated; R, right; s, synchronous.

Table 2. Characteristics of the patients treated for the contralateral adrenal metastasis published in the literature.

From our series of four patients, two are alive 141 and 24 months after adrenalectomy without signs of disease recurrence. Two patients died from multiple metastases 13 and 14 months after adrenalectomy, including the patient with synchronous contralateral adrenal metastasis.

For the entire group of patients, the 5 and 10 years disease–specific survival rates were 61.5 % and 25.6%, respectively. The 5-year overall survival for metastatic (N+ and M+) disease was significantly worse as compared with the non-metastatic disease (6.25% and 72.8%, respectively) (p=0.0001).

There was no statistically significant difference when the survival of patients with solitary adrenal lesions was compared to that of the patients with organ–confined primary RCC. Furthermore, no differences in survival have been detected between the patients with synchronous or metachronous adrenal metastasis (p=0.346 for overall survival; p=0.256 for disease-specific survival). With multivariate statistical analysis the presence of solitary adrenal metastases was not predictive of the clinical prognosis of the patients following adrenalectomy.

The biggest number of the patients with contralateral adrenal metastasis from RCC reported in the literature is 11 [30]. This number is small for making the strong conclusions. Majority of the available studies indicate that the surgical treatment of the complication is worthwhile in selected patients [22, 23]. One study demonstrated that patients in whom RCC metastases (both synchronous and metachronous) were clinically confined to the adrenal gland had statistically better survival rates than those with diffuse metastasis [31]. In about one-third of the RCC patients with isolated adrenal metastasis, surgical resection of the metastasis led to an apparently curative outcome [32]. The longest disease-free survival after removing a contralateral adrenal metastases form RCC is 12.1 years [41], and the longest overall survival is 14.3 years [20]. In accordance with the literature, we didn't find statistically significant survival difference between the patients with localized RCC and solitary contralateral adrenal metastasis. Furthermore, with multivariate statistical analysis the presence of solitary adrenal metastases was not predictive of the clinical prognosis of the patients following adrenalectomy.

The exact reason why do these patients survive longer remains unclear. The several possible explanations exist. It has been speculated that this is a localized disease and that complete removal of the tumor improves prognosis. Another explanation is that the patient's immune system can probably inhibit microscopic disease after tumor debulking. Finally, it has been postulated that this may be a naturally selected group of patients with slow-growing cancer which is not very aggressive and does not metastasize readily [19].

2. Conclusion

In conclusion, the solitary contralateral adrenal metastasis from RCC is an extremely rare clinical complication that can occur very late after the radical nephrectomy. The increased use of radiological diagnostic tests like: ultrasound, CT and/or MRI has led to more efficient detection of these lesions. Aggressive surgery remains the treatment of choice in these cases improving prognosis in some of the patients. There is no doubt that the existing data are limited and we need more studies to define the optimal management strategy in the patients with contralateral adrenal metastasis from RCC.

Author details

Archil Chkhotua*, Laurent Managadze and Ambrosi Pertia

*Address all correspondence to: achkhotua@gmail.com

National Centre of Urology, Tbilisi, Georgia

References

[1] Siegel R, Ward E, Brawley O, Jemal, A. Cancer Statistics, 2011. CA Cancer J Clin 2011; 61(4): 212–236.

[2] Pantuck AJ, Zisman A, Belldegrun AS. The changing natural history of renal cell carcinoma. Journal of Urology 2001; 166(5): 1611-1623.

[3] Kozlowski JM. Management of distantsolitary recurrence in the patient with renal cancer: contralateral kidney and other sites. Urologic Clinics of North America 1994; 21(4): 601–624.

[4] Sagalowsky AI, Kadesky KT, Ewalt DM, Kennedy TJ. Factors influencing adrenal metastasis in renal cell carcinoma. Journal of Urology 1994; 151(5): 1181-1184.

[5] Winter P, Miersch WD, Vogel J, Jaeger N. On the necessity of adrenal exstirpation combined with radical nephrectomy. Journal of Urology 1990; 144(4): 842-843.

[6] O'Brien WM, Lynch JH. Adrenal metastases by renal cell carcinoma. Incidence at nephrectomy. Urology 1987; 29(6): 605-607.

[7] Angervall L,Wahlqvist L. Follow up and prognosis of renal carcinomain a series operated by perifascial nephrectomy combined with adrenalectomy and retroperitoneal lymphadenectomy. European Urology 1978; 4(1): 13-17.

[8] Robey EL, Schellhammer PF. The adrenal gland and renal cell carcinoma: is ipsilateraladrenalectomy a necessary component ofradical nephrectomy? Journal of Urology 1986; 135(3): 453-455

[9] Saitoh H, Nakayama M, Nakamura K, Satoh T. Distant metastasis of renal adenocarcinoma in nephrectomized cases. Journal of Urology 1982; 127(6): 1092–1095.

[10] O'Dea MJ, Zincke H, Utz DC, Bernatz PE. The treatment of renal cell carcinoma with solitary metastasis. Journal of Urology 1978; 120(5): 540–542.

[11] Cheville JC, Blute ML, Zincke H, Lohse CM, Weaver AL. Stage pT1 conventional (clear cell) renal cell carcinoma: athological features associated with cancer specific survival. Journal of Urology 2001; 166(2): 453–456.

[12] Fourcar E, Dehner LP. Renal cell carcinoma occurring with contralateral adrenal metastasis. A clinical and pathological trap. Archives of Surgery 1979; 114(8): 959–963.

[13] Neal PM, Leach GE, Kaswick JA, Lieber MM. Renal cell carcinoma: recognition and treatment of synchronous solitary contralateral adrenal metastasis. Journal of Urology 1982; 128(1): 135–136.

[14] Previte SR, Willscher MK, Burke CR. Renal cell carcinoma with solitary contralateral adrenal metastasis: experience with 2 cases. Journal of Urology 1982; 128(1): 132–134.

[15] Hasegawa J, Okumura S, Abe H, Kanamori S, Yoshida K, Akimoto M. Renal cell carcinoma with solitary contralateral adrenal metastasis. Urology 1988; 32(1): 52–53.

[16] Lemmers M, Ward K, Hatch T, Stenzel P. Renal adenocarcinoma with solitary metastasis to the contralateral adrenal gland: report of 2 cases and review of the literature. Journal of Urology 1989; 141(5): 1177– 1180.

[17] Huisman TK, Sands JP Jr. Renal cell carcinoma with solitary metachronous contralateral adrenal metastasis: experience with 2 cases and review of the literature. Urology 1991; 38(4): 364–368.

[18] Dieckmann KP, Wullbrand A, Krolzig G. Contralateral adrenal metastasis in renal cell cancer. Scandinavian Journal of Urology and Nephrology 1996; 30(2): 139–143.

[19] Plawner J. Results of surgical treatment of kidney cancer with solitary metastasis to contralateral adrenal. Urology 1991; 37(3): 233–236.

[20] Elashry OM, Clayman RV, Soble JJ, McDougall EM. Laparoscopic adrenalectomy for solitary metachronous contralateral adrenal metastasis from renal cell carcinoma. Journal of Urology 1997; 157(4): 1217–1222.

[21] Kessler OJ, Mukamel E, Weinstein R, Gayer E, Konichezky M, Servadio C. Metachronous renal cell carcinoma metastasis to the contralateral adrenal gland. Urology 1998; 51(4): 539–543.

[22] Stein A, Mecz Y, Sova Y, Lurie M, Lurie A. Synchronous and metachronous contralateral adrenal metastases from primary renal cell carcinoma. Urology International 1997; 58(1): 58–60.

[23] Barnes RD, Abratt RP, Cant PJ, Dent DM. Synchronous contralateral adrenal metastasis from renal cell carcinoma: a 7 year survival following resection. The Australian and New Zealand journal of surgery 1995; 65(7): 540–541.

[24] Yamasaki Y, Koga S, Nishikido M, Noguchi M, Kanetake H, Saito Y. The role of surgery in renal cell carcinoma with solitary metachronous metastasis to contralateral adrenal gland. Anticancer Research 1999; 19(6C): 5575–5576.

[25] Mesurolle B, Mignon F, Travagli JP, Meingan P, Vanel D. Late presentation of solitary contralateral adrenal metastasis of renal cell carcinoma. European Radiology 1997; 7(4): 557–558.

[26] Turini D, Barbanti G, Beneforti P, Misuri D, Di Mauro F. Biological, diagnostic and therapeutic aspects of a case of renal cell carcinoma occurring with bladder and contralateral adrenal metastasis. Urology International 1988; 43(5): 293–296.

[27] Kim SH, Brennan MF, Russo P, Burt ME, Coit DG. The role of surgery in the treatment of clinically isolated adrenal metastasis. Cancer 1998; 82(2): 389–394.

[28] Sagalowsky AI, Molberg K. Solitary metastasis of renal cell carcinoma to the contralateral adrenal gland 22 years after nephrectomy. Urology 1999; 54(1): 162.

[29] Ertl CW, Darras FS. Solitary metachronous contralateral adrenal metastasis from renal cell carcinoma. Urology 1999; 54(1): 162.

[30] Lau WK, Zincke H, Lohse CM, Cheville JC, Weaver AL, Blute ML. Contralateral adrenal metastasis of renal cell carcinoma: treatment, outcome and a review. BJU International 2003; 91(9): 775–779.

[31] Antonelli A, Cozzoli A, Simeone C, Zani D, Zanotelli T, Portesi E, Cosciani Cunico S. Surgical treatment of adrenal metastasis from renal cell carcinoma: a single-centre experience of 45 patients. BJU International 2006; 97(3): 505–508.

[32] Utsumi T, Suzuki H, Nakamura K, Kim W, Kamijima S, Awa Y, Araki K, Nihei N, Naya Y, Ichikawa T. Renal cell carcinoma with a huge solitary metastasis to the contralateral adrenal gland: A case report. International Journal of Urology 2008; 15(12): 1077–1079.

[33] Mesurolle B, Mignon F, Travagli JP, Meingan P, Vanel D. Late presentation of solitary contralateral adrenal metastasis of renal cell carcinoma. European Radiology 1997; 7(4): 557–558.

[34] BloomDA, Kaufman JJ, Slith RB. Late recurrence of renal tubular carcinoma. Journal of Urology 1981; 126(4): 546-548.

[35] Campbell CM, Middleton, RG, Rigby 0F. Adrenal metastasis in renal cell carcinoma. Urology 1983; 21(4): 403-405.

[36] Ito A, Satoh M, Ohyama C, Saito S, Shintaku I, Nakano O, Aoki H, Hoshi S, Orikasa S. Adrenal metastasis from renal cell carcinoma: Significance of adrenalectomy. International Journal of Urology 2002; 9(3): 125–128.

[37] Korobkin M. CT characterisation of adrenal masses: the time has come. Radiology 2000; 217(3): 629–632.

[38] Pertia A, Nikoleishvili D, Trsintsadze O, Gogokhia N, Managadze L, Chkhotua A. Importance of cell cycle regulatory proteins and proliferation markers in conventional renal cell carcinoma. In: Watanabe HS. (ed.) Horizons in Cancer Research, Nova Science Publishers, Inc., New York, 2011 Vol. 42, pp. 191-205.

[39] Silverman, SG, Gan YU, Mortele KJ, Tuncali K, Cibas ES. Renal masses in the adult patient: the role of percutaneous biopsy. Radiology 2009; 240(1): 6-22.

[40] Stephenson AJ, Chetner MP, Rourke K, Gleave ME, Signaevsky M, Palmer B, Kuan J, Brock GB, Tanguay S. Guidelines for the surveillance of localized renal cell carcinoma based on the patterns of relapse after nephrectomy. Journal of Urology 2004; 172(1): 58–62.

[41] Yokoyam Sapienza P, Stipa F, Lucandri G, Baratti L, Delfino M, Mingazzini PL. Renal carcinoma with a solitary synchronous contralateral adrenal metastasis: a case report. Anticancer Res 1997; 17(1B): 743–747.

Chapter 9

Current Perspectives in Metastatic Renal Cell Carcinoma Treatment: The Role of Targeted Therapies

V. Michalaki, M. Balafouta, D. Voros and
C. Gennatas

Additional information is available at the end of the chapter

http://dx.doi.org/10.5772/54856

1. Introduction

Renal cell carcinoma (RCC) accounts for approximately 3% of adult malignancies and close to 90% of all renal neoplasms. Renal cell carcinomas, by definition, are tumors that originate in the renal cortex. These tumors are often asymptomatic, have diverse clinical manifestations, and can be associated with hereditary syndromes. Surgery is the treatment of choice for localized RCC. In localized RCC, partial nephrectomy for small tumors and radical nephrectomy for larger tumors continue to be the gold standard. Surgical practice has reduced morbidity and has advanced toward more limited and less invasive resection approaches. In addition, cytoreductive nephrectomy is often indicated before embarking on systemic treatment in patients with metastatic disease.

In recent years, there has been a shift from radical nephrectomy toward more nephron-sparing approaches. RCC still remains a predominantly surgical disease because RCCs are frequently characterized as tumors that are resistant to chemotherapy and radiation. However, advances in the treatment of metastatic RCC have evolved, primarily with biologic response modifiers.

The management of RCC has undergone the most significant transformation. Scientific understanding of the molecular basis of cancer and the role of growth factors have resulted in the identification of signaling pathways relevant in the pathogenesis of renal cell carcinoma. This knowledge provided the impetus for developing new drugs that target and inhibit these diff e rent pathways. Previously, systemic therapy for renal cancer has been limited to the use of interleukin-2 and the off-label use of interferon. These drugs formulated an immunotherapeutic approach to the treatment of advanced renal cancer. Translational research and participation of patients with advanced renal cell carcinoma in clinical trials have resulted in

INTECH
open science | open minds

© 2013 Michalaki et al.; licensee InTech. This is a paper distributed under the terms of the Creative Commons Attribution License (http://creativecommons.org/licenses/by/3.0), which permits unrestricted use, distribution, and reproduction in any medium, provided the original work is properly cited.

the approval of six systemic targeted therapies. These include sorafenib tosylate, sunitinib malate, temsirolimus, everolimus, bevacizumab in combination with interferon, and most recently, pazopanib. Each of these drugs has increased therapeutic options and appears to prolong survival for patients with advanced renal cancer.

2. Biologic basis of targeted therapy

Recent advancements in the understanding of the genetics of RCC have led to a new pathological classification of five different subtypes of RCCs: clear cell, papillary, chromophobe, collecting duct carcinoma (Bellini Duct tumor), and renal carcinoma unclassified (renal medullary carcinoma). This classification is primarily based on cytologic appearance and the cell origin in combination with growth pattern and genetic alterations [1].

The grading of RCC is based on the morphology of a neoplasm with hematoxylin and eosin (H&E) staining on microscopy. The most popular and widely used system for grading RCC is a nuclear grading system described by Fuhrman, Lasky, and Limas in 1982. This system categorizes RCC into one of four grades based on nuclear characteristics and has been shown to correlate with prognosis.

Adenocarcinomas represent the great majority (85%) of renal cell cancers. Adenocarcinomas may be subdivided into clear cell renal carcinomas, the most common form of kidney cancer; Many cases of clear cell carcinoma are linked to inactivation of the von Hippel-Lindau tumor suppressor protein (pVHL), [2]. VHL is a 213 amino acid protein that polyubiquinates hypoxia-inducible factor 1 alpha (HIF1alpha) which marks it for destruction by the cellular proteosome. Normally, low oxygen conditions allow HIF1alpha to accumulate and bind to HIF1beta thereby creating a complex that transcriptionally activates genes. In patients with aberrant VHL, HIF1alpha is left to accumulate freely without degradation even under normal oxygen conditions and thus the transcription of genes related to glucose metabolism, apoptosis, angiogenesis and endothelial stabilization are abnormally promoted. This disordered response to hypoxia activates over 100 HIF-responsive genes which include growth factors and their receptors such as VEGF, platelet-derived growth factor (PDGF), and transforming growth factor alpha/beta (TGF), [3].

1nactivation of the VHL gene is an early step in clear cell renal carcinogenesis, at least for those tumors associated with VHL disease. Subsequent studies have shown that VHL inactivation is also common in non-hereditary clear cell renal carcinoma. Approximately 50% of sporadic clear cell renal carcinomas harbor somatic mutations affecting the maternal and paternal VHL locus.

Another downstream effect of the VEGF receptor (VEGFR) pathway is the activation of PI3 kinase and Akt which in turn promote mTOR kinase [4]. mTOR is a central component of intracellular pathways that promote tumor growth and proliferation, cellular metabolism and is a mediator of the hypoxic response as an upstream activator of HIF1alpha. When mTOR and raptor combine to form an activated complex, they phosphorylate and thus activate the eukaryotic translation initiation factor 4E binding protein-1 (eIF-4BP1) and ribosomal S6 kinase (p70s6k). This leads to the synthesis of cellular proliferation proteins such as cyclin D1, angiogenesis mediators such as VEGF, and hypoxia response regulators such as HIF1alpha [5].

3. Targeted therapies

Systematic studies of cell lines in which pVHL or HIF status has been manipulated suggest that as many as 100 HIF-responsive genes might be dysregulated when pVHL is crippled [6]. A number of these genes encode proteins that are implicated in tumorigenesis. This makes them amenable to pharmacologic attack. Evidence now indicates that targeting these HIF-responsive genes can alter the natural history of human renal carcinoma.

Fortunately, a number of drugs have been identified that indirectly downregulate HIF protein levels. One such drug, rapamycin, inhibits mTOR, which plays a critical role in the regulation of protein translation. This in turn affects HIFα, which is very sensitive to changes in protein translation due in part to its high metabolic turnover rate. Inhibitors of mammalian target of rapamycin (mTOR) like rapamycin, downregulate HIF, [7].

4. Targeting HIF-responsive growth factors

4.1. Vascular endothelial growth factor

Clear cell renal carcinomas are notoriously angiogenic. Indeed, prior to the availability of computed tomography, renal angiograms were often used to diagnose these tumors. Renal carcinomas overproduce a variety of angiogenic moieties including vascular endothelial growth factor (VEGF), the product of a HIF-responsive gene. In addition to promoting angiogenesis, VEGF might suppress antitumor immune responses as well. It has also been suggested that VEGF has direct stimulatory effects on renal carcinoma cells, although these findings await further corroboration, [8, 9].

Several drugs that inhibit VEGF, or its kinase insert domain-containing receptor (KDR), have activity against clear cell renal carcinomas. In a randomized phase II study, patients with metastatic renal carcinoma who were treated with 10 mg/kg (but not 3 mg/kg) bevacizumab, a neutralizing antibody against VEGF, exhibited a significant delay in time-to-disease progression, [10]. Other unrelated KDR inhibitors such as SU11248 (sunitinib maleate), BAY43-9006 (sorafenib), and AG-013736 also appear to have significant activity against this tumor subtype, [11, 12].

5. VEGFR tyrosine kinase inhibitors

VEGF stimulates endothelial cell proliferation and survival. Immature blood vessels appear to be exquisitely sensitive to VEGF withdrawal. In contrast, mature blood vessels are less sensitive to VEGF withdrawal because their endothelial cells are responsive to additional survival factors such as platelet-derived growth factor (PDGF) released from surrounding pericytes. Ongoing efforts to improve our understanding of the basic biology of RCC have identified several potential targets for therapeutic modulation. One particularly promising area of investigation is the role of VEGF in the pathogenesis of renal cell carcinoma. VEGF is a tumor-secreted cytokine that plays an important role in both normal and tumor-associated angiogenesis. VEGF exerts its biologic effect by binding to cell surface VEGF receptors, thereby inducing dimerization and autophosphorylation of intracellular receptor tyrosine kinases, leading to activation of downstream signal transduction elements. There are several forms of VEGF receptors (VEGFR), but VEGFR-2 appears to be the main receptor responsible for the proangiogenic effects of VEGF. The relevance of VEGF to tumor biology is supported by the high incidence of von Hippel-Lindau tumor suppressor gene mutations in patients with RCC, which subsequently leads to increases in VEGF expression. Receptor tyrosine kinases (RTKs) play an integral role in the signaling cascade of VEGF and PDGF [12].

RTKs have an extracellular domain that binds to their respective ligand and an intracellular domain that holds the tyrosine kinase responsible for downstream signaling. Upon ligand binding, the RTKs dimerize or multimerize to induce a conformational change that allows ATP binding resulting in autophosphorylation and transphosphorylation. These tyrosine domains are then able to phosphorylate and activate various proteins in the downstream signal transduction cascade.

6. Sunitinib

Sunitinib is an oral drug with inhibitory activity against several related protein tyrosine kinase receptors, including the platelet-derived growth factor receptor (PDGFR)–ß, stem cell factor receptor (KIT), and Fms-like tyrosine kinase-3, as well as the vascular endothelial growth factor (VEGF) receptors 1, 2 and 3, [13]. Two initial phase II trials of sunitinib 50 mg/day for 4 weeks followed by 2 weeks rest in 169 metastatic renal cell carcinoma (RCC) patients who had failed previous cytokine-based therapy demonstrated an investigator-assessed objective response rate of 45%, a median duration of response of 11.9 months, and a median progression-free survival (PFS) of 8.4 months [14, 15]. Recently, a survival analysis of these patients was reported, suggesting a trend for improved median overall survival (OS) with sunitinib therapy (26.4 vs 21.8 months; hazard ratio: 0.821; 95% confidence interval: 0.673-1.001; P =.051.Based on these data, sunitinib has emerged as a frontline standard of care for patients with metastatic RCC. Common toxicities associated with sunitinib have included fatigue, hand-foot syndrome, diarrhea, mucositis, hypertension and hypothyroidism. Cardiotoxicity has been reported and thus monitoring may be required in patients with preexisting heart disease [16].

In a population-based retrospective analysis comparing patients treated in the IFN era (n=131) versus those treated in the sunitinib era (n=69), the patients treated with first-line sunitinib had an associated doubling in OS compared to those treated with interferon (17.3 versus 8.7 months, p=0.004) [17]. When adjusted for Memorial Sloan Kettering Cancer Center (MSKCC) prognostic criteria, the HR of death for sunitinib versus IFN was 0.049 (p=0.001). Even those patients classified as having a poor prognosis by MSKCC criteria had a survival advantage. Current treatment algorithm for patients with met (10.7 versus 4.1 months, p=0.0329), suggesting that use of sunitinib is beneficial in this population as well.

7. Sorafenib

Sorafenib is an oral multikinase inhibitor that inhibits vascular endothelial growth factor (VEGF) receptors 1-3, platelet-derived growth factor receptor (PDGFR)–ß, and the serine threonine kinase Raf-1 [18]. A phase III trial of sorafenib randomized 905 treatment-refractory metastatic RCC patients to sorafenib 400 mg orally twice daily or placebo [19]. In the sorafenib arm, a progression-free survival (PFS) advantage of 5.5 months vs 2.8 months was observed (hazard ratio for disease progression: 0.44; 95% confidence interval: 0.35-0.55; P <.01). The median overall survival was also increased for patients in the sorafenib group (19.3 vs 15.9 months) but did not reach prespecified statistical boundaries for significance. The common toxicities experienced with sorafenib are similar to sunitinib except that the hand-foot syndrome may be more pronounced and cardiotoxicity and fatigue appears to occur less frequently. Based on these data, sorafenib has been FDA approved and become a standard of care for second-line treatment of mRCC after immunotherapy failure. However, a smaller, randomized phase II of sorafenib vs interferon alfa-2b in 189 previously untreated metastatic RCC patients failed to demonstrate a PFS advantage over IFN. Compared with interferon alfa-2b, sorafenib did not significantly improve the median PFS (5.6 vs 5.7 months, respectively), [20]. Although the reason for the lack of significant effect when compared with interferon alfa-2b in the frontline setting remains unclear, one possibility is that it is because of a weaker inhibition of VEGF receptor compared with sunitinib. Although there may be patients in whom sorafenib is a preferred initial agent because of the toxicity profile or other considerations, sorafenib has largely been relegated to second-line and later therapy. The identification of those patients for whom sorafenib would be the preferred frontline treatment is needed.

8. Mammalian Target of Rapamycin (mTOR) inhibitors

Temsirolimus is an inhibitor of mammalian target of rapamycin (mTOR), a molecule implicated in multiple tumor-promoting intracellular signaling pathways.

Activation of the mTOR protein, through cellular stimuli-triggered activation of the PI3K/Akt pathway, can also result in HIF accumulation. mTOR phosphorylates and activates p70S6K, which results in enhanced translation of certain proteins, including HIF. Activated HIF translocates into the nucleus, where it triggers the transcription of a large number of hypoxia-inducible genes; among these are the growth factors vascular endothelial growth factor (VEGF) and PDGF. These growth factors interact with their respective cell-surface receptors, leading to cell migration, proliferation, and permeability. Temsirolimus and everolimus bind to the

FK506-binding protein; this resultant protein-drug complex inhibits the kinase activity of mTOR within the mTORC1 complex.

Temsirolimus was initially evaluated for patients with mRCC in a randomized phase II study of three different dose levels [21]. When patients were retrospectively stratified into MSKCC prognostic risk groups, the poor risk group appeared to have a better than expected OS, leading to further evaluation in this population.

The subsequent phase III trial with temsirolimus had a primary endpoint of OS. Six hundred and twenty-six previously untreated patients with poor prognostic criteria were randomized to temsirolimus 25mg IV weekly, IFN alpha 18 million units (MU) three times a week or temsirolimus 15 mg IV weekly plus IFN 6 MU three times a week [22]. To be considered poor risk, patients were required to have three or more of the following adverse risk features: Karnofsky performance status less than 80%, lactate dehydrogenase over 1.5 times the upper limit of normal, hemoglobin below the lower limit of normal, serum corrected calcium more than 10 mg/dl, time from first diagnosis of RCC to start of therapy of less than a year and three or more metastatic sites. Of patients included in this trial, 19% had nonclear cell or unknown histology. Temsirolimus monotherapy demonstrated an OS advantage compared to IFN alpha (10.9 months versus 7.3 months, log rank $p<0.008$). The objective response rates were 8.6% for temsirolimus and 4.8% for IFN, which was not statistically significant. The median PFS for the temsirolimus monotherapy arm and interferon arm was 3.8 months (95% confidence interval (CI): 1.9–2.2) and 1.9 months (95% CI: 3.6–5.2), respectively. Common side effects include fatigue, hypercholesteremia and hyperglycemia. Temsirolimus has become a first-line option for patients with metastatic RCC of any histologic subtype, appropriately applied to patients with poor prognostic criteria.

Another mTOR inhibitor, everolimus (RAD001) has recently been reported to improve progression-free survival in a phase III trial of patients with mRCC who had progressed on sunitinib, sorafenib or both [23]. These patients were randomized to receive either everolimus 10mg orally daily or placebo and were stratified by the number of previous tyrosine kinase inhibitors (TKI) and MSKCC 'previously treated' risk groups (one point each for anemia, hypercalcemia, and Karnofsky performance status <80; 0 points=favorable, 1 point=intermediate, 2 +points=poor risk group). The primary endpoint was PFS and in the everolimus and placebo groups it was 4.9 months and 1.87 months ($p<0.0001$), respectively. The PFS benefit was seen in all three MSKCC risk groups. Common side effects included asthenia, anemia and stomatitis. Up to 14% of patients experienced some form of pneumonitis. OS was 14.79 and 14.39 months ($p=0.117$) respectively, however crossover to everolimus was permitted in this study. One hundred and six patients randomized to placebo crossed over to receive everolimus after initial progression. For this group, the median PFS was 5.09 months, which is similar to the PFS of the original everolimus group. This is the first agent tested in a second-line trial after initial TKI failure to demonstrate benefit. US FDA approval has recently been granted.

9. Axitinib (AG013736)

AG013736 is another orally bioavailable small-molecule TKI of VEGFR-2 and PDGFR-B that has shown activity in metastatic RCC. Preclinical data from Inai and colleagues suggested that AG013736 inhibited angiogenesis and caused regression of existing tumor vessels.A phase II trial enrolled 62 treatment-refractory patients with RCC that had progressed on sorafenib [24]. They were treated with oral axitinib 5mg twice daily. Of 62 patients, 13 (21%) patients exhibited a partial response and the median PFS was 7.4 months. Another phase II trial with axitinib enrolled cytokine-refractory, nephrectomized patients and demonstrated a response rate of 44.2% and a median time to progression of 15.7 months (25]. Grade 1/2 toxicity included hypertension (33%), fatigue (29%), nausea (29%), diarrhea (27%), hoarseness (19%), anorexia (17%), and weight loss (15%). Grade 3/4 toxicity included hypertension (18%), diarrhea (6%), fatigue (6%), blister (4%), and limb pain (4%). These studies confirm that AG-013736 produces a substantial objective response rate in cytokine-refractory, metastatic RCC.

10. Pazopanib (GW786034)

Pazopanib hydrochloride is an oral, angiogenesis inhibitor targeting vascular endothelial growth factor receptor, platelet-derived growth factor receptor, and c-kit. In October 2009, the US Food and Drug Administration–approved pazopanib for the treatment of patients with advanced renal cell carcinoma. In the international, multicenter, randomized, double-blind trial, 435 patients were randomly assigned (2:1) to receive pazopanib (n = 290) or placebo (n = 145), [26]. The study demonstrated a median progression-free survival (the primary endpoint) of 9.2 months in the pazopanib arm vs 4.2 months in the placebo arm (hazard ratio [HR]: 0.46; P <.001). This effect was observed both in patients who had not received previous treatment (HR: 0.40) as well as patients pretreated with cytokine therapy (HR: 0.54). The median duration of responses was 13.5 months. The overall survival results were not mature yet and 40% of patients died by the time of final data cut-off. Based on this study, the recommended dose of pazopanib for the treatment of advanced renal cell carcinoma is 800 mg administered orally once daily without food (at least 1 hour before or 2 hours after a meal).

11. BAY 73-4506

BAY 73-4506 is an orally active, potent multikinase inhibitor targeting both tumor cell proliferation and tumor vasculature through inhibition of receptors of tyrosine kinases (VEGFR, KIT, RET, FGFR, and PDGFR) and serine/threonine kinases (RAF and p38MAPK). Previously untreated patients with predominantly clear cell RCC and measurable disease according to RECIST were enrolled in this multicenter, open-label, phase II study. Eligibility criteria included ECOG performance status 0–1, low or intermediate risk MSKCCC prognostic profiles, and adequate bone marrow and organ function. Treatment consisted of BAY 73-4506

160mg once daily on a 3 weeks on/1 week off schedule. The primary endpoint was overall response rate. Preliminary efficacy data of the 33 patients evaluable for response show a 27% partial response (PR) and a 42% stable disease (SD) rate [27].

12. Sequence of targeted therapy

Currently, we have the fortunate problem of having several agents demonstrating efficacy in the first- and second-line setting, with a number of other small molecule inhibitors that target VEGFR tyrosine kinase being evaluated in mRCC consistently showing activity. With similar mechanisms of action, clinical responses have been observed, including in patients that have previously received TKI therapy. Part of the challenge in moving forward is the lack of understanding of the biologic underpinnings of resistance to the currently approved agents and uniform clinical definitions of what truly constitutes treatment resistance.

Studies combining targeted therapies are being performed with the known caveat that combinations are associated with high financial cost and risk of increased toxicity due to additive and overlapping side effect profiles. Rational combinations of active agents continue to be evaluated. Currently, combinations of targeted therapy remain experimental and they should only be employed in the context of a clinical trial.

Targeted agents are also being studied in the adjuvant setting for patients with resected highrisk RCC. The Adjuvant Sorafenib or Sunitinib for Unfavorable Renal Carcinoma (ASSURE) intergroup trial randomizes high-risk nephrectomized patients to 1 year of sorafenib, sunitinib or placebo (estimated enrolment: 1332, primary endpoint: disease-free survival (DFS)) (NCT00326898). Other trials such as the phase III sunitinib versus placebo study for the treatment of patients at high risk of recurrent RCC (S-TRAC: estimated enrolment 236, primary endpoint: DFS) (NCT00375674) and the sorafenib versus placebo trial in patients with resected intermediate or high-risk RCC (SORCE: estimated enrolment 1656, primary endpoint: DFS) (NCT00492258) will further help elucidate the effect of these agents in the adjuvant setting.

13. Combination therapy

One of the next directions in the therapy of advanced RCC involves the combination of several targeted agents to better inhibit a single pathway at several different levels or inhibition at the same level of several pathways mediating different effects. As combinations of targeted agents undergo investigation, it will be critical for these combinations to demonstrate clinical benefit above and beyond those of sequential monotherapy with the same agents, in order to justify the added toxicity and risk. Thus, prospective data in this regard are critical, and some data have recently emerged.

http://dx.doi.org/10.5772/54856

Combinations of VEGF-targeting agents have undergone initial testing. Several combinations of these targeted agents were studied, including temsirolimus with either bevacizumab or sorafenib. Bevacizumab was also combined with sunitinib, and PTK787/ZK222584. These combinations have frequently demonstrated enhanced toxicity, preventing the use of the maximum single-agent doses. However, temsirolimus and bevacizumab in combination could be given at full doses of each agent without enhanced toxicity and with encouraging clinical activity.

The combination of sorafenib and bevacizumab showed preliminary evidence of antitumor activity, but the full doses of each agents were not reached due to dose-limiting toxicity related primarily to hand-foot syndrome, functional stomatitis, anorexia, and fatigue.

Additional preclinical data have described potentially favorable immunomodulation with sunitinib therapy. Such data may provide a rationale for combination strategies with immunotherapy to optimize antitumor effect.

At this point, such combinations cannot be recommended for routine use outside of a clinical trial setting.A greater understanding of the pleiotropic effects of targeted agents is needed to rationally build combinations.

14. Future directions and conclusions

Surgery is the mainstay of therapy across renal cell carcinoma stages, and surgical innovation has resulted in less invasive approaches to localized disease while preserving oncologic efficacy. Renal cell carcinoma has become a model for solid tumors in which a better understanding of biologic pathways has led to systemic therapies that have dramatically improved patient outcomes. Given the availability of multiple treatment options, each with a slightly different profile of risk and benefit, there are currently multiple options for therapy. The approach to treatment requires appreciation of the risks and benefits of each of these agents, as well as knowledge of the limitations of the current data.

The goal for every metastatic renal cell carcinoma patient upon presentation is to maximize overall therapeutic benefit, meaning delaying for as long possible a lethal burden of disease while maximizing quality of life and patient convenience.

Author details

V. Michalaki, M. Balafouta, D. Voros and C. Gennatas

Oncology Unit Areteion Hospital Univesity of Athens, Greece

References

[1] Campbell, S. C, & Lane, B. R. (2012). Malignant renal tumors. In A. Wein, L. Kavoussi, A. Novick, A. Partin, & C. Peters (Eds.), Campbell-Walsh urology (10th ed., Philadelphia: Elsevier Saunders., 1413-1474.

[2] Barrisford, G. W, Singer, E. A, Rosner, I. L, Linehan, W. M, & Bratslavsky, G. Familial renal cancer: molecular genetics and surgical management.Int J Surg Oncol. (2011).

[3] Rini, B. I, & Small, E. J. (2005). Biology and clinical development of vascular endothelial growth factortargeted therapy in renal cell carcinoma. J Clin Oncol , 23, 1028-1043.

[4] Altomare, D. A, & Testa, J. R. (2005). Perturbations of the AKT signaling pathway in human cancer. Oncogene , 24, 7455-7464.

[5] Hudson, C. C, Liu, M, Chiang, G. G, Otterness, D. M, Loomis, D. C, Kaper, F, et al. (2002). Regulation of hypoxia-inducible factor 1alpha expression and function by the mammalian target of rapamycin. Mol Cell Biol , 22, 7004-7014.

[6] Shen, C. Kaelin WG Jr. The VHL/HIF axis in clear cell renal carcinoma. Semin Cancer Biol. (2012).

[7] Medici, D, & Olsen, B. R. Rapamycin Inhibits Proliferation of Hemangioma Endothelial Cells by Reducing HIF-Dependent Expression of VEGF. PLoS One. (2012). e42913.., 1.

[8] Pal, S. K, Williams, S, Josephson, D. Y, Carmichael, C, Vogelzang, N. J, & Quinn, D. I. Novel therapies for metastatic renal cell carcinoma: efforts to expand beyond the VEGF/mTOR signaling paradigm. Mol Cancer Ther. (2012). Mar;, 11(3), 526-37.

[9] Hilmi, C, Guyot, M, & Pagès, G. VEGF spliced variants: possible role of anti-angiogenesis therapy. J Nucleic Acids. (2012).

[10] Bukowski, R. M, Kabbinavar, F. F, Figlin, R. A, Flaherty, K, Srinivas, S, Vaishampayan, U, et al. (2007). Randomized phase II study of erlotinib combined with bevacizumab compared with bevacizumab alone in metastatic renal cell cancer. J Clin Oncol , 25, 4536-4541.

[11] Choueiri, T. K, Plantade, A, Elson, P, Negrier, S, Ravaud, A, Oudard, S, et al. (2008). Efficacy of sunitinib and sorafenib in metastatic papillary and chromophobe renal cell carcinoma. J Clin Oncol , 26, 127-131.

[12] Christensen, J. G. (2007). A preclinical review of sunitinib, a multitargeted receptor tyrosine kinase inhibitor with anti-angiogenic and antitumour activities. Ann Oncol 18(Suppl 10): x, 3-10.

[13] Mendel, D. B, Laird, A. D, Xin, X, Louie, S. G, Christensen, J. G, Li, G, et al. (2003). In vivo antitumor activity of SU11248, a novel tyrosine kinase inhibitor targeting vascular endothelial growth factor and platelet-derived growth factor receptors: determination of a pharmacokinetic/pharmacodynamic relationship. Clin Cancer Res , 9, 327-337.

[14] Motzer, R. J, Hutson, T. E, Tomczak, P, Michaelson, M. D, Bukowski, R. M, Rixe, O, et al. (2007b). Sunitinib versus interferon alfa in metastatic renal-cell carcinoma. N Engl J Med , 356, 115-124.

[15] Motzer, R. J, Michaelson, M. D, Rosenberg, J, Bukowski, R. M, Curti, B. D, George, D. J, et al. (2007a). Sunitinib efficacy against advanced renal cell carcinoma. J Urol , 178, 1883-1887.

[16] Witteles, R. M, Telli, M. L, Fisher, G. A, & Srinivas, S. (2008). Cardiotoxicity associated with the cancer therapeutic agent sunitinib malate. J Clin Oncol 26: 9597.

[17] Heng, D. Y, Chi, K. N, Murray, N, Jin, T, Garcia, J. A, Bukowski, R. M, et al. (2009). A population-based study evaluating the impact of sunitinib on overall survival in the treatment of patients with metastatic renal cell cancer. Cancer , 115, 776-783.

[18] Ahmad, T, & Eisen, T. (2004). Kinase inhibition with BAY in renal cell carcinoma. Clin Cancer Res 10: 6388S-92S., 43-9006.

[19] Escudier, B, Eisen, T, Stadler, W. M, Szczylik, C, Oudard, S, Siebels, M, et al. (2007a). Sorafenib in advanced clear-cell renal-cell carcinoma. N Engl J Med , 356, 125-134.

[20] Escudier, B, Szczylik, C, Hutson, T. E, Demkow, T, Staehler, M, Rolland, F, et al. (2009a). Randomized phase II trial of first-line treatment with sorafenib versus interferon Alfa-2a in patients with metastatic renal cell carcinoma. J Clin Oncol , 27, 1280-1289.

[21] Atkins, M. B, Hidalgo, M, Stadler, W. M, Logan, T. F, Dutcher, J. P, Hudes, G. R, et al. (2004). Randomized phase II study of multiple dose levels of CCI-779, a novel mammalian target of rapamycin kinase inhibitor, in patients with advanced refractory renal cell carcinoma. J Clin Oncol , 22, 909-918.

[22] Hudes, G, Carducci, M, Tomczak, P, Dutcher, J, Figlin, R, Kapoor, A, et al. (2007). Temsirolimus, interferon alfa, or both for advanced renal-cell carcinoma. N Engl J Med , 356, 2271-2281.

[23] Kay, A, Motzer, R, Figlin, R, Escudier, B, Oudard, S, Porta, C, et al. (2009). Updated data from a phase III randomized trial of everolimus (RAD001) versus PBO in metastatic renal cell carcinoma (mRCC). Genitourinary Cancers Symposium, February Orlando., 26-28.

[24] Rini, B. I, Wilding, G, Hudes, G, Stadler, W. M, Kim, S, Tarazi, J. C, et al. (2007). Axitinib (AG-013736; AG) in patients (pts) with metastatic renal cell cancer (RCC) refractory to sorafenib. J Clin Oncol 25: 5032.

[25] Rixe, O, Bukowski, R. M, Michaelson, M. D, Wilding, G, Hudes, G. R, Bolte, O, et al. (2007). Axitinib treatment in patients with cytokine-refractory metastatic renal-cell cancer: a phase II study. Lancet Oncol , 8, 975-984.

[26] Sternberg, C. N, Szczylik, C, Lee, E, Salman, P. V, Mardiak, J, Davis, I. D, et al. (2009). A randomized, double-blind phase III study of pazopanib in treatment-naive and

cytokine-pretreated patients with advanced renal cell carcinoma (RCC). J Clin Oncol 27: 5021.

[27] Eisen, T, Joensuu, H, Nathan, P, Harper, P, Wojtukiewicz, M, Nicholson, S, et al. (2009). Phase II study of BAY a multikinase inhibitor, in previously untreated patients with metastatic or unresectable renal cell cancer. J Clin Oncol 27: 5033., 73-4506.

Chapter 10

New Systemic Treatment Approaches for Metastatic Renal Cell Carcinoma

Thean Hsiang Tan, Sina Vatandoust and
Michail Charakidis

Additional information is available at the end of the chapter

http://dx.doi.org/10.5772/55280

1. Introduction

Kidney cancer comprises 2-3% of all cancers according to Cancer Research UK statistics. (http://info.cancerresearchuk.org). Renal Cell Carcinomas (RCC) is the most common subtype (around 90%) with clear-cell variant constituting up to 75% of all RCCs. Non clear-cell variant are less common and consist of papillary (Type I and II; 10-15%), chromophobe (4%) and collecting duct (including the rare medullary variant; <1%). [1, 2] At initial diagnosis, one third of patients have evidence of distant metastases, and amongst patients who undergo curative nephrectomy, a third will have a recurrence within 5 years. Historically, treatment options have been limited in metastatic RCC, as cytotoxic chemotherapy is not effective in this disease and immunotherapy is of modest benefit. [1] The treatment outlook for metastatic RCC has changed in the past decade, with the introduction of new therapeutic agents which target molecular pathways involved in tumour angiogenesis.

2. Molecular pathogenesis

2.1. Clear- cell variants renal cell carcinoma

The discovery of von Hippel–Lindau (VHL) / hypoxia-inducible factor (HIF) oxygen-sensing pathway and its role in the pathogenesis of RCC (clear-cell as well as some of the non-clear-cell variant), has led to a new approach in the systemic therapy for RCC. [1, 3] Tumour suppressor gene VHL encodes the VHL protein (pVHL), which interacts with hypoxia-inducible factor (HIF) to regulate cellular response to oxygen deprivation. HIF is a gene

INTECH
open science | open minds

© 2013 Tan et al.; licensee InTech. This is a paper distributed under the terms of the Creative Commons Attribution License (http://creativecommons.org/licenses/by/3.0), which permits unrestricted use, distribution, and reproduction in any medium, provided the original work is properly cited.

transcription factor and consists of two subunits: HIF α-subunit and the HIF β-subunit (also known as aryl hydrocarbon receptor nuclear translocator (ARNT) protein). In the presence of normal oxygen tension (or normoxic state), HIF-α is hydroxylated. pVHL-E3 ubiquitin ligase complex targets the hydroxylated HIF-α for proteosomal degradation. [4] VHL protein functions as the substrate-recognition subunit of this complex. [5, 6]

VHL gene mutation or hypermethylation leads to intracellular accumulation of HIF-α subunits. [7] HIF-α subunits, after translocation into the nucleus, act in concert with the HIF-β subunits, and form transcriptional factor complexes that induce transcription of hypoxia-response genes. [8] The endpoint is an increase in the production of pro-angiogenic factors including vascular endothelial growth factor (VEGF), platelet-derived growth factor (PDGF) and transforming growth factor alpha and beta (TGF-α and TGF-β). [9] By increasing angiogenesis through VHL-HIF pathway the tumour increases its potential to survive and progress. [10]

2.2. Non clear-cell variant

Papillary carcinomas are commonly bilateral, multifocal and frequently present as small, early stage tumours. [11] They can be further subdivided histologically into papillary types I and II with underlying different genetics and molecular pathways. [12] Type I papillary renal cancers are linked to activating mutations of the methyl-nitroso-nitroguanidine induced (MET) oncogene. [13] The MET oncogene mutations activate the intracellular kinase domains and subsequently trigger the hepatocyte growth / MET pathway. [13] Type II papillary renal cancers on the other hand are associated with mutations of the fumarate hydratase (FH) tumour suppressor gene. [14] Mutational inactivation of the FH tumour suppressor gene leads to a pseudo-hypoxic state and up-regulation of the HIF α-subunits. The accumulation of fumarate is induced by the mutated FH enzyme. That in turn causes inhibition of HIF-prolyl hydroxylase(HPH), an enzymatic regulator of the intracellular HIF-α. Inactivation of the HPH disrupts the hydroxylation of HIF leading to failure of recognition by pVHL and subsequent VHL-dependent proteosomal degradation of HIFs. Accumulation of HIF leads to over-expression of pro-angiogenic factors and tumour proliferation. [15]

Chromophobe renal cell cancers accounts for 4% of all RCCs. [1] The exact pathogenesis is not established. It is thought that the VEGF-angiogenic pathway is implicated based on the elevated levels of VEGF and its receptors in this type of RCC. The KIT oncogene and the folliculin gene linked to the familial form of chromophobe/oncocytic RCC hybrid (Brit-Hogg-Dubé-Syndrome), are extra molecular targets identified in this variant [16, 17] Collecting duct RCC are very rare and the underlying pathogenesis has not been established. [18]

3. Systemic treatment of metastatic renal cell carcinoma

The current guidelines from the National Comprehensive Cancer Network Metastatic (NCCN) continue to identify nephrectomy as an important initial consideration, even in the context of metastatic disease. [19] The current recommendations are to consider patients for nephrectomy and/or oligmetastatectomy prior to initiation of systemic therapy whenever appropriate. [20]

The traditional teaching is that cytoreductive nephrectomy lead to improved outcome from systemic therapy. This is based on phase III data that showed an improvement in response to IFN-α following nephrectomy in the metastatic setting. In the era of targeted therapy / anti-VEGF therapies, the validity of this practice has been called into question. [20] Clinical trials are underway to address this very question.

Beyond surgery, the only systemic options available prior to the era of targeted therapy consisted of interleukin-2 (IL-2) and interferon-α (IFN-α). Other treatments that had been trialed included chemo- and hormonal therapy have all been discouraging. [21]

IFN-α classically caused flu-like syndrome, depression and in some cases suicidal ideation and is certainly onerous especially in the patients with poorer performance status. [1, 22] IL-2, the other cytokine has a small long term survival benefit of 4%. This is however at the cost of potentially life threatening toxicities such as hypotension, oliguria, capillary leak syndrome with secondary multi-organ failure, somnolence and confusion. [23] Not surprisingly, the underlying enthusiasm for cytokine agents as frontline therapy in metastatic RCC has been replaced by tyrosine kinase inhibitors / targeted therapy which has a more favourable toxicity profile. [24]

The targeted therapies used in metastatic RCC consist of 1. Anti-VEGFs, which are monoclonal antibodies that bind directly to VEGF and related peptides and therefore removing them from the circulation (bevacizumab) and 2. Small molecule tyrosine kinase inhibitors (SMTKIs) that target the down-stream tyrosine kinase signaling pathways, are involved in promotion of tumour angiogenesis, endothelial growth, proliferation and ultimately tumour survival and metastasis. [25] The SMTKIs that have been approved for use in 2012 include sunitinib, sorafenib, pazopanib and axitinib.

3.1. Small molecular tyrosine kinase inhibitors

3.1.1. Sunitinib

Sunitinib is a multi-kinase inhibitor targeting numerous VEGF receptors (VEGF-1, 2, 3) and additional tyrosine kinase receptors (PDGFR, c-Kit, FLT-3, CSF-1R, and RET) [26-29] Early trials showed sunitinib to be effective in patients with advanced malignancies including RCC. [30]

3.1.1.1. Sunitinib intermittent dosing

A phase II study of sunitinib in patients with cytokine-refractory metastatic RCC assessed the clinical efficacy and safety of sunitinib as second-line therapy. [31] Sixty three patients who previously failed cytokine-based therapy received 50mg of sunitinib for 4 weeks followed by a 2 week scheduled break, in a 6 week cycle. A partial response of 40% (n=25) (PR) and a stable disease response for ≥ 3 months in 27% (n=17) of the patients were reported. The median time to progression and survival were 8.7 months and 16.4 months respectively. [31]

A second but larger phase II trial of 106 patients similarly confirmed promising activities of sunitinib in cytokine refractory, metastatic RCC. An overall objective response of 44% was observed with 1% (n=1) of patients demonstrated a CR and 44% showed PR. [32] A further

22% (n=23) of patients showed SD for ≥ 3 months. The median response for the 46 responders was 10 months whilst the median progression free survival (PFS) was 8.3 months [32]

These results led to a phase III trial comparing sunitinib with INF-α that was deemed standard of care at the time for patients with metastatic clear cell RCC. [33] Seven hundred and fifty treatment naïve patients with clear-cell histology and good performance status (ECOG 0 or 1) were randomized in a 1:1 ratio to receive either sunitinib (dose as per earlier studies) or INF-α (9×10^6 units subcutaneously thrice weekly). [32, 34] The median duration of treatment was 6 months (1-15 months) in the sunitinib group and 4 months (1-13 months) in the IFN-α group. The median PFS assessed by an independent third-party review was 11 months in the sunitinib group and 5 months in the IFN-α group, corresponding to a hazard ratio (HR) of 0.42 (95% CI 0.32–0.54; $p < 0.001$). [33] The investigators' assessment showed similar results. An updated analysis published in 2009 has shown the ORR of 47% for sunitinib and 12% for IFN-α ($p < 0.000001$), with a median PFS of 11 months and 5 months, respectively, for sunitinib and IFN-α ($p < 0.000001$), similar to the original report. [35] These results were uniformly seen, regardless of the patients' age, gender and prognostic category. Patients on sunitinib also experienced a median OS in excess of 2 years. The OS was 26.4 months for sunitinib and 21.8 months for IFN-α ($p = 0.051$). [33] However, a dedicated exploratory analysis of patients on both treatment arms who did not receive post-study cancer treatment showed the median OS with sunitinib was twice as long as IFN-α (28.1 months versus 14.1 months respectively, p=0.003). [33] Based on these significant findings, sunitinib replaced IFN-α as first line treatment for stage IV RCC.

In a real-world setting, sunitinib has proven its efficacy in an expanded-access program, designed to allocate access to sunitinib in patients with metastatic RCC who would otherwise be excluded from clinical trials. [33, 36] Four thousand five hundred patients were enrolled in this international, open labeled study. The cohort importantly included older patients (≥ 65 years old; n=1414), those with poorer ECOG status (≥ 2; n=582), non clear-cell histology (n=288) and with brain metastases (n=320). [36] Patients with poor performance status and brain metastases prior to this had been excluded in all sunitinib trials.

The median number of treatment cycles and treatment duration were 5 cycles and 15.6 months respectively. 56% of patients received more than 6 months of sunitinib treatment. The survival data closely resembled the phase III study with an observed median PFS and OS of 10.9 months and 18.4 months respectively. [33] No differences were noted in median PFS and OS between patients with or without prior cytokine therapy. Importantly, the subgroup analysis of i. elderly patients demonstrated median PFS and OS of 11.3 and 18.2 months respectively. [33] ii. patients with poorer performance status, the median PFS and OS were 5.1 months and 6.7 months respectively and finally in patients with brain metastases with an overall poorer prognosis, a median PFS of 5.6 months and median OS of 9.2 months were observed. [33]

3.1.1.2. Sunitinib continuous dosing

The efficacy of continuous sunitinib dosing was examined in an open-label multicenter phase II trial. [37] In this study 107 patients were randomly assigned to either morning or evening daily dose of 37.5mg for a median duration of 8.3 months. 43% of patients had their dose reduced due to grade 3-4 adverse events. The ORR was 20% with a median duration of response of 7.2 months. The median PFS observed was 8.2 months and the OS was 19.8 months. Tolerability and QOL between the morning and evening dose were similar. However, grade 3 diarrhea, fatigue and hand-foot syndrome were more common in the evening dosing patients. The continuous schedule may benefit patients who are not able to tolerate the intermittent sunitinib 50mg regimen. [33]

Another trial assessing continuous vs. intermittent sunitinib dosing was the EFFECT phase II study. In this trial patients with locally recurrent clear-cell RCC or metastatic RCC, treatment naïve patients, were randomly assigned to standard dosing (50mg/day; 4 weeks on, 2 weeks off) and continuous dosing (37.5mg/day). The intermittent schedule when compared with the continuous schedule showed a trend to improved ORR (32.2% vs. 28.1%; p=0.444) and median PFS (8.5 months vs. 7.0 months; p=0.070). No difference were noted between the median OS (23.1 months vs. 23.5 months, p=0.615). [38] Interestingly the median OS was lower than the phase III sunitinib vs. INF-α trial which had a median OS of 26 months. The phase III trial had a higher number of patients with better baseline prognostic features (better performance status and more patients had underwent nephrectomy), which may account for better survival results. [33, 38]

3.1.2. Sorafenib

Sorafenib (Nexavar, BAY 43-9006) is an oral multi-kinase inhibitor that targets multiple non-receptor as well as receptor kinases. These include BRAF and CRAF, non-receptor serine threonine kinases which belong to the RAF/Mek/ERK signaling pathway and also receptor tyrosine kinases including VEGFR2, VEGFR3, PDGFR, fetal liver tyrosine kinase 3 (FLT-3)… and c-kit. [2] In a phase II randomized discontinuation trial of patients with metastatic RCC who had failed previous systemic therapies, sorafenib at a dose of 400 mg BD showed significant disease-stabilizing activity. [39] In another phase II trial, patients with metastatic RCC on sorafenib (initial starting dose of 400mg BD and escalating to 600mg BD on progression) were compared with INF-α in the first line setting. PFS was similar in both arms, although in the sorafenib arm, patients experienced greater rates of tumour size reduction, superior quality of life and better treatment tolerance. [40] Subsequently in a phase 3 trial (TARGET) 903 patients with metastatic clear-cell RCC who had progressed on previous treatment were randomized to receive either placebo or sorafenib (400mg BD). Compared with the placebo group, the sorafenib group demonstrated a higher ORR (57% vs. 34%) and PFS was significantly longer (5.5 months vs. 2.8 months; HR=0.44; p<0.01). [41] This improvement was independent of age (over or under 70 years), prognostic risk, prior cytokine therapy, and previous cardiovascular disease. [41] In this trial, patients in the placebo arm crossed over to sorafenib when progression of disease was diagnosed. In the first interim analysis, a trend towards better OS was noted in patients taking sorafenib, and this was unchanged in the final analysis (17.8 vs. 15.2 months, respectively, HR= 0.88; p = 0.146). [42] After censoring for the patients who had crossed over on progression from the placebo arm, the OS was significantly longer in the sorafenib arm (17.8 vs. 14.3 months; HR = 0.78; p = 0.029). [41] Sorafenib has also been accessed in a real-world setting through open-label expanded access studies in Europe (The European Advanced Renal Cell Carcinoma Sorafenib (EU-ARCS) and North America

(NA-ARCCS). Both studies showed that sorafenib provides similar benefits in first- and second- or later line patient populations and the safety profile was similar to that reported in clinical trials. [43-45] Ongoing clinical trials comparing sorafenib with other treatment options in the first line setting are currently being undertaken. [46]

The role of sorafenib as second line treatment for advanced RCC has also generated significant interest. Sorafenib was compared directly with temsirolimus in the INTORSECT trial. [47] This is the first head-to-head trial comparing a VEGF inhibitor to an mTOR inhibitor. This trial enrolled 551 patients with advanced RCC with good performance status who had progressed after first-line sunitinib therapy. The median PFS with temsirolimus was 4.28 months and 3.91 months with sorafenib. The median OS for temsirolimus cohort was 12.7 months compared to 16.6 months in the sorafenib arm. These results highlighted that temsirolimus did not show superiority over sorafenib in the primary end-point of PFS and the secondary end-point of OS. [47] To date, sorafenib is considered a reasonable first-line treatment option especially in elderly patients or patients with cardiovascular diseases or other co-morbidities. [46, 48]

3.1.3. Pazopanib

Pazopanib is an oral tyrosine kinase inhibitor that targets VEGF-1, -2, and -3 receptors, PDGF-α and -β receptors, and c-kit. [49] A phase II study enrolled 225 patients with metastatic RCC: (69% were treatment naïve, and 31% had received previous treatment with cytokine- or bevacizumab-containing regimen). In this study, the ORR was 35%, median duration of response was 68 weeks and median PFS was 52 weeks. This trial showed durable activity and tolerability of pazopanib in patients with advanced RCC. (Hutson *et al*, 2010) In a phase III study, 435 patients with locally advanced, and/or metastatic RCC were randomized to receive oral pazopanib or placebo (54% were treatment naïve and 46% were cytokine pretreated). The PFS was significantly prolonged with pazopanib compared with placebo (median PFS 9.2 vs. 4.2 months; HR=0.46; 95% CI, 0.34 to 0.62; $p < 0.0001$), with similar results shown in both the Treatment naïve subpopulation (median PFS 11.1 v 2.8 months; HR, 0.40; 95% CI, 0.27 to 0.60; $P < .0001$), and the cytokine-pretreated subpopulation (median PFS, 7.4 v 4.2 months; HR, 0.54; 95% CI, 0.35 to 0.84; $p < 0.001$). In the pazopanib arm, the ORR was 30% compared with 3% in the placebo arm ($p < 0.001$). The median duration of response was longer than 1 year. [50] The final median OS were 22.9 vs. 20.5 months in the pazopanib and placebo arms respectively ($p=0.224$). The lack of significant difference could be due to the early, frequent, and prolonged crossover to pazopanib in patients originally randomized to placebo. [50, 51] Whilst the role of pazopanib as a frontline agent for metastatic RCC is being established, it remains unclear how it compares with sunitinib in terms of efficacy. This was addressed in an open-label study (COMPARZ) where pazopanib was compared head-to-head with sunitinib in 1100 patients with locally advanced and/or metastatic RCC. Pazopanib demonstrated similar efficacy or non-inferiority to sunitinib in terms of PFS with duration of more than 10 months. Both agents resulted in side-effects, however fatigue and skin ulcers occurred less frequently for pazopanib than with sunitinib. The quality of life (QoL) favoured pazopanib and demonstrated better tolerance for pazopanib than sunitinib. [52]

3.1.4. Axitinib

Axitinib, an oral agent that inhibits VEGF receptor-1, -2 and -3, is active in cytokine-refractory metastatic RCC. Two complete and 21 partial responses (ORR of 44.2%) were reported in 52 patients taking axitinib 5mg twice daily in a second line treatment study. The median response duration was 23 months and median OS was 29.9 months. [53] The 5 year survival rate was 20.6%. The ten patients surviving for more than five years had an ORR of 100% compared with 30% in <5 year survivors. They took axitinib for longer (median 5.8 years vs. 0.67 years) and were fitter, with baseline ECOG PS of 0 in 80% of the longer term survivors compared with 53% in <5 year survivors. [54]

In a phase II trial, 213 patients were allocated on axitinib 5mg BD for four weeks, after which some eligible patients were randomly assigned to further stepwise dose titration (5 to 7 to 10mg BD) according to tolerability of either axitinib or placebo. Individuals who did not meet the eligibility criteria were treated in a separate arm without dose titration. [55] The inclusion criteria for randomisation after the initial dose schedule of axitinib for 4 weeks were blood pressure ≤ 150/90 mmHg and less or equal to 2 concurrent anti-hypertensive medications. No grade 3 or 4 toxicities from the initial dose and no dose reductions required in the first 4 weeks of axitinib.

The most important outcomes of this study were a higher drug exposure, of more or equal 150 ng-h/ml serum concentration, and was associated with a higher RR (59% vs. 40%) and an improvement in PFS (14 vs. 11 months). Patients with a higher diastolic blood pressure (90mmHg) and an increase in diastolic blood pressure on day 15 of the first cycle had better outcomes in ORR and PFS. The final results of this phase II trial are pending and will determine if the titratrion strategy is associated with improved clinical outcomes

In a phase III second line treatment study (AXIS), 723 patients with progressive disease after one first line treatment (sunitinib, bevacizumab, temsirolimus or cytokines) randomly received axitinib at doses titrated from 5mg up to 10mg BD or sorafenib 400mg BD. [56] The ORR was 19.4% for axitinib vs. 9.4% for sorafenib (p=0.0001) and a significantly longer median PFS (6.7 versus 4.7 months, p<0.0001) was seen in patients on the axitinib arm. In patients who had previously received cytokines PFS with axitinib was 12.1 months vs. 6.5 months with sorafenib, which was significant (p<0.0001). This also occurred in those having prior sunitinib (4.8 vs. 3.4 months, p=0.0107). As part of the same trial, patient-reported kidney specific symptom and function assessments were secondary endpoints. [57] Outcomes were similar for both drugs during treatment, however due to the significantly longer PFS with axitinib, this delayed worsening of the composite endpoint of cancer symptoms, progression or death compared with sorafenib. [56]

3.2. Anti-VEGF

3.2.1. Bevacizumab

Bevacizumab is a humanized monoclonal antibody that inhibits the VEGF molecule and therefore targeting all the receptor to which it binds. [58]) A randomized, double-blind, phase

II trial of 116 patients (placebo controlled, low-dose 3mg/kg or high dose 10mg/kg) showed that bevacizumab significantly prolonged the time to progression of disease in patients with metastatic RCC. [59, 60]

In a phase III trial (AVOREN), 649 patients with previously untreated metastatic RCC were randomized to receive bevacizumab (10 mg/kg infusion) and interferon alfa-2a versus placebo and interferon alfa-2a (IFN). A significant improvement in PFS, (10.2 vs. 5.4 months) and also ORR (31% vs. 13%, respectively; $p < 0.0001$) was observed in the bevacizumab arm compared with the IFN-α monotherapy arm. [61] Final OS analysis of this trial showed a trend towards improved OS (Median OS was 23.3 months with bevacizumab plus IFN and 21.3 months with IFN plus placebo). Patients (> 55%) in both arms received at least one post-protocol anti-neoplastic treatment, which could confound the OS analysis. [61]

Another concurrent phase III trial (CALGB 90206) but in a non-blinded fashion, randomized 732 patients previously untreated metastatic RCC to receive bevacizumab and IFN-α versus monotherapy with IFN-α. In this trial, the median PFS was 8.5 months in patients receiving bevacizumab plus IFN compared with 5.2 months for IFN monotherapy ($p < 0.0001$) and the ORR was similarly higher in the bevacizumab plus IFN arm than in the IFN monotherapy arm (25.5% vs. 13.1%, respectively; $p< 0.0001$). [62] Final analysis of this trial showed a median OS time of 18.3 months (95% CI, 16.5 to 22.5 months) for bevacizumab plus IFN-alpha and 17.4 months (95% CI, 14.4 to 20.0 months) for IFN-alpha monotherapy (unstratified log-rank $p = 0.097$) Grade 3 and 4 toxicity (hypertension (HTN), anorexia, fatigue, and proteinuria) were significantly higher in the bevacizumab plus IFN-alpha arm. Patients who developed HTN on bevacizumab plus IFN-alpha had a significantly improved PFS and OS versus patients without HTN. [62]

Both of these trials showed clear benefits in the median PFS arms with an overlapping HR and doubling of PFS when comparing the placebo/IFN-α arm with bevacizumab/IFN-α arm. [63] The effects of crossover to the active bevacizumab arm in the AVOREN trial, as well as the permission of second-line therapies in both trials would account for the dilution of the actual OS benefit in both trials. [63] Based on the results of these trials, regulatory approval of bevacizumab plus IFN in advanced RCC has occurred in Europe in the United States.

3.3. mTOR inhibitors

The mammalian target of rapamycin (mTOR) pathway is regulated by the PTEN tumour suppressor gene. It plays a significant role in angiogenesis and regulation of cell cycle. [8] mTOR activity is dependent on different factors, in particular to cellular stresses such as hypoxia, heat shock, oxidative stress, DNA damage and finally a change in the pH or osmotic cell pressure. [8] The mTOR pathway is downstream to phosphoinositide 3-kinase and akt pathway which is dysregulated in many malignancies. [8, 64] Activation of this pathway promotes mRNA translation and subsequent entry into the G_1 phase of cell cycle. Another different but important function of mTOR is the production of HIF-1α which drives angiogenesis, survival and growth of malignant cells. The selective inhibition of this pathway by the mTOR inhibitors is facilitated by binding to the intracellular protein FK506 binding protein 12 (FKBP-12) resulting in inhibition of the kinase activity of the mTOR. [8] There are two mTOR inhibitors registered for the treatment of metastatic RCC, namely temsirolimus and everolimus.

3.3.1. Temsirolimus

Temsirolimus is an analogue to sirolimus (rapamycin) which has been used with success as an immunosuppressive agent in renal transplantation. [65] Temsirolimus is a parenteral preparation and is administered as a weekly intravenous infusion at 25mg. It is metabolised by CYP3A4 to active metabolite sirolimus and has a half-life of about 9 to 27 hours. [65]

Based on the encouraging results from Phase I and II trials of temsirolimus either alone, or in combination with IFN-α, an international multicentre phase III trial was conducted. [8, 66] Six hundred and twenty six treatment naïve patients with poor prognostic factors were randomised to temsirolimus (25 mg i.v. weekly), IFN-α (3×10^6 units, with an increase to 18×10^6 units s.c. thrice weekly) or the combination of temsirolimus (15 mg weekly) and IFN-α (6×10^6 thrice weekly). Patients were required to have least three the following 6 predictors short survival: a serum lactate dehydrogenase level of more than 1.5 times the upper limit of the normal range, a hemoglobin level below the lower limit of the normal range; a corrected serum calcium level of more than 10 mg per deciliter (2.5 mmol per liter), a time from initial diagnosis of RCC to randomization of less than 1 year, a Karnofsky performance score of 60 or 70, or metastases in multiple organs. An important characteristic of recruitment of this study is the inclusion of up to 20% of non clear-cell renal cell histological subtype. This is the only randomised study available to date for patients with non clear-cell histology. Patients who received temsirolimus monotherapy had a longer median OS (10.9 vs. 7.3 months; $p = 0.008$) and PFS (3.8 vs. 1.9months; $p<0.001$) compared with those who received INF-α alone. [65] Finally those in the combination treatment arm had the most grade 3 or 4 adverse events leading to more dose reductions and delays. The median PFS in the temsirolimus, combination treatment and IFN-α alone were 3.8, 3.7 and 1.9 months, respectively, and the median OS was 10.9 months, 8.4 months and 7.3 months. [65] In this trial, older patients and patients with a higher serum LDH (> 1.5 fold the upper limit of normal) had better OS. [65]

This trial did not address the role of temsirolimus as second-line agent in patients refractory to VGEF therapy. The only published prospective randomised trial looking at this cohort of patients was RECORD-1 which examined everolimus vs. placebo. [67] The data supporting the use of temsirolimus in second line treatment post VEGF agents are all derived from single institution case series which demonstrated only a modest PFS of ~4 months.

3.3.2. Everolimus

Everolimus is an oral mTOR inhibitor. It has activity against advanced clear-cell RCC in patients who have failed sorafenib, sunitinib or both. [67] In a double-blind, placebo controlled phase III trial (RECORD-1, in which 410 patients with advanced clear cell RCC who had progressed after sunitinib, sorafenib or both were randomized in a 2:1 ratio to everolimus 10 mg once daily or placebo with best supportive care. Independent of gender, age, previous treatment with sorafenib, sunitinib or both, prolongation of PFS (4.9 vs. 1.9 months; $p< 0.0001$)

was found with everolimus over placebo. [67] However there was no statistically significant difference for median OS (14.8 months vs. 14.4 months) as majority (80%) of patients in the placebo plus best supportive arm were allowed to cross over after the unbinding at the second interim analysis. RECORD-1 trial proved the efficacy of mTOR inhibitors following VGEF therapy and as such received FDA approval for patients who have progressed following sunitinib / sorafenib. [67]

4. New agents in clinical development

The results with early TKIs in metastatic RCC has led to a number of small molecules multi-targeted agents being investigated in phase II and III studies. [68] These include tivozanib which targets VEGFR -1, -2, and -3, PDGFR and c-kit, dovitinib (VEGFR -1, -2, -3 and PDGFR-beta) and regorafenib. [69]

4.1. Tivozanib

In a phase II study, two hundred and seventy two patients with advanced RCC treated who had not received prior VEGF targeted therapy received tivozanib. [70] Patients took tivozanib 1.5 mg daily for 16 weeks, and according to response were then stratified into stopping or continuing tivozanib. Those with stable disease were randomised between tivozanib and placebo (and this group could re-start tivozanib if they developed progressive disease, or completed the double blind phase). Overall, by week 16, 84% of patients demonstrated PR or SD, ORR was 30%, disease control rate (DCR) was 85% and median PFS 11.7 months. Best results were achieved in patients with clear-cell histology who had undergone a nephrectomy. These patients achieved an ORR of 36%, DCR of 88% and median PFS of 14.8 months. Commonest adverse effects included hypertension (45%) which was grade 3-4 in 12%, and dysphonia (22%). [70]

Twenty-eight patients with advanced RCC and clear-cell variant, who had failed up to one prior VEGF-targeted therapy, were treated in a phase Ib open-label study of tivozanib combined with temsirolimus. [71] Tivozanib was administered orally daily for 3 weeks on and 1 week off. Intravenous temsirolimus was given once weekly. A standard 3+3 dose escalation design was used at four levels from 0.5 mg to 1.5 mg per day and 15 to 25 mg per week of tivozanib and temsirolimus, respectively. Twenty-eight patients (26 male) of median age 62 years and Karnofsky Performance Status from 100 to 80 were participated in the study. Median duration of treatment was 21.1 weeks. PR was seen in 28%, SD in 64% and DCR (PR and SD > 24 weeks) in 48% of the treated population. Treatment-related adverse events seen in ≥ 10% of patients were: fatigue, decreased appetite, stomatitis, thrombocytopenia, diarrhea, nausea, constipation and dyspnea. There were no grade 4 events, and no dose limiting toxicities. [71]

Preliminary results of a phase III trial comparing tivozanib to sorafenib in stage IV RCC as first line treatment were made available at the ASCO 2012 annual meeting. [72] Tivozanib in comparison with sorefenib resulted in an improvement in PFS (HR 0.80; median 12 vs. 10 months respectively; p=0.04) and higher ORR (33 vs. 23%). Patients on tivozanib experienced a higher incidence of grade 3 or 4 hypertension (26 vs. 17%), higher rates of dysphonia (21 vs. 5 %) and back pain (14 vs. 7%). However, tivozanib had less diarrhea (24 vs. 38%), hand and foot syndrome (15 vs. 71%) and alopecia (2 vs. 21%). [72]

4.2. Dovitinib

The highest tolerated dose of dovitinib is 500 mg daily on a 5-day on/ 2 day off schedule in 28-day cycles. A phase II study of dovitinib in clear-cell metastatic RCC and in patients previously treated with a VEGFR inhibitor and/or mTOR inhibitor was reported in 2011. [73] In 51 patients overall responses were PR in 8%, and SD ≥ 4 months in 37%. Median PFS and OS were 6.1 and 16 months respectively. The most common adverse events were nausea (73%; grade 3:9%), diarrhea (64%; grade 3:9%), vomiting (56%; grade 3: 5%), decreased appetite (48%; grade 3:7%), asthenia (36%; grade 3:12%), and fatigue (36%; grade 3: 10%). An on-going phase 3 trials is comparing dovitinib with sorafenib in patients who have had one previous VEGF- and mTOR-targeted therapy.

4.3. Regorafenib

A phase II of regorafenib in previously untreated metastatic or unresectable RCC patients has recently been published. [69]. Forty-eight of 49 patients enrolled were available for assessment of tumour response. Nineteen of these had an objective response (partial); (39.6%, 90% CI 27.7-52.5). Side-effects were noted in 98% of patients, and 35% experienced serious drug-related events. Two patients had grade 4 adverse events related to treatment including two cardiac ischaemia or infraction, one hypomagnesaemia, and one chest/thoracic pain. The authors advise close monitoring. [69]

5. Combination therapy in metastatic RCC

With the increasing use of VEGF and mTOR inhibitors, it has been noted that patients eventually develop resistance / relapse after 6 months to 3 years of therapy. [25] This has been the driving force for the development of more novel anti-angiogenic agents or treatment strategies such as combination of the various targeted agents (combination of anti-angiogenic agents or with mTOR inhibitors, chemotherapy or immunotherapy). [74] Combination therapies may lead to a more complete blockade of aberrant signaling and potentially delay / prevent the development of resistance observed with single-agent treatment. [74] Unfortunately, this invariably leads to increased toxicities as experienced in some of the phase I trials. [75]

5.1. VEGF-ligands or receptor inhibitors / mTOR plus immunotherapy combination

Two single arm phase II studies using sorafenib in combination with standard dose IFN-α showed higher ORR (approximately 30%) and longer PFS (7 – 12 months) when compared with phase III data of sorafenib monotherapy. [76, 77] However, in a randomized phase II trial of sorafenib vs. sorafenib and low-dose IFN-α in patients with advanced RCC, no statistically significant difference in ORR and PFS was noted in the two arms. [78] These results should be interpreted cautiously given the small number of patients in these studies. [78]

Both AVOREN (n = 649) [79] and CALGB 90206 (n = 732) [80] compared bevacizumab / IFN-α combination with IFN-α demonstrated that the PFS interval was significantly longer with bevacizumab plus IFN-α than with the IFN-α alone (AVOREN: 10.2 months versus 5.4 months, respectively; p = 0.0001; CALGB 90206: 8.5 months versus 5.2 months, respectively; p < 0.0001). The ORRs were 31% with bevacizumab plus IFN-α and 13% with placebo plus IFN-α (p = 0.0001) in the AVOREN study. In the CALGB 90206 trial, the ORRs were 25.5% with bevacizumab plus IFN-α and 13.1% with IFN-α (p < 0.0001). [74, 79, 80] The design of these trials however did not have a bevacizumab monotherapy arm and therefore the clinical efficacy of bevacizumab monotherapy remained unanswered. In an open-label phase 2 study (TORAVA), 171 patients with metastatic RCC were randomly assigned (2:1:1) to receive the combination of bevacizumab (10 mg/kg every 2 weeks) and temsirolimus (25 mg weekly) or sunitinib (50 mg/day for 4 weeks followed by 2 weeks off) or the combination of IFN-α (9 x 10_6 IU three times per week) and bevacizumab (10 mg/kg every 2 weeks). PFS at 48 weeks was 29.5% (26 of 88 patients, 95% CI 20.0-39.1) in group A, 35.7% (15 of 42, 21.2-50.2) in group B, and 61.0% (25 of 41, 46.0-75.9) in group C. Median PFS was 8.2 months (95% CI 7.0-9.6) in group A, 8.2 months (5.5-11.7) in group B, and 16.8 months (6.0-26.0) in group C. The toxicity of the experimental regimen was high with over 50% of patients not able to tolerate the combination of bevacizumab and temsirolimus over several months. This combination failed to show any beneficial activity and was more toxic than the treatments used in the other arms, and therefore was not recommended as first line treatment in these patients. [81]

The combination of temsirolimus and IFN-α was studied in a phase III trial. Six hundred and twenty six patients were randomized to receive of IFN-α alone, temsirolimus alone, or a combination of the two drugs. Median OS times in the IFN-α arm, the temsirolimus arm, and the combination-therapy arm were 7.3, 10.9, and 8.4 months, respectively. Unlike temsirolimus alone, the combination of temsirolimus plus IFN-α did not improve OS. Therefore the temsirolimus / IFN-α combination is not recommended as standard practice for treatment of advanced RCC. [65]

Lastly, in a global, open-labelled multi-centre phase IIIb trial (INTORACT), temsirolimus and bevacizumab was compared with interferon and bevacizumab as first-line treatment in 791 patients with predominantly clear-cell metastatic RCC. [82] At the interim analysis, 489 patients were assessed PFS events. Median PFS with temsirolimus / bevacizumab combination was 9.1 month compared to 9.3 months in the interferon / bevacizumab group. The median OS was 25.8 months in the temsirolimus and 25.5 months for the interferon group. [82]

5.2. VEGF-ligands or receptor inhibitors / mTOR combination

Bevacizumab in combination with sorafenib and sunitinib has been evaluated in two phase I trials. In these trials although there were some promising results regarding the median time to progression and partial response rates in the combination arms, the adverse effects observed in the latter were prominent. [83, 84] The combination arm in both trials required dose reduction of both agents and resulted in a considerably lower maximum tolerated dose in contrast to the maximal tolerated dose of the single agent. Bevacizumab potentiated the side-effects of sorafenib such as hypertension and hand-foot syndrome; hematological, vascular toxicities (including microangiopathic hemolytic anaemia) and hypertension in the sunitinib combination. [75] Finally, a phase II study assessing the tolerability and efficacy of multiple combinations of currently available therapies, is being processed in the Eastern Cooperative Oncology BeST trial. The four arms are bevacizumab (10mg/kg), bevacizumab (5mg/kg) / temsirolimus (25 mg), bevacizumab (5mg/kg) and sorafenib (200mg twice daily)/ temsirolimus (25mg). [85]. The results are currently pending.

6. Sequencing therapy in metastatic RCC

Sequential use of targeted agents has several potential benefits. Firstly, this approach could lead to a treatment continuum, secondly, it provides patients the opportunity to receive full doses of the targeted agents without affecting tolerability and finally, sequential targeting of different molecular pathways could potentially overcome any resistance that would arise from single target inhibition. [86]

6.1. Anti-angiogenic therapy after immunotherapy

Few phase II trials using anti-angiogenic agents after progression on immunotherapy lead to promising results. [32, 59, 87] In a phase III trial (TARGET) patient who had progressed on cytokine therapy after receiving sorafenib, there was a notable doubling of PFS from 2.8 to 5.6 months. [41] Likewise, the utilization of axitinib post progression on cytokine in a phase II trial, lead to a TTP of 15.7 months. [77] There are no head-to-head data present to guide which agent is best utilized post cytokine therapy and a properly conducted phase III trial are required to share further insight into this treatment strategy.

6.2. mTOR blockade after anti-angiogenic therapy

In this strategy, the RECORD-1 trial investigated the efficacy of everolimus vs. placebo with best supportive care post progression on sunitinib, sorafenib or both. Seventy one per cent of patients included in the trial had received prior sunitinib treatment and 55% sorafenib therapy. Patient on everolimus achieved addition of 3-month in terms of PFS regardless of prior treatment. No overall survival benefit was observed due to large numbers of cross over from placebo to everolimus arm (80%). [67]

RECORD-3, a phase III clinical trial recently closed to patient recruitment, randomly assigned patients to either everolimus or sunitinib. Upon first sign of progression, patients would cross over to sunitinib if they were on everolimus and to everolimus if previously on sunitinib. The primary end point of this trial was to evaluate whether PFS post first-line treatment for patients who received everolimus will be non-inferior to patients who receive sunitinib. [52]

6.3. Serial anti-angiogenic agents

With the availability of multiple SMTKIs, an important focus ahead is in the identification of how to best utilize the TKIs in sequence. There is now increasing evidence supporting the sequential use of VEGF-targeted therapies.

In both phase II and III trials, axitinib has shown encouraging results in second-line setting in advanced RCC. [88] In an ongoing study, the Sequential Two-agent Assessment in Renal Cell Carcinoma Therapy (START), two hundred and forty treatment-naïve patients with clear-cell component metastatic RCC will be randomized into 6 arms to receive different 2-drug "sequences" of everolimus, bevacizumab, or pazopanib. The primary end point is the detection of the longest combination of the TTP. [89]

A retrospective study on RCC patients treated with sunitinib and sorafenib evaluated the effectiveness of switching from one TKI agent to the other after disease progression. In this study patients who received sunitinib followed by sorafenib experienced a shorter time to progression than patients who received sorafenib followed by sunitinib (risk ratio (RR) 3.0; p = 0.016). Similarly, the median OS was 102 weeks in patients who received sorafenib followed by sunitinib compared with 45 weeks in patients who received sunitinib followed by sorafenib (p = 0.061).[90]

An ongoing phase III trial (SWITCH trial) is currently being undertaken comparing sorafenib until progression followed by sunitinib and sunitinib until progression followed by sorafenib in the first line advanced RCC setting. The primary end point is the PFS and hopefully this trial will show further insight into which anti-VEGF treatment sequence will confer better clinical outcome in patients with metastatic RCC. [91]

7. Systemic treatment for non-clear cell renal cell carcinoma

With clear-cell RCC being the predominant histological subtypes and non clear-cell (papillary and chromophobe) being represented only in ~10% of clinical trials, there is consequently a paucity of data regarding treatment for advance non-clear-cell RCC. [92] Novel target therapies have demonstrated promising results in clear-cell histologies, however their activities remained undefined in the non-clear-cell counterpart. Majority of the data is derived from expanded access trials, retrospective series, and subset analyses of major trials. [93] Patients with non clear-cell RCC were both excluded from the landmark phase III trials of sunitinib and sorafenib. The largest non clear-cell series were derived from the sunitinib and sorafenib expanded access trials, which allowed entry of non-clear-cell histologies. Gore and colleagues demonstrated sunitinib activity in the multi-centre, international, non-randomised expanded access compassionate trial. Of the 4500 patients enrolled, approximately 10% (n=437) had non clear-cell histology (not further characterized) were evaluated. An ORR of 11% was demonstrated (N=48) with 46 partial responders and 2 complete responders. Fifty sever percent had stable disease (N=250) for a t least 3 months. [36] The median OS was reported as 13.4 months. The ORR was notable lower, 11% compared to the reported 42 to 47% in the phase III trial. The non-stringent reporting of disease progression and the reliance of local practice may well account for the discrepancy in the results.

The Advanced Renal Cell Carcinoma Sorafenib (ARCS) expanded access trial recruited patient with advanced RCC who were not eligible for other clinical trials. One hundred and fifty eight patients with papillary RCC were enrolled. Partial response of 3.4% and 5.6% were noted for patients with papillary and chromophobe RCC respectively. Eighty-seven patients (77.1% of the papillary RCC and 88.8% of the chromophobe RCC) demonstrated disease stability for a duration of more than 8 weeks. Despite only modest activity being noted, this trial has at least shared insight into the activity of sorafenib into the two most common non clear-cell variant. [44] Another trial that demonstrated TKI activity across the different histological subtypes were reported in a retrospective analysis of patients with metastatic papillary and chromophobe RCC who received either sunitinib and sorafenib as their initial frontline therapy. The reported ORR, PFS and OS were 10%, 8.9 months and 12.2 months respectively. A sub-analysis revealed a longer higher response rate for chromophobe variant (25%) compared to papillary variant (4.8%); ($p=0.007$). Similarly the PFS in the chromophobe population was longer (9.3 months) when compared with papillary population 6.6 months ($p=0.07$). There were no differences between the OS across both histologies. When stratified according to TKI type, the papillary population had a statistically longer PFS (11.9 months) with sunitinib compared to sorafenib (5.1 months; $p<0.001$). [3]

Temsirolimus has demonstrated promising activity in both clear-cell and non-clear-cell RCC. The phase III trial undertaken by Hudes and colleagues, examined the efficacy of temsirolimus, IFN-α or combination of both in patients with poor MSKCC prognostic features. [65] Although majority of patients had clear-cell histology, approximately 20% of non-clear-cell variant were included in the clinical trial. An improvement in median OS and median PFS were seen in temsirolimus arm, across all histologies with a significant advantage in hazard ratio for OS in the temsirolimus. An updated sub-analysis of the study showed a hazard ratio of 0.55 and 0.36 for median OS and PFS respectively, clearly favouring temsirolimus over IFN-α monotherapy and IFN-α / temsirolimus combination arms. [94] The analysis also showed that 75% of the non clear-cell variant consisted of papillary subtype. This has led to subsequent FDA approval of temsirolimus as treatment for non-clear-cell histology in advanced RCC.

Everolimus through RECORD-1 trial has reported efficacy in patient who progressed on one or two line of TKI. This has led to the development of an open-label, single arm, multi-centre phase II examining the efficacy of everolimus as first-line systemic therapy for patients with advanced papillary RCC. [8] This trial will stratify the histology into type I and II, and recruitment will hopefully show further insight into the treatment of papillary variant of RCC.

Epidermal growth factor receptor (EGFR) has been investigated as potential therapeutic target in metastatic RCC. Erlotinib, an anti-EGFR was examined in a phase II study of treatment naïve patients with locally advanced or metastatic papillary RCC. [95] Fifty two patients were registered and 45 were evaluable. The ORR was reported as 11% and the disease control rate was 64% with 5 partial responders and 24 patients with stable disease. The six month PFS was 30% and median survival of 27 months was documented. [95]

Collecting duct tumour is a very aggressive but rare variant of aggressive but rare variant of RCC. The largest data is derived from a phase II multi-centre trial of 23 treatment naïve patients who received platinum based chemotherapy with gemcitabine. The choice of chemotherapy is that of a platinum doublet based on some similarities to transitional cell carcinoma of the bladder. The ORR was 26% with a median PFS and OS of 7.1 months and 10.5 months respectively.[18] There is no data to support the use of TKI in this variant of tumour.

8. Side effects of targeted therapies used in renal cell carcinoma

The increasing use of novel anti-VEGF agents, and for longer periods of time for the treatment of RCC has raised challenges in the management of the associated toxicities or adverse effects. There are supportive interventions developed for their prevention and control. [96]

It has been identified in clinical trials and post marketing surveillance that the treatment toxicities associated with the new targeted therapies against cancer differ significantly from the toxicities seen with conventional chemotherapy. [96, 97]

Many of the anti-VEGF agents share similar toxicities, including hypertension, fatigue, gastrointestinal, skin and bone marrow effects. The mTOR inhibitors have unique adverse effects, which include metabolic alterations (hypercholesterolnaemia, hyperglycermia), gastrointestinal alterations and interstitial pneumonitis. Hypothyroidism is seen uniquely in patients on sunitinib, potentially sorafenib and pazopanib. [96]

8.1. Hyperension

Arterial hypertension is commonly observed as an adverse event in patients treated with inhibitors of the VEGF pathway. [96, 98] The most common implicated anti-VEGF agents include axitinib, bevacizumab, sorafenib, sunitinib and pazopanib. [33, 41, 51, 99, 100] Prompt identification of arterial hypertension is essential to prevent serious consequences such as strokes and heart failure. [101, 102] The regular use of ambulatory BP monitoring may be valuable for early detection and accurate assessment of blood pressure (BP) changes. [103] Hypertension has occurred whether or not the patient has a history of high blood pressure, however incidence may be higher in patients with pre-existing cardiovascular disease. [33, 41, 50, 99] There are pre-existing algorithms to treat hypertension associated with targeted therapies [96] but it falls on the clinician's discretion to individualise treatment accordingly. [98] For example, the use of angiotensin-converting enzyme (ACE) inhibitor is a logical choice if bevacizumab is the underlying cause as they may improve the associated proteinuria. [104] Angiotensin II inhibitors, diuretics, dihydropyridine calcium channel blockers (CCBs), and β-blockers are also considered as appropriate anti-hypertensive agents.

8.1.1. Hypertension as a biomarker

Hypertension induced by sunitinib and bevacizumab is associated with improved clinical outcomes, supporting its use as an efficacious biomarker. In a retrospective analysis which included pooled efficacy and safety data (n=544, n=4917) from four trials of patients with metastatic RCC treated with sunitinib 50mg/d (4 week on / 2 week off), it was observed that patients who had a systolic BP ≥to 140mmHg and a diastolic blood pressure of ≥ 90mmHg had better outcomes compared to those without treatment induced hypertension The ORR were 54.8% in the treatment induced hypertension cohort vs. 8.7% in the normotensive patients. The median PFS was 12.5 vs. 2.5 months in the hypertensive and normotensive respectively and similarly the median OS was 30.9 months in the hypertensive group vs. 7.2 months in the normotensive group. [105] The rates of AEs were similar between patients with and without hypertension. However patients with high BP experienced more frequent renal adverse events (5% vs. 3%). [105] More importantly, no difference in outcome (PFS and ORR) was noted regardless of whether patients received treatment for their hypertension. [105]

Treatment induced arterial hypertension is also correlated with good clinical outcomes in patients treated with bevacizumab for metastatic colorectal cancer [106] but this has not been investigated widely in metastatic RCC.

8.2. Fatigue

Fatigue is a very frequent side-effect seen with the targeted agents used in metastatic RCC [74, 96, 107] The incidence of fatigue in phase III studies ranged from 14% to 51% for all grades and up to 11% for grade 3–4.

There is no direct treatment available to alleviate treatment induced fatigue. Monitoring and treating patients for any aggravating or reversible factors (i.e. anaemia, anxiety, hypothyroidism, depression may help. If grade 3–4 fatigue persists, dose reduction or cessation of the treatment should be considered. [96, 108]

8.2.1. Fatigue as a biomarker

Fatigue is another potential biomarker in patients with metastatic RCC treated with sunitinib. A retrospective analysis of pooled data from 770 patients who received sunitinib in 5 clinical trials for metastatic RCC revealed that the development of grade 1-2 fatigue was linked with significantly longer time to progression and improved overall survival. [109]

8.3. Hand and foot syndrome as biomarker

In a retrospective registry of metastatic RCC, 705 and 365 patients treated with sunitinib and sorafenib respectively were assessed for outcomes of the disease in those who developed hand and foot syndrome. In the sunitinib group, the median OS was 43 months for those with the hand and foot syndrome vs. 31 months (p=0.027) in those without. The PFS in patients with the dermatological toxicity was 20.8 months vs. 11.1 months (p=0.007) in those without. In the sorafenib group, no differences was noted in median OS for those that did and did not experience hand foot syndrome (27.9 vs. 24.6 months (p=0.244). The PFS was 12.2 vs. 8.8 months (p=0.050) with a difference of 3.4 months in those that experienced hand foot syndrome. In multivariable cox regression analysis, hand and foot syndrome was associated with longer OS in the sunitinib group. In sorafenib, the survival benefits were less convincing. [110]

8.4. Other biomarkers

Emerging data has also shown that other adverse effects such as hypothyroidism, myelosuppression in addition to the aforementioned hypertension and hand foot syndrome were biomarkers for tumour control and OS when sunitinib is the agent in use. [111, 112] In mTOR inhibitors, serum LDH, elevated cholesterol and pneumonitis have been studied as predictive biomarkers. [113-115]

9. Quality of life in patients with renal cell carcinoma receiving targeted

9.1. Therapy

Quality of life (QoL) has been evaluated in a series of trials of patients taking novel targeted agents for RCC. Questionnaires used have included the Functional Assessment of Cancer Therapy-General (FACT-G), the FACT Kidney Symptom Index-15 item (FKSI-15), the FACT-Kidney Symptom Index-Disease related Symptoms (FKSI-DRS), the European Organization for Research and Treatment of Cancer Quality of Life Questionnaire (EORTC QLQ-C30 and the Euro QOL 5D (Index and Visual Analogue Scale) utility score (EQ-5D) Index.

One of the important outcomes was that newer treatment approaches may be better tolerated with improved QOL compared to the older generation agents. Sunitinib has shown meaningful differences, both in kidney cancer related symptoms and overall QOL over IFN-α. [33] This is not unexpected given the more difficult toxicity profile of sunitinib.

Sorafenib, on the contrary revealed no worst QoL score based on the FACT-G or FKSI-15 undertaken in the TARGET trial. On the other hand, targeted therapies compared to placebo were not revealing worse scores in the QOL questioners. Interestingly, qualitative assessment of one's ability to enjoy life, concerns for well-being, fevers, dyspnea and cough were reported less in the patients on sorafenib. [116]

Pazopanib unexpectedly did not have a clinically different QoL compared with placebo, despite the adverse events that a clinician may expect with pazopanib. [50, 100]

In the AXIS trial where axitinib was compared head-to-head with sorafenib, patient-reported kidney-specific symptom and function assessments were secondary endpoints that were examined. [57] Overall, patients on the axitinib treatment arm reported comparable outcomes to that of sorafenib. The PFS benefit seen by axitinib is associated with a delay in worsening of the composite endpoint of advanced RCC symptoms, progression, or death with sorafenib. [57]

PSICES is a small but important randomized trial comparing patient's preference for pazopanib or sunitinib for first-line treatment of metastatic RCC. The rationale of this trial was to select the more tolerable agent with the recent approval of numerous TKIs as front-line agents. [117] One hundred and sixty nine patients with metastatic RCC were randomly assigned to blinded treatment of pazopanib for 10 weeks with a wash out prior to 50mg of sunitinib for 10 weeks, and vice versa (4 weeks of sunitinib followed by 2 weeks break before 10 weeks of pazopanib). Fifty four and sixty patients first received pazopanib and sunitinib respectively. The patience preference when assessed at 22 weeks revealed 70% of patients preferred pazopanib, 22% preferred sunitinib, and 8% expressed no preference. The magnitude of difference was 49.3% between pazopanib and sunitinib. Fewer patients received pazopanib required a dose reduction (13% vs. 20%), prematurely discontinued treatment during the first study period (14% vs. 8%), or prematurely discontinued treatment during the second period (15% vs. 31%). [117, 118]

10. Conclusion

The discovery of anti-angiogenic (small molecule tyrosine kinase inhibitors and anti-VEGF agents) agents has altered the treatment landscape for patients with metastatic RCC. Their effective anti-neoplastic activities have provided hope of survival beyond six month, in contrast to that traditionally gained from IFN-α therapy. Different treatment strategies are being investigated vigorously, either in combination or in sequence with the aim of improving the pre-existing survival and response rates. Whilst the treatment algorithm for advanced clear-cell variant of renal cell carcinoma is constantly evolving with increasing treatment options, the non clear-cell counterpart remains an area in need of significant research. With improved understanding of the various molecular pathways, options for non clear-cell variants would hopefully become more established. The recognition of the potentially serious side-effects of targeted agents begs for vigilance in the clinician's part to improve treatment adherence and compliance. Close monitoring of these toxicities will also allow for better identification of their role as bio-markers of efficacy. The ultimate goal is to have an effective agent that leads to durable response with a tolerable side-effect profile.

Acknowledgements

We wish to express our gratitude to Ms. Judith Lees, Senior Cancer Pharmacist, RAH Cancer Centre, for assistance with new drugs information.

Author details

Thean Hsiang Tan, Sina Vatandoust and Michail Charakidis

RAH Cancer Centre, Royal Adelaide Hospital, Adelaide, Australia

References

[1] Cohen HT, McGovern FJ. Renal-cell carcinoma. N Engl J Med. 2005 Dec 8;353(23): 2477-90

[2] Wilhelm SM, Adnane L, Newell P, Villanueva A, Llovet JM, Lynch M. Preclinical overview of sorafenib, a multikinase inhibitor that targets both Raf and VEGF and PDGF receptor tyrosine kinase signaling. Mol Cancer Ther. 2008 Oct;7(10):3129-40

[3] Choueiri TK, Plantade A, Elson P, Negrier S, Ravaud A, Oudard S, et al. Efficacy of sunitinib and sorafenib in metastatic papillary and chromophobe renal cell carcinoma. J Clin Oncol. 2008 Jan 1;26(1):127-31

[4] Haase VH. Renal cancer: oxygen meets metabolism. Exp Cell Res. 2012 May 15;318(9):1057-67

[5] Ohh M, Park CW, Ivan M, Hoffman MA, Kim TY, Huang LE, et al. Ubiquitination of hypoxia-inducible factor requires direct binding to the beta-domain of the von Hippel-Lindau protein. Nat Cell Biol. 2000 Jul;2(7):423-7

[6] Kamura T, Sato S, Iwai K, Czyzyk-Krzeska M, Conaway RC, Conaway JW. Activation of HIF1alpha ubiquitination by a reconstituted von Hippel-Lindau (VHL) tumor suppressor complex. Proc Natl Acad Sci U S A. 2000 Sep 12;97(19):10430-5

[7] Maxwell PH, Wiesener MS, Chang GW, Clifford SC, Vaux EC, Cockman ME, et al. The tumour suppressor protein VHL targets hypoxia-inducible factors for oxygen-dependent proteolysis. Nature. 1999 May 20;399(6733):271-5

[8] Amato R. Everolimus for the treatment of advanced renal cell carcinoma. Expert Opin Pharmacother. 2011 May;12(7):1143-55

[9] Kim WY, Kaelin WG. Role of VHL gene mutation in human cancer. J Clin Oncol. 2004 Dec 15;22(24):4991-5004

[10] Vaupel P. The role of hypoxia-induced factors in tumor progression. Oncologist. 2004;9 Suppl 5:10-7

[11] Beck SD, Patel MI, Snyder ME, Kattan MW, Motzer RJ, Reuter VE, et al. Effect of papillary and chromophobe cell type on disease-free survival after nephrectomy for renal cell carcinoma. Ann Surg Oncol. 2004 Jan;11(1):71-7

[12] Furge KA, MacKeigan JP, Teh BT. Kinase targets in renal-cell carcinomas: reassessing the old and discovering the new. Lancet Oncol. 2010 Jun;11(6):571-8

[13] Choi JS, Kim MK, Seo JW, Choi YL, Kim DH, Chun YK, et al. MET expression in sporadic renal cell carcinomas. J Korean Med Sci. 2006 Aug;21(4):672-7

[14] Linehan WM, Pinto PA, Srinivasan R, Merino M, Choyke P, Choyke L, et al. Identification of the genes for kidney cancer: opportunity for disease-specific targeted therapeutics. Clin Cancer Res. 2007 Jan 15;13(2 Pt 2):671s-9s

[15] Isaacs JS, Jung YJ, Mole DR, Lee S, Torres-Cabala C, Chung YL, et al. HIF overexpression correlates with biallelic loss of fumarate hydratase in renal cancer: novel role of fumarate in regulation of HIF stability. Cancer Cell. 2005 Aug;8(2):143-53

[16] Pavlovich CP, Walther MM, Eyler RA, Hewitt SM, Zbar B, Linehan WM, et al. Renal tumors in the Birt-Hogg-Dube syndrome. Am J Surg Pathol. 2002 Dec;26(12):1542-52

[17] Yamazaki K, Sakamoto M, Ohta T, Kanai Y, Ohki M, Hirohashi S. Overexpression of KIT in chromophobe renal cell carcinoma. Oncogene. 2003 Feb 13;22(6):847-52

[18] Oudard S, Banu E, Vieillefond A, Fournier L, Priou F, Medioni J, et al. Prospective multicenter phase II study of gemcitabine plus platinum salt for metastatic collecting duct carcinoma: results of a GETUG (Groupe d'Etudes des Tumeurs Uro-Genitales) study. J Urol. 2007 May;177(5):1698-702

[19] National Comprehensive Cancer Network guidelines 1.2012 kidney cancer. Available from: http://wwwnccnorg/professionals/physician_gls/defaultasp.Accessed February 1, 2012

[20] Posadas EM, Figlin RA. Systemic therapy in Renal Cell Carcinoma: Advancing Paradigms. Oncology. 2012;26(3):1-18

[21] Yagoda A, Bander NH. Failure of cytotoxic chemotherapy, 1983-1988, and the emerging role of monoclonal antibodies for renal cancer. Urol Int. 1989;44(6):338-45

[22] Motzer RJ, Bander NH, Nanus DM. Renal-cell carcinoma. N Engl J Med. 1996 Sep 19;335(12):865-75

[23] Fyfe G, Fisher RI, Rosenberg SA, Sznol M, Parkinson DR, Louie AC. Results of treatment of 255 patients with metastatic renal cell carcinoma who received high-dose recombinant interleukin-2 therapy. J Clin Oncol. 1995;13:688-96

[24] Tan TH, Pranavan G, Haxhimolla HZ, Yip D. New systemic treatment options for metastatic renal-cell carcinoma in the era of targeted therapies. Asia Pac J Clin Oncol. 2010 Mar;6(1):5-18

[25] Jonasch E, Hutson TE, Harshman LC, Srinivas S. Advanced Renal Cell Carcinoma: Overview of Drug Therapy fro the Practicing Physician. J Clin Oncol. 2011;ASCO Education Book:145-51

[26] Abrams TJ, Murray LJ, Pesenti E, Holway VW, Colombo T, Lee LB, et al. Preclinical evaluation of the tyrosine kinase inhibitor SU11248 as a single agent and in combination with "standard of care" therapeutic agents for the treatment of breast cancer. Mol Cancer Ther. 2003 Oct;2(10):1011-21

[27] Kim DW, Jo YS, Jung HS, Chung HK, Song JH, Park KC, et al. An orally administered multitarget tyrosine kinase inhibitor, SU11248, is a novel potent inhibitor of thyroid oncogenic RET/papillary thyroid cancer kinases. J Clin Endocrinol Metab. 2006 Oct;91(10):4070-6

[28] Mendel DB, Laird AD, Xin X, Louie SG, Christensen JG, Li G, et al. In vivo antitumor activity of SU11248, a novel tyrosine kinase inhibitor targeting vascular endothelial

growth factor and platelet-derived growth factor receptors: determination of a pharmacokinetic/pharmacodynamic relationship. Clin Cancer Res. 2003 Jan;9(1):327-37

[29] Murray LJ, Abrams TJ, Long KR, Ngai TJ, Olson LM, Hong W, et al. SU11248 inhibits tumor growth and CSF-1R-dependent osteolysis in an experimental breast cancer bone metastasis model. Clin Exp Metastasis. 2003;20(8):757-66

[30] Faivre S, Delbaldo C, Vera K, Robert C, Lozahic S, Lassau N, et al. Safety, pharmacokinetic, and antitumor activity of SU11248, a novel oral multitarget tyrosine kinase inhibitor, in patients with cancer. J Clin Oncol. 2006 Jan 1;24(1):25-35

[31] Motzer RJ, Bukowski RM. Targeted therapy for metastatic renal cell carcinoma. J Clin Oncol. 2006;24:5601-8

[32] Motzer RJ, Michaelson MD, Rosenberg J, Bukowski RM, Curti BD, George DJ, et al. Sunitinib efficacy against advanced renal cell carcinoma. J Urol. 2007 Nov;178(5): 1883-7

[33] Motzer RJ, Hutson TE, Tomczak P, Michaelson MD, Bukowski RM, Rixe O, et al. Sunitinib versus interferon alfa in metastatic renal-cell carcinoma. N Engl J Med. 2007 Jan 11;356(2):115-24

[34] Desai J, Gurney H, Pavlakis N, McArthur GA, Davis ID. Sunitinib malate in the treatment of renal cell carcinoma and gastrointestinal stromal tumor: Recommendations for patient management. Asia-Pac J Clin Oncol. 2007;3:167-76

[35] Motzer RJ, Hutson TE, Tomczak P, Michaelson MD, Bukowski RM, Oudard S, et al. Overall survival and updated results for sunitinib compared with interferon alfa in patients with metastatic renal cell carcinoma. J Clin Oncol. 2009 Aug 1;27(22):3584-90

[36] Gore ME, Szczylik C, Porta C, Bracarda S, Bjarnason GA, Oudard S, et al. Safety and efficacy of sunitinib for metastatic renal-cell carcinoma: an expanded-access trial. Lancet Oncol. 2009 Aug;10(8):757-63

[37] Escudier B, Roigas J, Gillessen S, Harmenberg U, Srinivas S, Mulder SF, et al. Phase II study of sunitinib administered in a continuous once-daily dosing regimen in patients with cytokine-refractory metastatic renal cell carcinoma. J Clin Oncol. 2009 Sep 1;27(25):4068-75

[38] Motzer R, Hutson TE, Olsen MR, Hudes G, Burke JM, Edenfield WJ, et al. Randomized phase II multicentre study of the efficacy and safety of sunitinib on the 4/2 versus continuous dosing schedule as first-line therapy of metastatic renal cell carcinoma: renal EFFECT Trial. Journal of Clinical Oncology. 2011;29:(suppl 7; abstrc LBA308)

[39] Ratain MJ, Eisen T, Stadler WM, Flaherty KT, Kaye SB, Rosner GL, et al. Phase II placebo-controlled randomized discontinuation trial of sorafenib in patients with metastatic renal cell carcinoma. J Clin Oncol. 2006 Jun 1;24(16):2505-12

[40] Escudier B, Szczylik C, Hutson TE, Demkow T, Staehler M, Rolland F, et al. Randomized phase II trial of first-line treatment with sorafenib versus interferon Alfa-2a in patients with metastatic renal cell carcinoma. J Clin Oncol. 2009 Mar 10;27(8):1280-9

[41] Escudier B, Eisen T, Stadler WM, Szczylik C, Oudard S, Siebels M, et al. Sorafenib in advanced clear-cell renal-cell carcinoma. N Engl J Med. 2007 Jan 11;356(2):125-34

[42] Escudier B, Eisen T, Stadler WM, Szczylik C, Oudard S, Staehler M, et al. Sorafenib for treatment of renal cell carcinoma: Final efficacy and safety results of the phase III treatment approaches in renal cancer global evaluation trial. J Clin Oncol. 2009 Jul 10;27(20):3312-8

[43] Beck J, Bajetta E, Escudier B. A large open label, non comparative Phase III study of the multi-targeted kinase inhibitor sorafenib in European patients with advanced renal cell carcinoma. Presented at. 2007;ECCO(BArcelona, Spain.)

[44] Beck J, Procopio E, Verzoni S, Bajetta E, Escudier B. Large open label non-comparative clinical experience trial of the multi-targeted kinase inhibitor sorafenib in European patients with advanced RCC J Clin Oncol. 2008;26((Suppl.)):(Abstract 1621)

[45] Beck J, Procopio G, Bajetta E, Keilholz U, Negrier S, Szczylik C, et al. Final results of the European Advanced Renal Cell Carcinoma Sorafenib (EU-ARCCS) expanded-access study: a large open-label study in diverse community settings. Ann Oncol. 2011 February 15, 2011;22(8):1812-3

[46] Escudier B, Szczylik C, Porta C, Gore M. Treatment selection in metastatic renal cell carcinoma: expert consensus. Nat Rev Clin Oncol. 2012 Jun;9(6):327-37

[47] INTORSECT Trial: Phase III, randomized, open-label, multi centre study comparing temsirolimus with sorafenib as second line. . ESMO 2012: Conference proceedings, Sept 28 - Oct 2, 2012 Vienna Convention Centre, Vienna, Austria 2012

[48] Bellmunt J, Fishman M, Eisen T, Quinn D. Expert opinion on the use of first-line sorafenib in selected metastatic renal cell carcinoma patients. Expert Rev Anticancer Ther. 2011 Jun;10(6):825-35

[49] Hutson TE, Davis ID, Machiels JP, De Souza PL, Rottey S, Hong BF, et al. Efficacy and safety of pazopanib in patients with metastatic renal cell carcinoma. J Clin Oncol. 2010 Jan 20;28(3):475-80

[50] Sternberg CN, Davis ID, Mardiak J, Szczylik C, Lee E, Wagstaff J, et al. Pazopanib in locally advanced or metastatic renal cell carcinoma: results of a randomized phase III trial. J Clin Oncol. 2010 Feb 20;28(6):1061-8

[51] Rini B, Al-Marrawi MY. Pazopanib for the treatment of renal cancer. Expert Opin Pharmacother. 2011 May;12(7):1171-89

[52] NCT00720941 Cgi. Pazopanib Versus Sunitinib in the Treatment of Locally Advanced and/or Metastatic Renal Cell Carcinoma (COMPARZ) *[cited 21 July 2011]*. 2011:Available from: http://clinicaltrials.gov/ct2/show/NCT00720941

[53] Rixe O, Bukowski RM, Michaelson MD, Wilding G, Hudes GR, Bolte O, et al. Axitinib treatment in patients with cytokine-refractory metastatic renal-cell cancer: a phase II study. Lancet Oncol. 2007 Nov;8(11):975-84

[54] Motzer RJ, de La Motte Rouge T, Harzstark AL, michaelson MD, Liu G, Gruenwald V, et al. Axitinib second-line therapy for metastatic renal cell carcinoma (mRCC): Five-year (yr) overall survival (OS) data from a phase II trial. J Clin Oncol. 2011;29:(suppl; abstr 4527)

[55] Rini B, Grunwald V, Fishman MN. Axitinib for first-line metastatic renal cell carcinoma (mRCC): Overall efficacy and pharmacokinetic (PK) analyses from a randomized phase II study of Clinical Oncology. 2012;30:(suppl; abstr 4503)

[56] Rini BI, Escudier B, Tomczak P, Kaprin A, Hutson TE, Szczylik C, et al. Axitinib versus sorafenib as second-line therapy for metastatic renal cell carcinoma (mRCC): Results of phase III AXIS trial. J Clin Oncol 2011;29:(suppl; abstr 4503)

[57] Cella D, Escudier B, Rini BI, Chen HX, Bhattacharyya JC, Tarazi JC, et al. Patient-reported outcomes (PROs) in a phase III AXIS trial of axitinib versus sorafenib as second-line therapy for metastatic renal cell carcinoma (mRCC) J Clin Oncol. 2011;29 (suppl) abstr 4504

[58] Gommersall L, Hayne D, Lynch C, Joseph JV, Arya M, Patel HR. Allogeneic stem-cell transplantation for renal-cell cancer. Lancet Oncol. 2004 Sep;5(9):561-7

[59] Yang JC, Haworth L, Sherry RM, Hwu P, Schwartzentruber DJ, Topalian SL, et al. A randomized trial of bevacizumab, an anti-vascular endothelial growth factor antibody, for metastatic renal cancer. N Engl J Med. 2003 Jul 31;349(5):427-34

[60] Presta LG, Chen H, O'Connor SJ, Chisholm V, Meng YG, Krummen L, et al. Humanization of an anti-vascular endothelial growth factor monoclonal antibody for the therapy of solid tumors and other disorders. Cancer Res. 1997 Oct 15;57(20):4593-9

[61] Escudier B, Bellmunt J, Negrier S, Bajetta E, Melichar B, Bracarda S, et al. Phase III trial of bevacizumab plus interferon alfa-2a in patients with metastatic renal cell carcinoma (AVOREN): final analysis of overall survival. J Clin Oncol. 2007 May 1;28(13): 2144-50

[62] Rini BI, Halabi S, Rosenberg JE, Stadler WM, Vaena DA, Archer L, et al. Phase III trial of bevacizumab plus interferon alfa versus interferon alfa monotherapy in patients with metastatic renal cell carcinoma: final results of CALGB 90206. J Clin Oncol. 2010 May 1;28(13):2137-43

[63] McDermott DF, George DJ. Bevacizumab as a treatment option in advanced renal cell carcinoma: an analysis and interpretation of clinical trial data. Cancer Treat Rev. 2010 May;36(3):216-23

[64] Beuvink I, Boulay A, Fumagalli S, Zilbermann F, Ruetz S, O'Reilly T, et al. The mTOR inhibitor RAD001 sensitizes tumor cells to DNA-damaged induced apoptosis through inhibition of p21 translation. Cell. 2005 Mar 25;120(6):747-59

[65] Hudes G, Carducci M, Tomczak P, Dutcher J, Figlin R, Kapoor A, et al. Temsirolimus, interferon alfa, or both for advanced renal-cell carcinoma. N Engl J Med. 2007 May 31;356(22):2271-81

[66] Hidalgo M, Buckner JC, Erlichman C, Pollack MS, Boni JP, Dukart G, et al. A phase I and pharmacokinetic study of temsirolimus (CCI-779) administered intravenously daily for 5 days every 2 weeks to patients with advanced cancer. Clin Cancer Res. 2006 Oct 1;12(19):5755-63

[67] Motzer RJ, Escudier B, Oudard S, Hutson TE, Porta C, Bracarda S, et al. Efficacy of everolimus in advanced renal cell carcinoma: a double-blind, randomised, placebo-controlled phase III trial. Lancet. 2008 Aug 9;372(9637):449-56

[68] Fisher R, Pickering L, Larkin J. New targeted therapies for renal cell carcinoma. Expert Opin Investig Drugs. 2011 Jul;20(7):933-45

[69] Eisen T, Joensuu H, Nathan PD, Harper PG, Wojtukiewicz MZ, Nicholson S, et al. Regorafenib for patients with previously untreated metastatic or unresectable renal-cell carcinoma: a single-group phase 2 trial. Lancet Oncol. 2012 Oct;13(10):1055-62

[70] Nosov D, Bhargava P, Esteves WB, Strahs AL, Lipatov ON, Lyulkp OO, et al. Final analysis of the phase II randomized discontinuation trial (RDT) of tivozanib (AV-951) versus placebo in patients with renal cell carcinoma (RCC). J Clin Oncol 2011;29: (suppl; abstr 4503)

[71] Kabbinavar FF, Srinivas S, Hauke RJ, Amato RJ, Esteves WB, Cotreau MM, et al. Results from a phase I trial of tivozanib (AV-951) combined with temsirolimus therapy in patients (pts) with renal cell carcinoma (RCC). J Clin Oncol 2011;29((suppl)):abstr 4549

[72] Motzer R, Nosov D, Eisen T, Bondarenko I, Lesovoy V, Lipatov ON, et al. Tivozanib versus sorafenib as initial targeted therapy for patients with advanced renal cell carcinoma: Results from a phase III randomized, open-label, multicenter trial. J Clin Oncol 30, 2012).

[73] Angevin E, Grünwald V, Castellano DE, Lin CC, Gschwend JE, Harzstark AL, et al. A phase II study of dovitinib (TKI258), an FGFR- and VEGFR-inhibitor, in patients with advanced or metastatic renal cell cancer (mRCC). J Clin Oncol 2011;29((suppl)): (abstr 4551)

[74] Hutson TE. Targeted therapies for the treatment of metastatic renal cell carcinoma: clinical evidence. Oncologist. 2011;16 Suppl 2:14-22

[75] Feldman DR, Baum MS, Ginsberg MS, Hassoun H, Flombaum CD, Velasco S, et al. Phase I trial of bevacizumab plus escalated doses of sunitinib in patients with metastatic renal cell carcinoma. J Clin Oncol. 2009 Mar 20;27(9):1432-9

[76] Gollob JA, Rathmell WK, Richmond TM, Marino CB, Miller EK, Grigson G, et al. Phase II trial of sorafenib plus interferon alfa-2b as first- or second-line therapy in patients with metastatic renal cell cancer. J Clin Oncol. 2007 Aug 1;25(22):3288-95

[77] Ryan CW, Goldman BH, Lara PN, Jr., Mack PC, Beer TM, Tangen CM, et al. Sorafenib with interferon alfa-2b as first-line treatment of advanced renal carcinoma: a phase II study of the Southwest Oncology Group. J Clin Oncol. 2007 Aug 1;25(22): 3296-301

[78] Jonasch E, Corn P, Pagliaro LC, Warneke CL, Johnson MM, Tamboli P, et al. Upfront, randomized, phase 2 trial of sorafenib versus sorafenib and low-dose interferon alfa in patients with advanced renal cell carcinoma: clinical and biomarker analysis. Cancer. 2010 Jan 1;116(1):57-65

[79] Escudier B, Pluzanska A, Koralewski P, Ravaud A, Bracarda S, Szczylik C, et al. Bevacizumab plus interferon alfa-2a for treatment of metastatic renal cell carcinoma: a randomised, double-blind phase III trial. Lancet. 2007 Dec 22;370(9605):2103-11

[80] Rini BI, Halabi S, Rosenberg JE, Stadler WM, Vaena DA, Ou SS, et al. Bevacizumab plus interferon alfa compared with interferon alfa monotherapy in patients with metastatic renal cell carcinoma: CALGB 90206. J Clin Oncol. 2008 Nov 20;26(33): 5422-8

[81] Negrier S, Gravis G, Perol D, Chevreau C, Delva R, Bay JO, et al. Temsirolimus and bevacizumab, or sunitinib, or interferon alfa and bevacizumab for patients with advanced renal cell carcinoma (TORAVA): a randomised phase 2 trial. Lancet Oncol. 2011 Jul;12(7):673-80

[82] INTORACT trial: global phase IIIb, randomized, open-label, multi-centre study, comparing temsirolimus plus bevacizumab with interferon pluas bevacizumab as first line treatment in clear cell metastatic renal cell carcinoma. ESMO 2012: Conference proceedings, Sept 28 - Oct 2, 2012. Vienna Convention Centre, Vienna, Austria. 2012

[83] Sosman JA, Flaherty KT, Atkins MB, McDermott DF, Rothenberg WL, Vermeulen WL, et al. Updated results of phase I trial of sorafenib (S) and bevacizumab (B) in patients with metastatic renal cell cancer (mRCC). J Clin Oncol. 2008;26 (May 20 Suppl):Abstr 5011

[84] Azad NS, Posadas EM, Kwitkowski VE, Steinberg SM, Jain L, Annunziata CM, et al. Combination targeted therapy with sorafenib and bevacizumab results in enhanced toxicity and antitumor activity. J Clin Oncol. 2008 Aug 1;26(22):3709-14

[85] NCT00378703 Cgi. Bevacizumab, Sorafenib, and Temsirolimus in Treating Patients With Metastatic Kidney Cancer (BeST) *[cited 16 Dec 2010]*. 2006:Available from http://clinicaltrials.gov/ct2/show/NCT00378703

[86] Bellmunt J. Future developments in renal cell carcinoma. Ann Oncol. 2009 May;20 Suppl 1:i13-7

[87] Motzer RJ, Michaelson MD, Redman BG, Hudes GR, Wilding G, Figlin RA, et al. Activity of SU11248, a multitargeted inhibitor of vascular endothelial growth factor receptor and platelet-derived growth factor receptor, in patients with metastatic renal cell carcinoma. J Clin Oncol. 2006 Jan 1;24(1):16-24

[88] Dutcher JP, Wilding G, Hudes GR, Stadler WM, Kim S, Tarazi JC, et al. Sequential axitinib (AG-013736) therapy of patients (pts) with metastatic clear cell renal cell cancer (RCC) refractory to sunitinib and sorafenib, cytokines and sorafenib, or sorafenib alone. J Clin Oncol. 2008;26(May 20 suppl):abstr 5127

[89] NCT1217931 Cgi. Sequential Two-agent Assessment in Renal Cell Carcinoma Therapy *[cited 17 May 2011]*. 2011:Available from: http://clinicaltrials.gov/ct2/show/NCT01217931?term=NCT&rank=1

[90] Dudek AZ, Zolnierek J, Dham A, Lindgren BR, Szczylik C. Sequential therapy with sorafenib and sunitinib in renal cell carcinoma. Cancer. 2009 Jan 1;115(1):61-7

[91] NCT00732914 Cgi. Sequential Study to Treat Renal Cell Carcinoma *[cited 18 Oct 2010]*. 2010:Available from: http://clinicaltrials.gov/ct2/show/NCT00732914?term=NCT&rank=1

[92] Motzer RJ, Bacik J, Mariani T, Russo P, Mazumdar M, Reuter V. Treatment Outcome and Survival Associated With Metastatic Renal Cell Carcinoma of Non–Clear-Cell Histology. J Clin Oncol. 2002 May 1, 2002;20(9):2376-81

[93] Tazi el M, Essadi I, Tazi MF, Ahellal Y, M'Rabti H, Errihani H. Advanced treatments in non-clear renal cell carcinoma. Urol J. 2011 Winter;8(1):1-11

[94] Schmidt LS, Warren MB, Nickerson ML, Weirich G, Matrosova V, Toro JR, et al. Birt-Hogg-Dube syndrome, a genodermatosis associated with spontaneous pneumothorax and kidney neoplasia, maps to chromosome 17p11.2. Am J Hum Genet. 2001 Oct;69(4):876-82

[95] Gordon MS, Hussey M, Nagle RB, Lara PN, Jr., Mack PC, Dutcher J, et al. Phase II study of erlotinib in patients with locally advanced or metastatic papillary histology renal cell cancer: SWOG S0317. J Clin Oncol. 2009 Dec 1;27(34):5788-93

[96] di Lorenzo G, Porta C, Bellmunt J, Sternberg C, Kirkali Z, Staehler M, et al. Toxicities of targeted therapy and their management in kidney cancer. Eur Urol. 2011 Apr;59(4):526-40

[97] Ravaud A. Treatment-Associated Adverse Event Management in the Advanced Renal Cell Carcinoma Patient Treated with Targeted Therapies. Oncologist. 2011;16(suppl 2):32-44

[98] Izzedine H, Ederhy S, Goldwasser F, Soria JC, Milano G, Cohen A, et al. Management of hypertension in angiogenesis inhibitor-treated patients. Ann Oncol. 2009 May;20(5):807-15

[99] Rixe O, Billemont B, Izzedine H. Hypertension as a predictive factor of Sunitinib activity. Ann Oncol. 2007 Jun;18(6):1117

[100] Sternberg CN. Randomised, double-blind phase III study of pazopanib in patients with advaced/metastatic renal cell carcinoma (MRCC), ESMO: Pazopanib in advanced MRCC - late breaker published 11/10/2011 by cancer reported Jo Armstrong. 2010

[101] Khakoo AY, Kassiotis CM, Tannir N, Plana JC, Halushka M, Bickford C, et al. Heart failure associated with sunitinib malate: a multitargeted receptor tyrosine kinase inhibitor. Cancer. 2008 Jun;112(11):2500-8

[102] Bhojani N, Jeldres C, Patard JJ, Perrotte P, Suardi N, Hutterer G, et al. Toxicities associated with the administration of sorafenib, sunitinib, and temsirolimus and their management in patients with metastatic renal cell carcinoma. Eur Urol. 2008 May; 53(5):917-30

[103] Grunwald V, Heinzer H, Fiedler W. Managing side effects of angiogenesis inhibitors in renal cell carcinoma. Onkologie. 2007 Oct;30(10):519-24

[104] Keefe D, Bowen J, Gibson R, Tan T, Okera M, Stringer A. Noncardiac vascular toxicities of vascular endothelial growth factor inhibitors in advanced cancer: a review. Oncologist. 2011;16(4):432-44

[105] Rini BI, Cohen DP, Lu DR, Chen I, Hariharan S, Gore ME, et al. Hypertension as a biomarker of efficacy in patients with metastatic renal cell carcinoma treated with sunitinib. J Natl Cancer Inst. 2011 May 4;103(9):763-73

[106] Scartozzi M, Galizia E, Chiorrini S, Giampieri R, Berardi R, Pierantoni C, et al. Arterial hypertension correlates with clinical outcome in colorectal cancer patients treated with first-line bevacizumab. Ann Oncol. 2009 Feb;20(2):227-30

[107] Adams VR, Leggas M. Sunitinib malate for the treatment of metastatic renal cell carcinoma and gastrointestinal stromal tumors. Clin Ther. 2007 Jul;29(7):1338-53

[108] Ravaud A. How to optimise treatment compliance in metastatic renal cell carcinoma with targeted agents. Ann Oncol. 2009 May;20 (Suppl 1):i7-12

[109] Davis MP, Figlin R, Hutson TE. Asthenia and fatigue as potential biomarkers of sunitinib efficacy in metasatic renal cell carcinoma. Eur J Cancer. 2011;47:(Suppl 1):s135 (Abstract 1139)

[110] Poprach A, Pavlik T, Melichar B, Puzanov I, Dusek L, Bortlicek Z, et al. Skin toxicity and efficacy of sunitinib and sorafenib in metastatic renal cell carcinoma: a national registry-based study. Ann Oncol. 2012 Jun 13

[111] Schmidinger M, Vogl UM, Bojic M, Lamm W, Heinzl H, Haitel A, et al. Hypothyroidism in patients with renal cell carcinoma: blessing or curse? Cancer. Feb 1;117(3): 534-44

[112] Donskov F, Carus A, Barrios C. Neutropenia and thrombocytopenia during treatment as biomarkers of sunitinib efficacy in patients with metastatic renal cell carcinoma (mRCC). Eur J Cancer. 2011;47:(Suppl 1):S136 (Abstract 1141)

[113] Dadydeen DA, Jagannthan JP, Ramaiya NH. Pneumonitis associated with mTOR therapy in patients with metastatic renal cell carcinoma: Incidence, radiographic findings, and correlation witih clnical outcome. 2011 ASCO Annual Meeting Proceedings (Post Meeting Edition). J Clin Oncol. 2011;29:(15 Suppl): Abstract e15176

[114] Lee CK, Marschner IC, Simes RJ, Voysey M, Egleston B, Hudes G, et al. Increase in cholesterol predicts survival advantage in renal cell carcinoma patients treated with temsirolimus. Clin Cancer Res. 2012 Jun 1;18(11):3188-96

[115] Armstrong A, George D, Halabi S. Serum lactate dehydrogenase (LDH) as a biomarker for survival with mTOR inhibition in patients with metastatic renal cell carcinoma (RCC). 2010 ASCO Annual Meeting Proceedings (Post-Meeting Edition). J Clin Oncol. 2010;28:(15 Suppl): Abstract 4631

[116] Bukowski R, Cella D, Gondek K, Escudier B. Effects of sorafenib on symptoms and quality of life: results from a large randomized placebo-controlled study in renal cancer. Am J Clin Oncol. 2007 Jun;30(3):220-7

[117] Escudier B, Porta C, Bono P, De Giorgi U, Parikh O, Hawkins RE, et al. Patient preference between pazopanib (Paz) and sunitinib (Sun): Results of a randomized double-blind, placebo-controlled, cross-over study in patients with metastatic renal cell carcinoma (mRCC)—PISCES study, NCT 01064310. Journal of Clinical Oncology. 2012;30(18s):CRA4502

[118] Escudier B, Porta C, Bono P, De Giorgi U, Parikh O, Hawkins RE, et al. Patient preference between pazopanib (Paz) and sunitinib (Sun): Results of a randomized double-blind, placebo-controlled, cross-over study in patients with metastatic renal cell carcinoma (mRCC)—PISCES study, NCT 01064310. conference proceedings. 2012;Sept 26 - Oct 2, 2012. Vienna Convention Centre, Vienna, Austria

Changing Mechanisms of Action as a Strategy for Sequential Targeted Therapy of Metastatic Renal-Cell Carcinoma

Mirjana Rajer

Additional information is available at the end of the chapter

http://dx.doi.org/10.5772/55694

1. Introduction

Renal cell carcinoma (RCC) affects more than 200.000 people annually worldwide resulting in 102.000 deaths each year. Men are twice as frequently affected as women; population aged between 50 and 70 years is most frequently affected. Obesity, hypertension, tobacco smoking and certain occupational exposures have been shown to increase one's risk for developing RCC. Rarely RCC develops as a part of the familiar syndrome (e.g. von Hippel-Lindau) [1,2].

Treatment of renal cell carcinoma has changed dramatically over the past few years. Until 2005 cytokine therapy (interferon (IFN-α) or interleukin (IL-2)) was the only (IFN-α) or interleukin (IL-2) was the only available treatment for mRCC patients. Treatment with cytokines was associated with little clinical benefit together with substantial side effects; even treatment related deaths were not infrequent. Treatment options for second line therapy were very limited; patients could be treated only with another cytokine or best supportive care. Responses to second line cytokine therapy were modest. Fewer than 4% of patients had partial response and < 12% had stable disease [2,3].

Lack of effective therapy together with better knowledge about the cancer biology led to the development of new targeted agents. Since the start of the "targeted era" development of new therapies evolved swiftly. Better treatment results in the first line therapy are allied to the better outcome of the patients on subsequent lines of treatment. Prognosis of patients improved and mRCC is becoming more a chronic type of disease, rather than a rapidly progressing and fatal one [3].

Despite rapid progress in development of new treatments, many questions still remain unanswered. Patients on targeted therapies progress some time during their treatment and

INTECH
open science | open minds

© 2013 Rajer; licensee InTech. This is a paper distributed under the terms of the Creative Commons Attribution License (http://creativecommons.org/licenses/by/3.0), which permits unrestricted use, distribution, and reproduction in any medium, provided the original work is properly cited.

mRCC is considered an incurable disease [4]. In trying to overcome this, the mechanism of action and especially mechanisms of resistance to targeted therapies, need to be studied and explained even more in detail [3-7].

In this chapter evidence on sequential therapy after progression to the first line will be presented with the emphasis on changing mechanism of action. Additionally, mechanisms of resistance to targeted therapies and therapeutic options to overcome resistance will be discussed.

2. Molecular biology of renal cell carcinoma

Most of the knowledge about molecular biology comes from the studies of a hereditary form of renal cell carcinoma. Studies of families with inherited RCC over the past twenty years lead to the identification of five inherited renal cancer syndromes and their related genes. Description of all five syndromes is beyond the scope of this chapter; only Von Hippel-Lindau syndrome will be explored [2].

2.1. Von Hippel-Lindau tumor suppressor gene

The von Hippel-Lindau (VHL) disease is a rare, autosomal dominantly inherited disease. Individuals with this syndrome are predisposed to development of multiple benign and malignant tumors. Most common are clear cell renal tumors, retinal and central nervous system hemangioblastomas, pheocromocytomas, pancreatic neuroendocrine tumors, endolymphatic sac tumors and pancreatic and kidney cists. VHL occurs in 1 in 36.000 and symptomatic disease develops in 70% of affected persons by the age of 60 years. Bilateral RCC develop in 25-45% of VHL patients. VHL results from mutation in the von Hippel-Lindau gene on chromosome 3p25-26. The VHL gene discovered in 1993 is a tumor suppressor gene; both copies of gene must be inactivated for tumor initiation. Different germline mutations predisposing to VHL include; large deletions, protein-truncating mutations and missense mutations that exchange the amino acids in the VHL protein. More than 1000 different mutations have been identified until now. According to the type of mutation, patients are classified in different groups, predisposed to different types of tumors. Group of patients bearing deletions or nonsense mutations, most often develop RCC [2,8].

The research on VHL gave light to the inside of molecular biology of sporadic kidney cancer. It is known, that loss of VHL function, including somatic mutations and epigenetic defects, is found in 70–90% of the sporadic clear cell RCC [8]. The pathophysiologic mechanism of such strong association is currently not very understood [8,9].

The VHL protein pVHL has several functions. The most studied is its role in the regulation of hypoxia inducible factor (HIF1α), member of transcription factors family. At normal cellular oxygen levels, pVHL binds to HIF1α and causes its degradation. In low oxygen or in the case when VHL gene is mutated pVHL does not bind to HIF1α. Consequently HIF1α dimerise with HIF1β and activate the transcription of genes involved in vessel development (vascular endothelial growth factor, platelet-derived growth factor B, erythropoietin) and genes involved in glucose uptake and metabolism. Up-regulation of targeted genes involved in neovascularization by HIF1α offers the explanation of high vascularity of RCC [2,8]. Beside this, pVHL has numerous other functions in the processes of regulation of extracellular matrix, senescence, phosphorylation enhancers and other. The importance of many physiologically relevant functions of pVHL is at present difficult to interpret [8].

Besides VHL, six other genes have been found to predispose to RCC (MET, FLCN, FH, SDH, TSC 1 and TSC 2). These genes interact trough common nutrient and energy sensing pathways. Understanding of the molecular mechanisms by which these genes interact in these pathways has enabled the development of targeted therapies [2].

2.2. VEGF-R pathway

Loss of both alleles of VHL gene leads to up-regulated transcription of growth factors such as VEGF, PDGF and TGF-α. These factors bind to their tyrosine kinase receptors. This leads to downstream signalling and ultimately to effects such as increased angiogenesis, increased cell proliferation and decreased apoptosis. As described previously pVHL mutations are inevitably connected to flawed HIF inactivation which results in production of VEGF. VEGF is the most prominent angiogenesis regulator. Its function is mediated through two tyrosine kinase receptors VEGF-R1 and VEGF-R2 in vascular endothelial cells. VEGF in the beginning binds to VEGF-R2, which promotes endothelial cell proliferation, migration and vascular permeability. In the next step VEGF binds to VEGF-R1 to assist the organization of new capillaries [9].

2.3. mTOR pathway

mTOR is another regulator of HIF 1α, its signalling activity increases the cellular levels of HIF 1α, which worsens the already high levels of it because of absence of pVHL function. mTOR is a serine/threonine kinase that has a key function in apoptosis, cell growth and tumor proliferation. mTOR forms complexes with regulatory associated proteins named mTORC1 and mTORC2. mTORC 1 can be activated by growth factors including VEGFR, PDGFR, EGFR and IGFR and nutrients trough phosphatidylinositol-3 kinase/Akt (PI3K/Akt) pathway. Activated mTORC1 stimulate protein synthesis, entrance into G 1 phase, and proteins that regulate apoptosis [9].

3. Development of systemic therapy in mRCC

3.1. Chemotherapy

The successes on other solid tumors led researches to the assumption chemotherapy would be effective also in mRCC. Chemotherapeutic trials were conducted between 1983 and 1993. Different agents; bleomycin, cisplatin, 5-FU, gemcitabine and vinblastine have been tested. Results were disappointing; less than 10% of patients had clinical benefit in all of these trials. Response rates in the range of 10 to 15% have been achieved with combination of two agents.

Today chemotherapy has no role in the treatment of mRCC patients and is not part of the everyday clinical practice [2].

Several mechanisms have been discovered to be responsible to the resistance of RCC cells to chemotherapy. Beside increased detoxification, altered targets and impaired apoptosis pathways, increased expression of transporting proteins play an important role. P-glycoprotein is a 170-kD membrane glycoprotein that acts as a pump that expels chemicals like vinblastine out of the cell [2].

3.2. Cytokines

The interest in interferon in the treatment of RCC came when sporadic responses in patients with RCC on leucocyte interferon, were observed. Natural interferon produced from donor's leucocytes, was later substituted with recombinant. Different forms and dosages were tested and no major differences between them were observed. Uniformly response rates ranged from 0 to 29% with few complete and very few durable responses. Some trials suggested that certain group of patients have larger benefit (good performance status, prior nephrectomy and restricted metastases to the lungs), but this was not a uniform finding. Today interferon as mono-therapy is not widely used, because of the low efficacy coupled with high toxicity [2].

IL-2 was discovered in 1979 and it soon became clear that it could be effective in the treatment of RCC. Response rates of 33% have been reported in the initial trials. Later multicentric trials reported response rates in 7-19% of patients. In small number of patients responses were complete and durable; 7-9% of all patients did not relapse even after 10 years and these patients are considered to be cured from cancer. Unfortunately until today the selection of patients likely to have durable responses is not possible, because patient and tumor characteristics that predict best responses to IL-2 have not been identified yet [2]. Beside uncertain responses, unfavourable toxicity profile limits the use of IL-2. Patients treated with high doses of IL-2 may experience vascular leak syndrome, hypotension, multiorgan dysfunction and a variety of other toxicities. In the two decades, when IL-2 was the standard therapy of mRCC patients were selected on safety bases (performance status, co-morbidities), tumor histology (clear cell), risk scores (e.g. Memorial Sloan Kettering Cancer Center) and patient preferences [2,10].

3.3. VEGF targeted therapy

It is not surprising that several agents targeting VEGF demonstrate activity in RCC. As described in previous sub chapter there is direct link between VHL mutation and up regulation of angiogenesis- promoting proteins including VEGF and PDGF. VEGF is the main factor responsible for tumor angiogenesis and PDGF is signalling protein for perycites, structural supporting cells for blood vessels. VHL is mutated in most of the patients with RCC [2,10,11].

3.3.1. Sunitinib

Sunitinib is a potent multi-kinase inhibitor including platelet-derived growth factor receptor (PDGFR) α and β, stem cell factor receptor (c-KIT), FMS-like tyrosine kinase-3 (FLT-3), VEGF receptors 1,2,3, colony stimulating factor (CSF-1R) and neurotropic factor receptor. Large multicentric phase 3 trial in which 750 patients were randomized in a 1:1 fashion between treatment with IFN-α and sunitinib, demonstrated its superiority over IFN-α. Overall response rate was 31% in the sunitinib and 6% in the IFN group (p<0.0001).The median PFS in the sunitinib group was 11 and in IFN-α 5 months. Difference was observed also in overall survival (median 26.8 months in sunitinib and 21.8 months in the IFN group, p=0.051). The most common adverse events were fatigue, diarrhea, mucositis, hand-foot syndrome and hypertension [12,13]. Sunitinib was approved by FDA in 2007 and is today standard of care in the first-line treatment of mRCC [2,9].

3.3.2. Pazopanib

Pazopanib is an oral multitargeted tyrosine kinase inhibitor that targets VEGFR 1,2,3, PDGFR α and β and c-KIT. Approval of pazopanib in 2009 was based on a phase III trial in which 435 patients were randomized (2:1) to receive either pazopanib 800 mg once daily or placebo. The median PFS of 9.2 months in the pazopanib group was significantly longer than in placebo group where PFS was 4.2 months (p<0.0001). Main side effects were diarrhoea in half, hypertension in 40% and nausea, anorexia, vomiting and fatigue in 20% of patients [14]. Grade 3 hepatotoxicity was also reported. Pazopanib is recommended in the first line treatment of mRCC [2,14].

3.3.3. Bevacisumab

Bevacisumab is a recombinant monoclonal antibody that binds circulating VEGF protein and neutralizes it [15]. In the AVOREN trial 649 previously untreated patients were randomized to receive either bevacisumab every two weeks and IFN-α or placebo and IFN-α. Differences in PFS (10.2 vs. 5.4 months) and ORR (31 vs. 13%) were significantly better in bevacisumab group (p<0.0001 for both parameters) [16]. The second trial conducted by Cancer and Leukemia Group B was similar. PFS of 8.5 months in the bevacisumab was statistically significant better than in the IFN monotherapy group (PFS 5.2 months, p<0,0001). Differences were also demonstrated comparing ORR favoring bevacisumab group (25.5 vs. 13.1% p<0,0001). Fatigue, anorexia, hypertension and proteinuria were among the most common side effects and more prominent in the combination group [2,11,16,17].

3.3.4. Sorafenib

Sorafenib is a small molecule, oral multikinase inhibitor that inhibits VEGFR 1,2,3, PDGFR-β, RAF, serine/threonine intracellular kinase, FLT-3, cKIT and RET. Sorefenib was tested in a phase III trial (TARGET), 903 patients with mRCC resistant to standard therapy were randomized to receive sorafenib twice daily or placebo. PFS in the sorafenib group was 5.5 months and in placebo group 2.8 months (p<0.000001). Difference in OS did not reach statistical significance. Major side effects of sorafenib were rash, hand-foot syndrome, fatigue, diarrhoea and hypertension [18].

3.3.5. Axitinib

Axitinib is a second line inhibitor of VEGFR 1 and 2 and is approved in the second line treatment of mRCC. Axitinib was compared to sorafenib in a phase III trial (AXIX). 723 patients previously treated with suntinib, bevacisumab plus IFN, temsirolimus or cytokines that progressed, were randomized to receive axitinib or sorafenib 400 mg. Median PFS in the axitinib group was 6.7 months and was statistically significant better than in sorafenib group (4.7 months, $p<0.0001$). Patients in axitinib group had more hypertension, diarrhoea, dysphonia, fatigue and nausea, while patients in sorafenib had more hand foot syndrome, rash and alopecia [19].

3.4. mTOR targeted therapy

Abnormal functioning of signaling pathways contributes to many malignancies including RCC [20-22]. The mammalian target of rapamycin (mTOR) is a protein kinase that regulates cell growth, cell proliferation, cell motility, cell survival, protein synthesis, and transcription [2]. The disruption of mTOR signaling leads to suppression of the production of proteins that regulate progression of the cell trough the cell cycle and angiogenesis [22].

3.4.1. Temsirolimus

Temsirolimus, an mTOR inhibitor was approved for the treatment of mRCC in the 2007. Global Advance Renal Cell Carcinoma (ARCC) was a phase III trial of temsirolimus in previously untreated mRCC. Patients were randomized to receive either IFN-α, temsirolimus or both. PFS in the groups receiving temsirolimus was significantly longer than in the IFN group (3.7 months in temsirolimus groups vs. 1.9 months in the IFN group; $p=0.0019$). Patients treated with temsirolimus alone had better overall survival than patients treated with IFN alone (10.9 months vs. 7.3 months, $p=0.096$). Toxicity was greater in the combination group and included rash, stomatitis, pain, infection, peripheral edema, thrombocytopenia, hyperlipidemia, hypercholesterolemia and hyperglycemia [20].

3.4.2. Everolimus

Everolimus is an oral mTOR inhibitor approved for the treatment of mRCC in the second line after progression on sunitinib or sorafenib. Everolimus treatment was tested in phase III trial named RECORD-1. 410 patients which had progressed to previous treatment were randomly assigned to receive either everolimus or placebo. Median PFS in the everolimus group was 4.9 months, in placebo group 1.9 months ($p<0.001$). The median OS was not significantly different between the two groups (14.8 in everolimus and 14.4 in placebo group, $p=0.126$) The most common side effects of everolimus were stomatitis, rash, fatigue, asthenia and diarrhea [21,22].

Summary of phase III trials is presented in Tables 1 and 2.

	Author	Name	Treatment Arm	Prior Therapy
Sunitninib	Motzer et.al. (2007)		Sunitinib IFN-α	None
Pazopanib	Sternberg et.al. (2010)		Pazopanib Placebo	None or Cytokine
Bevacisumab	Escudier et.al. (2007)	AVOREN	Bevacisumab plus IFN-α Placebo plus IFN-α	None
Sorafenib	Escuder et.al. (2006)	TARGET	Sorafenib Placebo	Cytokine
Axitinib	Rini et.al. (2011)	AXIS	Axitinib Sorafenib	Sunitinib or Bevacisumab+IFN or temsirolimus or cytokines
Everolimus	Motzer et.al. (2008)	RECORD-1	Everolimus Placebo	Sunitinib or Sorafenib
Temsirolimus	Hudes et.al. (2007)	ARCC	Temsirolimus IFN-α Temsirolimus plus IFN-α	None

Table 1. Phase III trials of targeted agents in mRCC

4. Mechanism of resistance to targeted therapies

Large advances in treatment results achieved with targeted therapies in mRCC are remarkable, but still between a third and two-thirds of patients with mRCC have tumors refractory to anti-VEGF and mTOR inhibitors from the beginning of treatment and all patients develop drug resistance and relapse some time during the course of their disease. Research of the mechanisms of resistance is very important in planning the development of new targeted agents [3, 23,24]. Most of information about drug resistance in mRCC known today is from the preclinical studies or studies on patients with different types of cancer, where targeted therapies are being in clinical practice for longer time (e.g. breast cancer). This is partially due to the rapid approval of targeted agents in mRCC which surpassed understanding of the mechanisms of response and resistance [3].

Until now two types of resistance to targeted therapy have been determined, so called intrinsic and extrinsic resistance [3].

	Objective Response Rate	Progression Free Survival	Overall Survival	Most Common Adverse Events of Experimental Drug
Sunitninib	31% Sunitinib 6% IFN	11 months Sunitinib 5 months IFN P<0.0001	26.4 months Sunitinib 21.8 months IFN P=0.051	Diarrhea, fatique, nausea, stomatitis, vomiting
Pazopanib	30% Pazopanib 3% Placebo	9.2 months Pazopanib 4.2 months Placebo P<0.0001	21.1 months Pazopanib 18.7 months Placebo	Diarrhea, hypertension, hair color change, nausea, anorexia
Bevacisumab	31% Bev+IFN 13% Placebo+IFN	10.2 months Bev+IFN 5.4 months Placebo+IFN P<0,0001	23.3 months Bev+IFN 21.3 months Placebo +IFN P=0.13	Fatique, pyrexia, anorexia, bleeding, asthenia
Sorafenib	10% Sorafenib 2% Placebo	5.5 months Sorafenib 2.8 months Placebo P<0,01	17.8 months Sorafenib 15.2 months Placebo P=0.15	Diarrhea, rash, fatigue, hand-foot syndrome
Axitinib	19% Axitinib 9% Sorafenib	6.7 months Axitinib 4.7 months Sorafenib P<0.001	Not reported	Diarrhea, hypertension, fatigue, decreased apetite, nausea
Everolimus	1% Everolimus 0% Placebo	4.9 months Everolimus 1.9 months Placebo P<0,0001	14.8 months Everolimus 14.4 months Placebo P=0.177	Stomatitis, rash, fatigue, asthenia, diarrhea
Temsirolimus	8.6% Tem 4.8% IFN 8.1% Tem+IFN	3.7 months Tem 1.9 months IFN 3.7 months Tem+IFN P=0.0001 (between Tem and IFN)	10.9 months Tem 7.3 months IFN 8.4 months Tem+IFN P=0.08 (between Tem and IFN)	Asthenia, rash, anemia, nausea, anorexia

Table 2. Phase III trials of targeted agents in mRCC

4.1. Intrinsic resistance

Intrinsic resistance (primary resistance) occurs when tumor does not respond to the targeted therapy from the beginning of the treatment. Lack of the clinical benefit, even a short-lasting one is observed in these patients. Roughly 25% of patients are resistant to therapy; no response is detected on first evaluation after 2-3 months [23]. This type of resistance has not been explained entirely jet.

In the case of the resistance to VEGF inhibitors and TKI-s pre-existing pro-angiogenic factors, such as fibroblast growth factor-2 promote tumor angiogenesis. Pre-existence of pro-angiogenic factors compensate for the inhibition of VEGF signaling and thus allow angiogenesis to continue [3,23]. Pre-existing inflammatory cells may also contribute to the angiogenesis by expressing pro-angiogenic factors. In pre-clinical trials mRCC tumors that were not responsive to anti-VEGF antibody were associated with increase in infiltrating CD11b + GR1 + myeloid cells, which expressed several pro-angiogenic factors [23].

The proposed mechanisms of resistance to inhibitors of mammalian target of rapamycin (mTOR) include the presence of redundant signaling pathways, presence of KRAS or BRAF mutations, loss of phosphatase and tension homologue deleted on chromosome ten (PTEN), low cellular levels of p27 or 4E-bp1 and overexpression of eIF4E [3].

Intrinsic resistance to anti-angiogenic factors and mTOR inhibitors is widespread and leads to poor patient outcome. Alternative pathways should be considered in this patients such as targeting RAF and MEK or PI3K/AKT. Including patients with resistant tumors in clinical trials testing these new agents that target these pathways is strongly recommended [23].

4.2. Extrinsic resistance

All patients who initially have clinical benefit of targeted therapy eventually develop resistance to it and experience disease progression. This resistance, named extrinsic resistance (also known as secondary, evasive, acquired or adaptive resistance) has been explained more in detail [23]. TKI and VEGF inhibitors both target components of VEGF signaling pathway. Thus the mechanisms involved will affect any of these targeted agents. Extrinsic resistance results from the acquisition of adaptive mechanisms to the action of angiogenesis inhibitors which ultimately results in evasion of the angiogenesis and reemergence of tumor-related vasculature [3,25].

Sprouting of new vessels has been detected in Xenograft RCC tumors resected shortly after the start of sunitinib. The development of resistance is constantly preceded by restoration of blood flow, which suggests that new vasculature is less dependent (but not necessary independent) of VEGF [25].

4.2.1. Up-regulation of pro-angiogenic factors

Different pro-angiogenic factors involved in the mechanism of resistance to targeted agents have been recognized. In a mouse model of pancreatic neuroendocrine cancer, resistant tumors expressed high levels of FGF 1, 2, ephrin A1, angiopoetin and interleukin-8 [23,25]. Inhibition of these proteins was shown to inhibit tumor growth of resistant RCC-s [25].

Interleukin-8 (IL-8) is a potent pro-angiogenic factor. Up-regulation of IL-8 plays an important role in RCC resistance. In a xenograft model of RCC mimicking clinical resistance to sunitinib, increased IL-8 secretion from tumors was associated with reactivation of tumor angiogenesis and administration of IL-8 neutralizing antibody lead to re-sensitization to sunitinib. Elevated IL-8 expression was also found in patients with tumors who did not respond to sunitinib from the beginning [5,22]. IL-angiogenic signaling may functionally compensate for the inhibition of VEGF/VEGFR-mediated angiogenesis [5].

Angiopoetin 2 (Ang-2) is a plasma glycoprotein involved in angiogenesis and cancer neovascularization. It is thought to have a role in development of the resistance. Levels of Ang-2 decrease after the initiation of sunitinib treatment and increase after the resistance occurs [23].

Sphingosine kinase (S1P) is also supposed to play a role in the resistance. S1P is an enzyme that catalyzes the formation of sphingosine-1-phosphate which is associated with cell proliferation, survival and angiogenesis. Plasma levels of S1P decrease after the start of sunitinib treatment and increase again upon the development of resistance. In pre-clinical models administering neutralizing antibodies against S1P to mice, delayed the growth of sunitinib-resistant tumors [23].

4.2.2. Down-regulation of angiostatic factors

Down-regulation of angiostatic factors is another mechanism of resistance to TKI-s. Treatment with sunitinib and sorafenib results in the increased expression of several IFN-inducible genes including the angiostatic chemokines CXCL 10 and CXCL 11 and tumor suppressor genes. Following the development of resistance, the expression of IFN-γ and several of IFN-inducible genes is reduced. Down regulation of these factors is associated with the development of resistance to sunitinib and sorafenib [23].

4.2.3. Recruitment of bone marrow-derived cells

Recruitment of bone marrow-derived cells which can result in the development of new blood vessels is another possible mechanism of resistance. In pre-clinical studies recruitment of CD11b + GR1 + myeloid cells cells resulted in resistance development. There is also evidence that tumor vasculature can be protected from anti-angiogenic therapy by increased pericyte coverage [23].

4.2.4. Development of invasion without angiogenesis

Invasion of tumor in normal tissue and recruitment of normal tissue vasculature protect the tumors from anti-angiogenic therapy. It has been reported that the tumor of a patient experiencing disease progression during antiangiogenic therapy had invaded the surrounding tissue and there had been increase of the vascularization from the normal tissue to the center of the tumor [23].

4.2.5. Resistance to m-TOR inhibitors

Resistance to mTOR inhibitors is far less explained. It is supposed to be the result of activation of feedback loops that promote the activation of molecular signaling pathways of survival, increased activity of mTOR-complex 2, up-regulation of insulin-like growth factor and increase in the ERK/MAPK pathway signaling [4,24,25].

4.2.6. Reversible resistance

Preclinical studies revealed that resistance to VEGF targeted therapies can be reversible. Hammers and colleagues grafted skin metastases of mRCC patient who had become resistant to sunitinib into mice and these xenogafts regained sensitivity and responded to sunitinib. Histology of original skin metastasis and xenograft revealed that a reversible epithelial-to-mesenchymal transition could be responsible for acquired resistance to sunitinib. Zhang concluded that reversible changes in gene expression within the tumor cells and/or their microenvironment could be the possible mechanism of reversible resistance. He implanted sorafenib-resistant RCC into mice and after implantation tumors regained the sensitivity to sorafenib [4,25].

4.2.7. Mechanism of resistance to different targeted agents

In the case of sunitinib, the proposed mechanism of resistance is the activation or up-regulation of alternative angiogenic signals (e.g. FGF-s, ephrins, andiopoetins) while in the case of sorafenib this mechanism seem to be recruitment of pro-angiogenic bone marrow-derived cells and monocytes. Recruitment of perycites that help to maintain vessels permeable and functional and prevent endothelial cells from being affected by antiangiogenic therapies, is the proposed mechanisms of resistance to pasopanib. In the case of bevacisumab resistance the increased potential of tumor cells to invade without the need of neovascularization is supposed to be the mechanism [4,9,25].

5. Overcoming the resistance

Overcoming the resistance to first line therapy is one of the aims of administering the second line and beyond. Several factors play important role in selection of second line strategy: clinical evidence, toxicity issues and individual patient profile [4,25,26].

Sequential use of targeted agents is currently the standard of care for mRCC patients. This approach enables patients to get most benefit from these agents avoiding the excessive toxicity associated with combination therapy [26-28]. Targeted agent in the second line can have the same or different mechanism of action as first-line one. Limited data suggest that the use of a TKI after the failure of another TKI is reasonable and that there is not complete cross-resistance of these agents. The hypothesis behind this is that although TKIs share the same mechanism of action, their molecular targets are different. Despite this, the evidence of this approach is not strong; prospective, phase III trials are missing. Changing mechanism of action can have several advantages: greater chance of overcoming resistance while decreasing the probability of cumulative toxicity [4,25]. Toxicities of TKI-s and mTOR inhibitors for example, differ considerably. Frequent grade 3 toxicities encountered in patients on TKI-s are hand-foot syndrome, diarrhoea, fatigue, hypertension, neutropenia and leukopenia, while grade 3 toxicities in patients treated with mTOR inhibitors are rash, stomatitis, pneumonitis, anemia and infection [25-30].

5.1. TKI-s following cytokine therapy

The almost historical treatment strategy where changing of mechanism of action proved to be effective was TKI-s following cytokines. Currently this approach is not of clinical use anymore, because most of the patients get molecular targeted agent in the first line; however it is likely that some patients will have been treated with a cytokine previously. Phase III trials demonstrated that this approach is effective and safe and become a basis of approval of sunitinib and pazopanib in the first line treatment [3].

5.2. Combinations of targeted agents

Combinations of targeted agents could be in theory effective mechanism to overcome the resistance because we could combine agents with different mechanisms of action. However combining these therapies may increase the incidence of side effects if the combination drugs are not selected carefully [29]. Most of patients do not tolerate full doses of two VEGF inhibitors at the same time. That is the reason why administering combination therapy long enough to surpass the clinical benefit of subsequent mono-therapy is not possible [25].

Combinations of VEGF-TKI and mTOR inhibitors also lead to unacceptable toxicity. In a trial of Patel et.al, combination of temsirolimus and sunitinib lead to dose limiting toxicity in 2 of 3 patients [31]. Data suggest that the side effects and tolerability of combinations correlate with the total number of inhibited targets. This is the explanation why some combinations with VEGF specific agent bevacisumab may be tolerated (e.g. bevacisumab plus everolimus). At present combination of targeted agents in the treatment of mRCC is not recommended in clinical practice mainly because of excessive toxicity [23,29].

5.3. Second VEGF-TKI after the first line VEGF-TKI

Retrospective and prospective phase II trials showed that treatment with second TKI could be beneficial in patients that progressed on first TKI. At first sight this may seem not logical, but variations in kinase targets and interaction may avoid resistance. However definitive data from phase III trials on this topic are still missing. Benefit of the second TKI after the first TKI may be dependent on its relative potency and selectivity profile [9]. Most of the results from retrospective and small prospective trials suggest that patients with mRCC who progress on sorafenib could benefit from sunitinib. Conversely the use of sorafenib after sunitinib or bevacisumab showed limited efficacy [9,27].

Sabin et.al. evaluated 68 patients treated with sunitinib and sorafenib consequently. ORR was better when the patients received sorafenib first; 15% in the group that received sunitinib followed by sorafnib group and 9% in the group that received sorafenib after sunitinib. Median PFS in the first group was 12.4 months (6 months on sorafenib and 6.4 months on sunitinib) and 8.9 months in the second group (5 months on sunitinib and 3.9 months on sorafenib) [26]. Porta et.al evaluated retrospectively 99 patients treated with sunitinib followed by sorafenib (SuSo) and 90 patients treated with sorafenib followed by sunitnib (SoSu). The median PFS of second line treatment in the first group (SuSo) was 7.9 months and in the second group was 4.2 months (SoSu) [32]. Clinical trial in progress NCT00732914 with the aim to evaluate if total PFS of sorafenib followed by sunitinib is superior compared to sunitinib followed by sorafenib is expected to give some additional light to this issue [3].

AXIS trial directly compared the efficacy and safety of axitinib to sorafenib after progression on sunitinib, bevacisumab, temsirolimus or cytokines. In the subpopulation of patients who previously received sunitinib, median PFS was 4.8 months with axitinib and 3.4 months with sorafenib (p=0,001). Shorter median PFS in both arms receiving first line sunitinib compared to those receiving cytokines (median PFS 12.1 in axitinib and 6.5 moths in sunitinib) suggest that at least partial cross-resistance with sequential TKI-s [3,9,19].

Reduced clinical efficacy of second line therapy as a result of cross resistance is key concern associated with the sequential administration of agents targeting the same molecular pathways. Two prospective trials showed that because of the cross-resistance, sorafenib had limited efficacy in patients who progressed on sunitinib or bevacisumab [27].

Another concern about using sequential VEGF-TKI therapies is toxicity. Although they may differ in toxicity profiles, all TKI-s share similar targets and exhibit class effect toxicities like hypertension, hand foot syndrome and rash [9]. Current data suggest that Switching to agents with different mechanisms of action in the second line therapy may provide superior efficacy and reduced cumulative toxicity [27].

5.4. VEGF-TKI after first line anti VEGF

Very limited data are available on the use of TKI-s after progression on bevacisumab and no clinical trial is currently ongoing to address this issue. Only two minor prospective trials conducted by Garcia and Rini evaluated the use of sunitinib or sorafenib in patients with bevacisumab-refractory mRCC [3].

In a phase II trial of Garcia, 48 patients were enrolled. After progression on treatment with sunitinib or bevacisumab, patients received twice daily 400 mg of sorafenib. One unconfirmed objective partial response was observed and the tumor burden reduction rate was 30%. The median PFS was 4.4 months. There was no association of PFS and tumor shrinkage with response to prior therapy. Most treatment-related adverse events were of mild-to-moderate intensity, and included fatigue, hypertension, diarrhoea, and hand-foot syndrome [33].

Rini et.al. conducted a phase II multicentric trial in which patients with mRCC and disease progression after bevacizumab-based therapy received oral sunitinib 50 mg once daily in 6-week cycles on a 4/2 schedule (4 weeks with treatment followed by 2 weeks without treatment). Sixty-one patients were enrolled. The ORR was 23.0%, median PFS was 30.4 weeks and median OS was 47.1 weeks. Most treatment-related adverse events were of mild-to-moderate intensity and included fatigue, hypertension, and hand-foot syndrome. Results from measuring different VEGF-s in the plasma suggest that sunitinib could inhibit some of the signaling factors involved in bevacisumab resistance [34].

5.5. mTOR inhibitor after first line VEGF-TKI

Another approach in patients who progress on first line TKI-s is to switch to a second line therapy with an agent with different mechanism of action like mTOR inhibitor [3,9]. On theoretical basis mTOR inhibitors could overcome the resistance to VEGF-TKIs. VEGF-TKIs increase tumor hypoxia which results in up-regulation of proangiogenic factors and increase potential of metastases. mTor inhibition decreases translation of proangiogenic factors and tumors that have become resistant to VEGF-TKI may respond to treatment with mTOR inhibitor [27]. The evidence of effectiveness of this approach comes from preclinical data. Trial conducted by Larkin and colleagues compared treatment with sunitinib, sunitinib followed by sorafenib or sunitinib followed by everolimus in mice implanted with murine RCC. Sunitinib followed by everolimus was associated with reduced primary tumor weight and volume in a greater extend compared to tumors treated with sunitinib and sunitinib followed by sorafenib. The conclusion was that sequential therapy with sunitinib followed by everolimus is associated with significant anti-tumor and anti-metastatic effect [35].

Everolimus was approved in the second line therapy on results of RECORD-1 trial. In this double blind, phase III trial, patients who had progressed on first line sunitinib, sorafenib or both were randomized to everolimus or placebo. Patients receiving everolimus had longer PFS compared to placebo (4.9 vs. 1.9 months, $p<0.001$). The clinical benefit of everolimus was observed regardless if the patients received previously one or two consequent TKI-s. In the subgroup of patients who received one TKI, median PFS in everolimus group was 5.4 months, and in group who received two TKI-s 4 months. This was statistically significant longer than in placebo groups, where PFS was 1.9 and 1.8 months respectively [8,20,36-38].

Prospective head to head trials to compare mTOR inhibitors and VEGF-TKI-s in the second line of treatment in patients who progressed on the first line VEGF-TKI-s have not been done. Di Lorenzo and colleagues indirectly compared survival benefit in patients on everolimus or sorafenib in the second line. Median overall survival was 81.5 weeks for patients receiving everolimus and 32.0 weeks for sorafenib [37].

The optimal sequencing of sunitinib and everolimus is currently being evaluated in the RECORD-3 trial and furthermore the everolimus plus bevacisumab in the second line after progression on TKI-s is currently being compared to everolimus plus placebo in the NCT01198158 trial [3].

The efficacy and safety of temsirolimus after progression on TKI-s are expected to be revealed in an ongoing trial NCT00474786, a phase III trial comparing temsirolimus vs. sorafenib in the second line treatment in patients who have failed on first-line sunitinib. Results from small population in retrospective and prospective phase II trial presented on ASCO 2010 suggest, that temsirolimus is safe and effective in pretreated patients, especially those with good performance status and good prognostic factors [3].

Regarding toxicity mTOR inhibitors and VEGF-TKIs block different molecular mechanisms, the toxicity profiles are usually not overlapping. In the RECORD-1 trial patients could tolerate treatment with everolimus after progression on VEGF-TKIs. Stomatitis, infection, asthenia and fatigue were the most common side effects reported on everolimus therapy. Common toxicities encountered in the treatment with VEGF-TKIs such as hypertension or hand-foot syndrome, were not frequent [3,19].

5.6. Alternative scheduling and dosage

A different approach to overcome the resistance can potentially be the change in scheduling and/or dosage of the targeted agent in usage. Sunitinib is approved in intermittent schedule of 4 weeks on drug and 2 weeks off drug. Continuous low-dose therapy has been shown to be a feasible treatment option in first and second line of treatment [37,38]. Comparison between the two scheduling is currently not very well determined, but clinical and toxicological differences may in future be important issue in treatment individualization. Another option is re-challenge with the same drug after discontinuation period on disease progression. The basis for this approach comes from pre-clinical data that indicate that resistance to sorafenib is reversed by re-implantation of resistant tumors in untreated mice [23].

The question of optimal treatment dosage becomes particularly relevant on disease progression. Meta-analysis of patients with solid tumors receiving sunitinib revealed that patients receiving higher dose, had longer time to progression compared to patients who received less sunitinib. Additionally patient receiving higher dose had more complete or partial remissions and greater decrease in tumor size. In the trial comparing sorafenib with IFN-α, patients in the sorafenib group received higher dose of sorafenib (600 mg BID) after progression on 400 mg BID. Reduction of tumor size was observed. Suggested clinical benefit of increased dose after progression is outweighed by increased toxicity. Most of patients do not tolerate dosage increase [22].

5.7. Intrinsic resistance

Prognosis of patients who progress early in the course of first line therapy VEGF targeted therapy is poor. No available agents seem to alter the course of their disease and give them clinical benefit. 86 patients with rapid progression after first line therapy were evaluated in a retrospective trial. PFS after second line therapy with treatment with different VEGF-TKI was 2 months and after second line therapy with mTOR 0.9 months (p=0.536). Larger retrospective trial in which 272 patients were included showed similar results. All patients had rapid disease progression after first line VEGF-TKIs. The response rates, PFS and OS of those receiving second-line VEGF-targeted therapy compared with mTOR inhibitors were 10 vs 6%, 2.8 vs.2 months and 7.9 vs. 4.7 months. Differences were not statistically significant [9].

6. Third line and beyond

Small prospective and retrospective trials suggest that changing the mechanism of action in the third line may restore the sensitivity to the initial treatment [3,9,27,32,39,40]. In the ASCO meeting in 2010 Ferrari presented the results of a prospective trial that compared the administration of everolimus or temsirolimus as third line therapy to good performance status patients resistant to TKI-s. Median PFS was 6 months and disease control was achieved in 39% of patients. These results suggest that treatment with mTOR inhibitor in the third line and further than, could be a potential promising treatment option [40].

Another trial conducted by Di Lorenzo et.al. evaluated sorafenib treatment in the third line after treatment with sunitinib and mTor inhibitor. Of the 34 patients eligible, 23.5% responded to third line sorafenib. Desease control was 44%, median PFS was 4 and median OS was 6 months. 47% of patients that responded to first line therapy, responded to third-line sorafenib while of patients who did not respond to first-line, did not respond also to third-line sorafenib.

The most common 3/4 grade side effects of third line sorafenib were hand-foot syndrome, anemia, fatigue, diarrhea and neutropenia. These results show that sorafenib could be considered in the third line treatment in mRCC patients after the failure on sunitinib and mTOR inhibitor [41]. Blesious retrospectively evaluated 105 patients in the RECORD-1 trial of whom 36 received a VEGF-TKI after receiving everolimus. Patients that received sunitinib, sorafenib and dovitinib had median PFS of 8 months, 5.3 months and 12.0 months. A partial response was reported in 8.6% of patients and 68.8% of patients had stable disease. Median OS was 29.1 months [42].

In a trial of Grunwald efficacy of VEGF-targeted therapies in patients after everolimus-resistant patients who had progressed on a previous TKI was explored. Patients received sunitinib, sorafenib, dovitinib or bevacisumab/ IFN therapy after failure of everolimus. Of the 40 patients included 10% had partial response and 55% had stable disease. Median PFS was 5.5 months. Authors conclude that VEGF targeted therapy show promising activity in everolimus resistant metastatic RCC [43].

Porta et. al. evaluated retrospectively the overall PFS benefit of the sequence VEGF-TKI, mTor inhibitor, VEGF-TKI sequence. The sequence of sorafenib-mTOR-sunitinib (14 patients) was compared to the sequence sunitinib-mTOR-sorafenib (26 patients). No significant difference in PFS was found between the two groups (21.9 months vs 22.8 months). The median PFS for the three lines of treatment were 11.7 months-5.1 months-9.1 months for the group sorafenib-mTOR-sunitinib and 14.4 months-4.3 months-3.9 months for sunitinib-mTOR-sorafenib group [44].

The results of these trials suggest that re-challenging strategy of VEGF-TKI in the third line of treatment after progression on VEGF-TKI in the first and mTOR inhibitors in the second may be a successful treatment approach. The other observation of these trials is that some patients have minor benefit from the VEGF-TKI inhibitors in the third compared to the benefit in the first line. The explanation for this is that probably partial cross-resistance to the VEGF-TKIs accounts at least to some extent for this. One possible strategy to overcome this resistance is to use the third-line agent with the ability to broadly inhibit multiple angiogenic pathways in addition to VEGF signaling [9].

Even if no clinical guidelines exist for the fourth-line targeted therapy, some reports suggest that patients may gain clinical benefit from the sequences of targeted agents with different mechanisms of action. 48 months of PFS was achieved in an mRCC patient treated with four lines of targeted therapies (sunitinib, everolimus, sorafenib, temsirolimus). Despite intensity, treatment was well tolerated and no cumulative toxicity was present. This case study advocates that sequential use of sunitinib, everolimus, sorafenib and temsirolimus and show that this could be effective treatment approach with good toxicity profile [45].

Metastatic RCC patients can get benefit from multiple lines of targeted therapy. Resistance to VEGF-TKIs and mTOR inhibitors seem to be at least partially reversible and re-challenging with the inhibitors from the same group in subsequent lines of therapy may be a therapeutic option if toxicity does not limit it. Tailoring treatment to the particular patient is of utmost importance [3,9,27,32].

7. Future directions

The current practice of delivery of sequential monotherapy targeted agents is empirical and mainly based on non-comparative clinical trials. In treatment refractory patients often practical issues like route of delivery or physician familiarity with the drug prevail over the scientific evidence in selecting treatment. Deeper understanding of the biology of response and resistance to targeted agents will elucidate future way in treatment of mRCC patients. New multi-targeted inhibitors are being rapidly developed and their role in overcoming resistance will become clear in the next few years. Together with the developments of these new drugs, finding predictive biomarkers of these new and "old" therapies is one of the major research goals [25].

7.1. New targeted agents

Dovitinib is an investigational multi-target inhibitor of FGF receptors 1-3, PDGF receptor, VEGFrs 1-3 and c-KIT. One of the mechanisms of resistance to VEGF-TKI seems to be hypoxia-mediated induction of FGF signaling. Dovitinib was tested in a phase II trial in which patients with mRCC who failed prior treatment with VEGF-TKI or mTOR inhibitor or cytokines. Median PFS and OS were 5.5 months and 11.8 months in all patients and 6.1 months and 10.2 months in patients treated with previous VEGF-TKI or mTOR inhibitor. The main grade 3 toxicities of dovitinib were nausea/vomiting in 15%, fatigue in 13.6%, asthenia in 13.5%, diarrhoea in 10.2% and hypertension in 10.2% of patients. Grade 4 hypertriglicemia occurred in 8.5% of patients [46].

Tivozanib is a potent selective long half-life tyrosine kinase inhibitor targeting VEGFR 1-3. 517 patients were included in a phase III trial published by Motzer et.al at ASCO 2012. Patients were randomized to receive either tivozanib or sorafenib. Median PFS was 11.9 months for tivozanib and 9.1 months for sorafenib (p=0.042). Overall response rate was 33% in tivozanib and 23% in sorafwnib group (p=0.014). Adverse events grade 3 for tivozanib were hypertension, diarrhea, fatigue, neutropenia and hand-foot syndrome [47].

7.2. Biomarkers

Predictive biomarkers could help clinicians to determine the best treatment approach [48,49]. Multiple candidate biomarkers of biological tumor activity as well as treatment response and patient prognosis are being evaluated [49]. However up to date, none of them showed potential in clinical use. VHL gene status did not correlate with PFS or OS. The reason for this may be that almost all RCC cancers have VHL silencing and so this marker cannot be selective enough. Biomarkers in the peripheral blood have also been tested. Results of some trials showed that patients with mRCC and elevated expression of angiogenic factors have greater benefit from VEGF-targeted therapies, although other trials yielded inconsistent results. Other types of predictive markers, like changes in the tumor blood flow measured by MRI during treatment with targeted agents are being explored [25,48,49].

8. Conclusion

Despite great improvement in treatment outcomes with targeted agents in mRCC, the fact remains that complete remissions are rarely achieved and most patients progress and develop resistance to the treatment. Many questions are still open and at least some of them are expected to be solved with the on-going and future clinical trials. Intrinsic and extrinsic tumor resistances are major obstacles in successful long term tumor control and one of the major questions is the optimal sequencing of treatment. Use of sequential therapy with changing mechanisms of action is a rational approach to overcome this resistance.

Author details

Mirjana Rajer

Address all correspondence to: mrajer@onko-i.si

Institute of Oncology Ljubljana, Slovenia

References

[1] Kumar PS, Figlin RA. Targeted therapies for renal cell carcinoma: understandidg their impact on survival. Targeted Oncology 2010; 5(2): 131-138.

[2] Mabrouk Y, Belhadj O, Rini BI. Cancer of the kidney. In: DeVita VT, Lawrence TS, Rosenberg SA. (eds.) Cancer principles and practice of oncology. Philadelphia: LWW; 2011.p 1161-1182.

[3] Larriba JLG, Espinosa ICG, Garcia-Donas J, Lopez M, Meana A, Puente J, Bellmunt J. Sequential therapy in metastatic renal cell carcinoma: pre-clinical and clinical rationale for selecting a second- or subsequent-line therapy with a different mechanism of action. Cancer Metastasis Review 2012; 31 Suppl 1:S11-17.

[4] Calvo E, Maroto P, Garcia X, Climent MA, Gonzales-Larriba JL, Esteban E. Update from the Spanish oncology genitourinary group on the treatment of advanced renal cell carcinoma: focus on special populations. Cancer Metastasis Review 2010;29 Suppl 1:11-20.

[5] Huang D, Ding Y, Zhou M, Rini BI, Petillo D, Qian CN, et.al. Interleukin-8 mediates resistance to antiangiogenic agent sunitinib in renal cell carcinoma. Cancer Research 2010; 70(3): 1063-1071.

[6] Kirkali Z, Tüzel E. Systemic therapy of kidney cancer: tyrosine kinase inhibitors, antiangiogenesis or IL-2? Future Oncology 2009; 5(6): 871-888.

[7] Guillot A, Levy A, Pacaut C, Collard O, Massard C, Merrouche Y, et.al. Reapprasal of the role of bevacisumab in the terapeutic strategy in advanced renal cell carcinoma. Clinical Genitourinary Cancer 2012; 10(3): 147-152.

[8] Hsu T. Complex cellular functions of the von Hippel–Lindau tumor suppressor gene: insights from model organisms. Oncogene. 2012; 31(18): 2247-2257.

[9] Oudart S, Elaidi RT. Sequential therapy with targeted agents in patients with advanced renal cell carcinoma: Optimizing patient benefit. Cancer treatments Review 2012; 38(8): 981-987.

[10] Porta C, Szczylik C, Escudier B. Combination or sequencing strategies to improve the outcome of metastatic renal cell carcinoma patients: a critical review. Critical Reviws in Oncology/ Hematology 2012; 82(3): 323-337.

[11] NCCN clinical practice guidelines. Kidney cancer: http://www.nccn.org (accessed November 2012)

[12] Motzer RJ, Hutson TE, Tomczak P, Michaelson MD, Bukowski RM, Rixe O, et.al. Sunitinib versus interferon alfa in metastatic renal-cell carcinoma. New England Journal of Medicine 2007; 356(2): 115-124.

[13] Motzer RJ, Hutson TE, Tomczak P, Michaelson MD, Bukowski RM, Rixe O, et.al. Overall survival and updated results for sunitinib compared with interferon alfa in patients with metastatic renal cell carcinoma. Journal of Clinical Oncology 2009; 27(22): 3584-3590.

[14] Sternberg CN, Davis ID, Mardiak J, Szczylik C, Lee E, Wagstaff J, et.al. Pazopanib in locally advanced or metastatic renal cell carcinoma: results of a randomized phase III trial. Journal of Clinical Oncology 2010; 28(6): 1061-1068.

[15] Guillot A, Levy A, Pecaut C, Collard O, Massard C, Merrouche Y et.al. Reappraisal of the reole of bevacisumab in the therapeutic strategy in advanced renal cell carcinoma. Clinical Genitourinary Cancer 2012; 10(3): 147-152.

[16] Escudier B, Pluzanska A, Koralewski P, Ravaud A, Bracarda S, Szczylik C, et.al. Bevacisumab plus interferon alfa-2a for treatment of metastatic renal cell carcinoma: a randomised, double-blind phase III trial. Lancet 2007; 370(9605): 2103-2111.

[17] Rini BI, Halabi S, Rosenberg JE, Stadler WM, Vaena DA, Archer L. Phase III trial of bevacizumab plus interferon alfa versus interferon alfa monotherapy in patients with metastatic renal cell carcinoma: final results of CALGB 90206. Journal of Clinical Oncology 2010; 28(13): 2137-2143.

[18] Escudier B, Eisen T, Stadler WM, Szczylik C, Oudard S, Siebels M, et.al. Sorafenib in advanced clear-cell renal-cell carcinoma. New England Journal of Medicine 2007; 356(2): 125-134.

[19] Rini BI, Escudier B, Tomczak P, Kaprin A, Szczylik C, Hutson TE, et.al. Comparative effectiveness of axitinib versus sorafenib in advanced renal cell carcinoma (AXIS): a randomised phase 3 trial. Lancet 2011; 378(9807): 1931-1939.

[20] Hudes G, Carducci M, Tomczak P, Dutcher J, Figlin R, Kapoor A et.al. Temsirolimus, interferon afa or both for advanced renal-cell carcinoma. New England Journal of Medicine 2007; 356(22): 2271-2281.

[21] Motzer RJ, Escudier B, Oudard S, Hutson TE, Porta C, Bracarda S, et.al. Efficacy of everolimus in advanced renal cell carcinoma: a double-blinf, randomised, placebo-controled phase III trial. Lancet 2008; 372(9637): 449-456.

[22] Motzer RJ, Escudier B, Oudard S, Hutson TE, Porta C, Bracarda S, et.al. Phase III trial of everolimus for metastatic renal cell carcinoma: final results and analysis of prognostic factors. Cancer 2010; 116(18): 4256-4265.

[23] Ravaud A, Gross-Goupil M. Overcoming resistance to tyrosine kinase in renal cell carcinoma. Cancer Treatment Review 2012; 38(8): 996-1003.

[24] Fisher R, Larkin J, Swanton C. Delivering preventive, predictive and personalised cancer medicine for renal cell carcinoma: the challenge of tumour heterogeneity. The EPMA journal 2011; 3(1): 1.

[25] Rini. New strategies in kidney cancer: therapeutic advances itough understanding the molecular basis of response and resistance. Clinical Cancer Research 2010; 16(5): 1347-1354.

[26] Dutcher JP, Mourad WF, Ennis RD. Integrating innovative therapeutic strategies into the management of renal cell carcinoma. Oncology (Williston Park) 2012; 26(6): 526-530.

[27] Larkin J, Swanton C, Pickering L. Optimizing treatment of metastatic renal cell carcinoma by changing mechanism of action. Expert Review Anticancer Therapy 2011; 11(4): 639-649.

[28] Singer EA, Gupta GN. Targeted therapeutic strategies for the management of renal cell carcinoma. Current Opinion in Oncology 2012; 24(3): 284-290.

[29] Bellmunt J. Future developments in renal cell carcinoma. Annals of Oncology 2009; 20 Suppl 1:i13-17.

[30] Schmidlinger M, Bellmunt J. Plethora of agents, plethora of targets, plethora of side effects in metastatic renal cell carcinoma. Cancer Treatment Reviews 2010; 36(5): 416-424.

[31] Patel PH, Senico PL, Curiel RE, Motzer RJ. Phase I study combining treatment with temsirolimus and sunitinib malate in patients with advanced renal cell carcinoma. Clinical Genitourinary Cancer 2009; 7(1): 24-27.

[32] Porta C, Szczylik C, Escudier B. Combination or sequencing strategies to improve the outcome of metastatic renal cell carcinoma patients: a critical review. Crit Rev Oncol Hematol. 2012 Jun; 82(3): 323-337.

[33] Garcia JA, Hutson TE, Elson P, Cowey CL, Gilligan T, Nemec C, et.al. Sorafenib in patients with metastatic renal cell carcinoma refractory to either sunitinib or bevacizumab. Cancer. 2010; 116(23): 5383-5390.

[34] Rini BI, Michaelson MD, Rosenberg JE, Bukowski RM, Sosman JA, Stadler WM, et.al. Antitumor activity and biomarker analysis of sunitinib in patients with bevacizumab-refractory metastatic renal cell carcinoma. Journal of Clinical Oncology 2008; 26(22): 3743-3748.

[35] Larkin J, Esser N, Calvo E, Tsuchihashi Z, Fiedler U, Graeser R, et.al. Efficacy of sequential treatment with sunitinib-everolimus in an orthotopic mouse model of renal cell carcinoma. Anticancer Ressearch 2012; 32(7): 2399-2406.

[36] Calvo E, Escudier B, Motzer RJ, Oudard S, Hutson TE, Porta C, et.al. Everolimus in metastatic renal cell carcinoma: Subgroup analysis of patients with 1 or 2 previous vascular endothelial growth factor receptor-tyrosine kinase inhibitor therapies enrolled in the phase III RECORD-1 study. European Journal of Cancer 2012; 48(3): 333-339.

[37] Barrios CH, Hernandez-Barajas D, Brown MP, Lee SH, Fein L, Liu JH, et.al. Phase II trial of continuous once-daily dosing of sunitinib as first-line treatment in patients with metastatic renal cell carcinoma. Cancer 2012; 118(5): 1252-1259.

[38] Escudier B, Roigas J, Gillessen S, Harmenberg U, Srinivas S, et.al. Phase II study of sunitinib administered in a continuous once-daily dosing regimen in patients with cytokine-refractory metastatic renal cell carcinoma. Journal of Clinical Oncology 2009; 27(25): 4068-4075.

[39] Di Lorenzo G, Casciano R, Malangone E, Buonerba C, Sherman S, Willet J, et.al. An adjusted indirect comparison of everolimus and sorafenib therapy in sunitinib-refractory metastatic renal cell carcinoma patients using repeated matched samples. Expert Opinion in Pharmacotherapy 2011; 12(10): 1491-1497.

[40] Ferrari VD, Fogazz Gi, Valcamonico F, Amoroso V, Procopio G, Nonnis D, et.al. III-IV line of target therapy in advanced renal cell carcinoma (RCC). Journal of Clinical Oncology 2010; 28 (Suppl); Abstract e15148.

[41] Di Lorenzo G, Buonerba C, Federico P, Rescigno P, Milella M, Ortega C, et.al. Third-line sorafenib after sequential therapy with sunitinib and mTOR inhibitors in metastatic renal cell carcinoma. European Urology 2010; 58(6): 906-911.

[42] Blesius A, Beuselinck B, Chevreau C, Ravaud A, Rolland F, Oudard S et.al. Are TKIs still active in patients treated with TKI and everolimus? Experience from 36 patients treated in France in the RECORD 1 trial (abstract). ESMO 2012.

[43] Grunwald V, Seidel C, Ganser A, Busch J, Weikert S. Treatment of everolimus-resistant metastatic renal cell carcinoma with VEGF-targeted therapies. British Journal of Cancer 2011; 105(11): 1635-1639.

[44] Porta C, Paglino C, Procopio G. Optimizing the sequential treatment of metastatic renal cell carcinoma- a retrospective mulnicenter analysis of 40 patients treated with either sorafenib, an mTOR inhibitor and sunitinib, or sunitinib, an mTOR and sorafenib. European Journal of Cancer 2011; 47(Suppl 1):Abstract 7131.

[45] Oudard S. More than 4 years of progression-free survival in a patient with metastatic renal cell carcinoma treated sequentially with sunitinib, everolimus, sorafenib and temsirolimus. Anticancer Research 2010; 30(12): 5223-5226.

[46] Angevin E, Grunwald V, Ravaud A. A phase II study of dovitinib (TKI258) an FGFR- and VEGFR inhibitor in patients with advanced or metastatic renal cellcancer. Journal of Clinical Oncology 2011; 29(Suppl): Abstract 4551.

[47] Motzer RJ, Nosov D, Eisen T, Bondarenko IN, Lipatov ON, et.al. Tivozanib versus sorafenib as initial targeted therapy for patients with advanced renal cell carcinoma: Results from a phase III randomized, open-label, multicenter trial. Journal of Clinical Oncology 2012; 30(Suppl); Abstract 4501.

[48] Hernandez-Yanez M, Heymach JV, Zurita AJ. Circulating biomarkers in advanved renal cell carcinoma: clinical applications. Current Oncology Repports 2012; 14(3): 221-229.

[49] Yuasa T, Takahashi S, Hatake K, Yonese J, Fukui I. Biomarkers to predict response to sunitinib therapy and prognosis in metastatic renal cell cancer. Cancer Science 2011; 102(11): 1949-1957.